人工関節周囲感染対策における国際コンセンサス

— 204の設問とコンセンサス

International Consensus on Periprosthetic Joint Infection

Chairmen : Javad Parvizi MD, FRCS
Thorsten Gehrke MD

監訳 田中　栄
　　　齋藤知行

編集 山田浩司

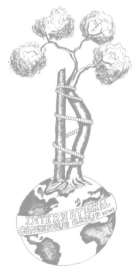

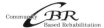

Authorized translation of English edition
"Proceedings of the International Consensus Meeting on Periprosthetic Joint Infection" by Javad Parvizi, Thorsten Gehrke
ⒸFirst Japanese Edition 2016 by CBR-PUBLISHERS, INC, Tokyo

序文

"Le hasard ne favorise que les esprits préparés.（幸運は用意された心にのみ宿る）" 〜 Louis Pasteur 〜

　そもそも初めから感染を起こそうと思って手術に臨む外科医はいないでしょう．なかでも患者さんの QOL や ADL を高める目的で行われる人工関節置換術において，感染症（人工関節周囲感染）はその目的を大きく損なう合併症であり，患者さんにとっても臨床医にとっても最も忌むべきもの，何としても避けるべき合併症であると言えます．しかし一方で，現状では人工関節周囲感染を完全になくすことができないのも事実であり，われわれは常に感染に対する対策を考えておかなければいけません．問題は，人工関節周囲感染は比較的稀であるうえに，個々に異なった背景や入りくんだ病態を示すため，大規模な無作為試験が行いにくく（そのような試験になじまず），きちんとしたエビデンスを提示するのが困難なことです．また仮にそのようなエビエンスがあったとしても，医療は日々前進しており，昨日の真実が本日の真実とは限りません．

　本書のもとになった International Consensus on Periprosthetic Joint Infection は，The Rothman Institute の Parvizi 教授らが中心となって，人工関節周囲感染に関する国際的なコンセンサスを得るために以前から行っておられる取り組みです．今回は 80 か国，50 以上の学会から整形外科医のみならず，感染症専門医，リウマチ専門医，放射線科専門医，病理学や薬学の研究者など 300 名を超える専門家が集まって，長い時間をかけて多くの論文を吟味して作成されたコンセンサスであり，まさに「臨床医および患者にとって有益な最高の研究を統合したもの[1]」です．今回多くの方々の努力によって，その日本語バージョンを皆さまにお届けできることになりました．なかでも編集を担当していただいた関東労災病院の山田浩司先生には，獅子奮迅の活躍をしていただき，本書発刊に大変ご尽力いただきました．この場を借りて感謝申し上げます．

本書には，人工関節周囲感染に関する最新かつ最高のエッセンスが詰まっています．皆さまの臨床現場に必ずやお役に立てるものと信じております．

---

1) Sackett DL, Strauss SE, Richardson WS, Rosenberg W, Haynes RB. Evidence-based medicine: how to practice and teach EBM. 2nd ed. Edinburgh: Churchill-Livingstone, 2000.

2016年3月

東京大学医学部整形外科　教授
田中　栄

序文

　人工関節周囲感染（Periprosthetic Joint Infection：PJI）は最も重篤な術後合併症であり，世界的な人工関節の普及とともにその問題が徐々に顕在化してきました．ある一定の確率で発生するPJIは人工関節の件数に比例し増加し，米国では再置換術の原因として上位を占め，医療経済的にも大きな社会問題となりつつあります．したがって，PJIの診断基準の確立と治療の標準化は喫緊の課題であると言えます．急性炎症で発生する例では診断が容易ですが，臨床症状や炎症反応に乏しい遅発性感染などはその診断が困難な例もあり，発生様式に多様性があることもこの病態の診断や治療に難渋する要因でもあります．確定診断には血液生化学的な検査や通常の細菌培養に加えていくつかの補助診断も必要となり，これらの点においても標準化が求められています．

　PJIの診断と治療に関して世界的な基準を設立する目的で，2013年のMusculoskeletal Infection Society（MSIS）総会でInternational Consensus Meeting on PJIが開催されました．世界80カ国の50を超える学術団体から，整形外科医，放射線医，病理医さらに内科医を含む342名の専門医に会議開催前に複数の質問に対して回答を求め，会自体で討論し一定のコンセンサスを得る方式で進められました．予防教育，周術期の対策，周術期や術後抗菌薬投与，手術環境，人工関節の選択，診断，術後管理，遅発性感染の予防など多岐にわたり，PJIに関するほぼすべての事項を網羅する内容でした．本会議で提案された成果は出版され，複数の診断法をもとに提唱されたPJIの診断基準は，現在多くの論文で採用されつつあります．

　実臨床に役立つ本書の内容をすべての整形外科の先生方に知っていただくために，分担執筆された先生方に早速，翻訳作業に取り組んでいただき，このたび，日本語版の発刊に至りました．本書を一度繙いていただくと，直ちにその特徴に気がつかれると思います．PJIに関することがらを章立てし，各章は質問とその回答という形式で記述されています．本書を読むこと

により，日常診療での疑問に対する回答や参考意見が得られることになります．しかもそれらの回答が多くの文献に基づき，現時点で世界的にも合意の得られた，最も信頼の高い内容となります．PJI は発生を予防することが肝要で十分に対策を講じる必要があり，また適切な初期対応が病態を重篤化させないために最も重要ですから，多くの先生方に本書を携帯していただき，ぜひ活用していただきたいと考えております．

末筆となりましたが，本書の翻訳作業にご尽力いただいた先生方に深謝いたします．

2016 年 3 月

横浜市立大学医学部整形外科　教授

齋藤知行

監訳・編集・訳者一覧

監訳

田中　栄　　東京大学医学部　整形外科　教授
齋藤知行　　横浜市立大学医学部　整形外科　教授

編集

山田浩司　　関東労災病院　整形外科・脊椎外科

訳者

西野仁樹　　東京大学医学部　整形外科（Workgroup1）
苅田達郎　　東京都立多摩総合医療センター　整形外科　部長（Workgroup2）
中元秀樹　　横浜労災病院　整形外科（Workgroup3）
時村文秋　　東京都健康長寿医療センター　整形外科　外科総括部長（Workgroup4）
木幡一博　　東京都立多摩総合医療センター　整形外科（Workgroup5）
吉井祥二　　関東労災病院　整形外科・脊椎外科　部長（Workgroup6）
小林直実　　横浜市立大学医学部　整形外科　講師（Workgroup7）
中嶋香児　　関東労災病院　整形外科・脊椎外科（Workgroup8）
兵頭　晃　　関東労災病院　整形外科・脊椎外科　部長（Workgroup9）
崔　賢民　　横浜市立大学医学部　整形外科（Workgroup10）
小林秀郎　　横浜市立大学医学部　整形外科（Workgroup11）
稲葉　裕　　横浜市立大学医学部　整形外科　准教授（Workgroup12）
大野久美子　東京大学医学部　整形外科（Workgroup13）
松下和彦　　川崎市立多摩病院　整形外科　部長（Workgroup14）
西川洋生　　昭和大学医学部　整形外科（Workgroup15）

Contents

序文 ……………………………………………………………………………………………… iii
序文 ……………………………………………………………………………………………… v
監訳・編集・訳者一覧 ………………………………………………………………………… vii

第 1 章 リスクの軽減と教育 …………………………………………………………… 1

Q1A 待機的な人工関節全置換術（TJA）後の，手術部位感染（SSI）あるいは人工関節周囲感染（PJI）発症の重要なリスクファクターにはどのようなものがあるか？ ……………………………………… 1

Q1B 待機的な TJA 後の，SSI あるいは PJI 発症の潜在的リスクファクターにはどのようなものがあるか？ ………………………………… 1

Q2 待機的人工関節置換術を受ける患者に対する口腔衛生の役割とは何か？ ……………………………………………………………… 2

Q3A メチシリン耐性黄色ブドウ球菌（MRSA）およびメチシリン感受性黄色ブドウ球菌（MSSA）のスクリーニングはどのようなプロセスを経るべきか？ ………………………………………………… 2

Q3B MRSA および MSSA 除菌を目的とした治療法として何が推奨されるか？ ……………………………………………………………… 2

Q4 医療従事者に対して MRSA や MSSA のスクリーニングを行うべきか？ ……………………………………………………………… 3

Q5 待機的人工関節置換術を受ける患者に対してルーチンの尿検査の役割は？ ……………………………………………………………… 3

Q6 待機的な TJA の前に疾患修飾薬は中止すべきか？ ………………… 3

Q7 感染性の関節炎に罹患したことのある患者においては，続発性の PJI リスクを最小化するためにどのような対策をとるべきか？ ……………………………………………………………… 4

第 2 章 周術期の皮膚準備 ……………………………………………………………… 15

Q1A 術前の皮膚除菌は有用か？ ………………………………………… 15

Q1B 術前皮膚除菌を行う場合は，どのような薬剤を使用し，周術期のどのタイミングで行うべきか？ ……………………………… 15

Q2 術前の術野消毒で推奨すべき薬剤はあるか？ ……………………… 15

Q3A 剃毛の適切な方法は？ ……………………………………………… 16

Q3B 剃毛はいつ行うべきか？ …………………………………………… 16

- **Q4** 皮膚病変のある患者に対して，どのように対応すべきか？ ……………… 16
- **Q5A** 術者と助手はどのように手洗いをするべきか？ …………………… 17
- **Q5B** 術者と助手は手洗いをする時にどの薬剤を使用すべきか？ ………………… 17

第 3 章 周術期抗菌薬投与 …………………………………………… 23

- **Q1** 抗菌薬の術前投与として適切なタイミングはいつか？ ………… 23
- **Q2** 予防抗菌薬投与で通常使用すべき適切な抗菌薬はあるか？ ………………… 23
- **Q3** 心臓の人工弁などの人工物が体内に存在する患者に対して，どの予防抗菌薬を使用すべきか？ ………………………………………… 23
- **Q4** セファロスポリンが投与できないとき，どのような抗菌薬を予防抗菌薬として使用すべきか？ ……………………………………… 24
- **Q5A** アナフィラキシー型のペニシリンアレルギー患者では，どの抗菌薬を投与するべきか？ ……………………………………………… 24
- **Q5B** アナフィラキシー型でないペニシリンアレルギーの場合，予防抗菌薬として使用すべき抗菌薬は何か？ ……………………… 24
- **Q6** バンコマイシンの予防的投与の適応は？ ………………………………… 25
- **Q7** バンコマイシンのルーチン使用を正当化できる医学的根拠は存在するか？ ………………………………………………………… 25
- **Q8** 抗菌薬の併用療法をルーチンで行うことは推奨できるか？（セファロスポリンとアミノグリコシド，もしくはセファロスポリンとバンコマイシン） ………………………… 25
- **Q9** 尿検査で異常所見を呈した患者，および/あるいは尿路カテーテルが留置されている患者では，どのような抗菌薬を予防的に投与すべきか？ …………………………………………………………… 26
- **Q10** 他の関節の感染治療を受けた患者では，術前に予防抗菌薬として使用する抗菌薬を変えるべきか？ …………………………… 26
- **Q11** 尿路カテーテル，あるいは術後ドレーンが留置されている間，術後の予防抗菌薬投与は継続するべきか？ ……………………………… 26
- **Q12** 手術部位感染（SSI）や PJI 予防のために最適な術後予防抗菌薬投与期間は？ ………………………………………… 27
- **Q13** 感染の疑いがある患者では，培養結果が出るまでどの抗菌薬を投与するべきか？ ………………………………………………………… 27
- **Q14** （二期的再置換術の）第二期の手術を行う場合は，どの抗菌薬が予防抗菌薬投与として適切か？ ……………………………………… 27

- **Q15** 長時間手術では，抗菌薬の術中追加投与はどのタイミングで行うべきか？ ……… 28
- **Q16** 予防抗菌薬投与は体重により投与量を調整するべきか？ ……… 28
- **Q17A** MRSA 保菌者では，予防抗菌薬としてどの抗菌薬が推奨されるか？ ……… 29
- **Q17B** MRSA の既往のある患者では，再度スクリーニングを行うべきか？ また，このような患者では，どのような抗菌薬を予防的に投与するべきか？ ……… 29
- **Q18** 腫瘍，もしくは腫瘍以外で メガプロステーシス を使用する大規模な整形外科的再建の場合，どの抗菌薬が推奨されるか？ ……… 29
- **Q19** 塊状他家骨移植（bulk allograft）で再建を行った患者では，予防的に投与する抗菌薬は変更するべきか？ ……… 30
- **Q20** コントロール不良な糖尿病患者，免疫不全疾患や自己免疫性疾患の患者では，予防抗菌薬投与は異なった抗菌薬を選択するべきか？ ……… 30
- **Q21A** 術前の予防抗菌薬は，初回人工関節置換手術と再置換手術では異なった抗菌薬を使用するべきか？ ……… 30
- **Q21B** 術前の予防抗菌薬は股関節と膝関節では異なる抗菌薬を使用するべきか？ ……… 31
- **Q22** カルバペネム耐性腸球菌や多剤耐性アシネトバクター保菌患者では，どの抗菌薬が予防抗菌薬投与として最も適しているか？ ……… 31

第 4 章 手術環境 ……… 49

- **Q1** 手術創内の細菌量は，手術部位感染（SSI）のしやすさと直接相関するか？ ……… 49
- **Q2** 手術室環境内の汚染細菌量は，SSI のしやすさと直接相関するか？ ……… 49
- **Q3** 待機的人工関節置換術を行う場合の手術室は，層流換気を備えている（バイオクリーンルームである）必要があるか？ ……… 49
- **Q4** 人工関節全置換術（TJA）で全身排気スーツを必ず着用するべきとする十分な医学的根拠はあるか？ ……… 50
- **Q5** 手術室の人の出入りでは，どのような対策をとるべきか？ ……… 50
- **Q6** 手術室のライトは，目線より上の物を触れないようにするためにフットペダルで操作できるようにするべきか？ ……… 50
- **Q7** 紫外線照射（ultraviolet（UV）light）は TJA 後の感染予防に有用か？ ……… 51

- **Q8** （夜間や週末の）使用されていない手術室で，殺菌用や滅菌用UVライトは手術室環境の清潔度に違いをもたらすか？ 51
- **Q9** 患者や手術室スタッフは手術室内空気汚染を助長しないようにマスクを使用するべきか？ 51
- **Q10** 手術室スタッフはどのような術衣を使用するべきか？ 52
- **Q11** 手術室での電子機器（携帯電話，ノート型パソコン，タブレットや音楽関係の器具）の使用に対してどのような規制を設けるべきか？ 52
- **Q12** 手術時間の延長は人工関節周囲感染（PJI）リスクを助長するか？ 52
- **Q13** 待機的 TJA の前に 既感染，不潔や汚染手術が入らないようにするべきか？ 53
- **Q14** 感染性合併症を予防するために患者体温管理は重要か？ 53
- **Q15** 温風式加温（FAW）ブランケットは SSI リスクを助長するか？ 53
- **Q16** 手術室スタッフは患者周囲におかれている医療機器などを触った際に，都度手指をアルコール製剤で消毒する必要があるか？ 54
- **Q17** 患者への診察，手技や手術台への移動などを行う際に遵守すべき手指衛生や手袋使用法のガイドラインは何か？ 54
- **Q18** TJA では汚染予防のため 3 重手袋を着用するべきか？ 54
- **Q19** 手術中はどの程度の頻度で手袋を交換するべきか？ 54
- **Q20** 器械台はいつ広げるべきか？ 55
- **Q21** 器械台は使用していない間は滅菌ドレープやタオルで覆うべきか？ 55
- **Q22** 皮膚を切開後，さらに深層の切開のためにメス刃は交換するべきか？ 55
- **Q23** 電気メスの先端は TJA 中に交換するべきか？ もし交換するとしたら，どのような頻度で交換するべきか？ 56
- **Q24** 吸引の先は，手術中定期的に交換するべきか？ もし交換するとしたら，どのような頻度で行うべきか？ また，吸引の先は大腿骨の髄腔内に入れるべきか？ 56
- **Q25** 膿盆は汚染源として知られているが，使用するべきか？ 56
- **Q26** 使い捨ての手術器具やカッティングガイドは，術野汚染リスクや PJI リスクを改善するか？ 56
- **Q27** 粘着ドレープは有用か？ 有用であるならば，どのようなタイプのドレープを使用するべきか（ヨード含有か，非含有か）？ 57

- **Q28** 術中，創縁や皮下脂肪にタオルや他の滅菌材料を当て，確実に創縁にクリップすることで，術野汚染や SSI は減少するか？ 57
- **Q29** どのようなドレープを使用すべきか（再利用可能なものか使い捨てか）？ 57
- **Q30** 術野の消毒前後に使用される粘着型 U 型ドレープは術野から非消毒エリアを効果的に遮るか？ 58
- **Q31** 洗浄は有効か？ どのような洗浄方法が良いか（高パルス，低パルス，もしくは バルブ）？ 58
- **Q32** どのような洗浄液を使用すべきか？ 抗菌薬を洗浄液に加えるべきか？ 58
- **Q33** 感染予防のための創内に自己血製剤を術中投与することに意味はあるか？ 59
- **Q34** ステープル，あるいは縫合糸の種類は感染イベントに影響するか？ もしするならば，感染を予防するうえで最良の閉鎖法は何か？ 59
- **Q35** 手術用安全チェックリストを使用したり，タイムアウトを行うことは人工関節患者の SSI 割合に影響を及ぼすか？ 59

第 5 章 血液保全 81

- **Q1** 輸血は手術部位感染（SSI）や人工関節周囲感染（PJI）のリスクの増大と関連するか？ 81
- **Q2** 人工関節全置換術（TJA）における同種血輸血の必要性をあらわす指標は何か？ 81
- **Q3A** PJI に対する人工関節置換術において，出血と同種血輸血を少なくする麻酔法は？ 81
- **Q3B** PJI の症例に対して脊髄麻酔は行うべきでないとするエビデンスはあるか（感染拡大のリスクがありうるため）？ 82
- **Q4A** 術中洗浄式自己血回収装置，術後非洗浄式自己血回収装置，バイポーラシーラーおよび希釈式自己血輸血法などの補助技術により PJI の術中出血量は減少するか？ 82
- **Q4B** 術中洗浄式自己血回収装置，術後非洗浄式自己血回収装置，バイポーラシーラーおよび希釈式自己血輸血法などの補助により TJA 中の出血は減少するか？ 82
- **Q5A** ドレーン留置は SSI や PJI に影響するか？ 83
- **Q5B** ドレーン抜去のタイミングは？ 83
- **Q6A** トラネキサム酸（TA）使用で PJI 治療を目的とした手術中の出血は減少するか？ 83
- **Q6B** TA の局所投与は静脈内投与に比べて有用か？ 83

Q7	多血小板血漿（PRP）やフィブリン糊のような薬剤で出血は減少するか？	84
Q8	PJI治療での二期的再置換術の第二期における自己血回収（術中および術後）は有用か？	84
Q9	PJI治療のための二期的再置換術の第一期と第二期の手術の間でのエリスロポエチン，造血薬などの薬剤の投与は有用か？	84
Q10	自己完結型の吸引装置は汚染の原因になるか？	85
Q11	PJI治療のための二期的再置換術において第二期の術前自己血貯血は有用か？	85

第 6 章　人工挿入物の選択 …… 95

Q1	人工挿入物の種類は，手術部位感染（SSI）あるいは人工関節周囲感染（PJI）の発生に影響を与えるか？	95
Q2A	抗菌薬含有セメントは待機的初回人工関節全置換術（TJA）後のPJI発生を減少させるか？	95
Q2B	抗菌薬含有セメントは待機的人工関節再置換術後のPJI発生を減少させるか？	95
Q3	人工股関節全置換術（THA）における摺動面のタイプはSSIやPJIの発生に影響を与えるか？	96
Q4	人工挿入物のサイズ（異物素材の大きさ）はTJA後のSSI発生に影響するか？	96
Q5	TJA後のSSIやPJIの発生に関して，様々な種類のセメント間で差はあるか？	96
Q6	抗菌薬の溶出に関して各セメント間で差はあるか？	96
Q7	セメントレス人工関節の種類でSSIやPJIの発生に差はあるか？	97
Q8	TJAの際，創部への抗菌薬パウダー（例えば，バンコマイシン）の使用は有用か？	97
Q9	感染後の骨欠損の再建に同種骨を用いた場合と金属補填材を用いた場合でSSIやPJIの発生に差があるか？	97
Q10	PJIの発生を最小限にするのに，人工挿入物表面の改良は有用か？	98
Q11	SSIやPJI予防のための新しい展開はあるか？	98

第 7 章　人工関節周囲感染の診断 …… 107

Q1A	人工関節周囲感染（PJI）の診断基準は？	107
Q1B	PJIの診断基準における留意事項は？	107

- **Q2** PJIの診断に関して，米国整形外科学会（AAOS）のアルゴリズムに賛同するか？ ... 108
- **Q3A** 急性発症のPJI診断における赤血球沈降速度（ESR），血清C反応タンパク（CRP），多形核好中球の割合（PMN%），白血球（WBC）数のカットオフ値は？ ... 109
- **Q3B** 遅発性PJIの診断におけるESR，CRP，PMN%，WBC数のカットオフ値は？ ... 110
- **Q3C** 炎症性関節症におけるPJIに関するESR，CRP，PMN%，WBC数のカットオフ値は？ ... 110
- **Q4** 関節液細胞数を分析するにあたり，変動を最小限に抑えるために重要な点は？ ... 111
- **Q5** 通常の培養はどのくらいの期間行うべきか？ ... 111
- **Q6A** PJIが疑われる症例において，通常の抗酸菌（AFB）や真菌検査は必要か？ ... 111
- **Q6B** 無菌ゆるみが疑われる場合，通常のAFBや真菌検査は必要か？ ... 112
- **Q7A** PJIまたは無菌性ゆるみが疑われる症例において，細菌培養のために必要な組織検体数は？ ... 112
- **Q7B** 培養検体はどのように採取すべきか？ ... 112
- **Q7C** すべての症例において，培養のための検体採取に先立って，抗菌薬の使用は控えるべきか？ ... 112
- **Q8** PJI診断において通常検査として超音波処理を行う必要があるか？ あるなら，どの患者群に適用されるべきか？ ... 113
- **Q9** PJI診断に，ポリメラーゼ連鎖反応（PCR）などの分子生物学的手法が果たす役割はあるか？ もしあれば，どのような患者に対して行うべきか？ ... 113
- **Q10** PJI診断に，画像診断法が果たす役割はあるか？ ... 113

第8章 術後創管理 ... 125

- **Q1A** 人工関節全置換術（TJA）後の創に対する最適なドレッシング材は何か？ ... 125
- **Q1B** 銀含浸ドレッシング材の使用は手術部位感染（SSI）や人工関節周囲感染（PJI）を減少させるか？ ... 125
- **Q2** TJA後どのような状態を創から浸出が持続していると考えるべきか？ ... 125
- **Q3A** TJA後の浸出が続く創に対処するための非外科的治療法は？ ... 126
- **Q3B** TJA後の浸出が続く創に対処するための外科的治療法は？ ... 126

- Q3C 創から浸出が持続している患者に経口あるいは静脈内抗菌薬投与を行うべきか? ……… 126
- Q4 TJA 後に浸出が持続する創に対する再手術の適応は? ……… 126
- Q5 SSI 軽減のためどのようにして再手術前に患者状態を改善できるか? ……… 127
- Q6 TJA 後に浸出が持続する創に対して I&D を行う際,術中培養は採取されるべきか? ……… 127
- Q7 TJA の I&D の際に,皮膚切開前の周術期抗菌薬投与は控えるべきか? ……… 127
- Q8 TJA 後,SSI と PJI のリスクを軽減するための最適な創閉鎖法は? ……… 128

第 9 章 スペーサー ……… 135

- Q1 人工膝関節周囲感染に対する治療で,インプラントを抜去してから再置換を行うまでの待機期間において,非人工関節型スペーサーと人工関節型スペーサーに機能的な差はあるか? ……… 135
- Q2 TKA の治療において非人工関節型スペーサーもしくは人工関節型スペーサーを使用することで,再置換術後少なくとも 2 年以降の機能的予後に差はあるか? ……… 135
- Q3 人工股関節周囲感染に対する治療でインプラントを抜去してから再置換を行うまでの待機期間中,非人工関節型スペーサーと人工関節型スペーサーに機能的な差はあるか? ……… 136
- Q4 THA の治療において,非人工関節型スペーサーもしくは人工関節型スペーサーを使用することで,再置換術後少なくとも 2 年以降における機能的予後に差はあるか? ……… 136
- Q5 膝および股関節の人工関節周囲感染(PJI)の治療に対し,非人工関節型スペーサーと人工関節型スペーサーでは,再置換術の手技上の難易度に差はあるか? ……… 136
- Q6 膝関節の人工関節型スペーサーと非人工関節型スペーサーでは,感染制御に関して差はあるか? ……… 137
- Q7 股関節の人工関節型スペーサーと非人工関節型スペーサーの使用では,感染制御に関して差はあるか? ……… 137
- Q8 膝関節に使用される人工関節型スペーサーの種類の違いにより,感染制御に関して差はあるか? ……… 137
- Q9 非人工関節型スペーサーや人工関節型スペーサーの使用において禁忌はあるか? ……… 137
- Q10 膝の手術において,製品として市販されているスペーサーと術者が手作りした可動性のあるスペーサーでは,機能的予後に差はあるか? ……… 138

- **Q11** 膝関節の手術で，製品として市販されているスペーサーと術者が手作りした可動性のあるスペーサーでは，感染制御率に差はあるか？ ……………………………………………………………… 138
- **Q12** 股関節の手術で，製品として市販されているスペーサーと術者が手作りした可動性のあるスペーサーでは，機能的予後に差はあるか？ ……………………………………………………………… 139
- **Q13** 股関節の手術で，製品として市販されているスペーサーと術者が手作りした可動性のあるスペーサーでは，感染制御率に差はあるか？ ……………………………………………………………… 139
- **Q14** どの抗菌薬を使用し，どのくらいの量をセメントスペーサーに加えるべきか？ ………………………………………………………… 139
- **Q15** 高用量の抗菌薬含有セメントスペーサーを準備するのに，最適な方法は（混合の仕方，抗菌薬を加えるタイミングと方法，多孔性）？ ……………………………………………………… 142

第10章 洗浄デブリドマン …………………………………………… 153

- **Q1A** 洗浄デブリドマン（I&D）はどの段階で考慮されるべきか？ …………………………………………………………………… 153
- **Q1B** 晩期の血行性感染に対する治療として，I&D を行ってもよいか？ …………………………………………………………………… 153
- **Q2** I&D の禁忌は？ ……………………………………………………… 153
- **Q3A** 人工膝関節全置換術（TKA）後の血腫に対して I&D を施行する際，深筋膜を切開するべきか？ ………………………………… 154
- **Q3B** 人工股関節全置換術（THA）後の血腫に対して I&D を施行する際，深筋膜を切開するべきか？ ………………………………… 154
- **Q4** I&D は，人工関節周囲感染（PJI）でどのように行うべきか？ … 154
- **Q5** モジュラーパーツは I&D の際に常に交換するべきか？ ……… 155
- **Q6** I&D の適応を決める際に有用な分類システム（例：Tsukayama 分類）はあるか？ ………………………………… 155
- **Q7** I&D は緊急処置なのか？ それとも術前に患者を最良な状態にしてから望むべきか？ …………………………………………… 155
- **Q8** 関節鏡検査は I&D において何かしら意味があるか？ ………… 155
- **Q9** インプラント抜去を行う前の I&D は，何度まで行うのが妥当か？ ………………………………………………………………… 156
- **Q10** I&D 施行中に細菌培養用のサンプルを採取するべきか？ もしそうであればどこからどのくらい採取するべきか？ …… 156

- Q11 I&D 後の患者に抗菌薬の長期投与は行うべきか？ もしそうであれば，その適応，抗菌薬のタイプ，投与量と治療期間は？ ... 156
- Q12 I&D 後の関節内局所抗菌薬投与は有用か？ 有用であるとすればその適応は？ ... 157
- Q13 吸収性抗菌薬含有剤（硫酸カルシウム など）は有用か？ 有用であるとすれば，その適応は？ ... 157

第11章 抗菌薬治療と再置換術のタイミング ... 165

- Q1 人工関節周囲感染（PJI）の人工関節抜去後の初期治療で，経口抗菌薬治療は点滴の代わりとなりうるか？ ... 165
- Q2 初期の抗菌薬点滴加療後に経口抗菌薬治療は適切か？ ... 165
- Q3 感染インプラント抜去後の適切な抗菌薬投与期間はどれくらいか？ ... 165
- Q4 抗菌薬投与期間はどのように決定するべきか？（炎症マーカー，臨床所見など） ... 166
- Q5 再置換術前に抗菌薬の休薬期間は必要か？ ... 166
- Q6 感染インプラント抜去後の点滴抗菌薬治療にリファンピンを併用することは，ブドウ球菌感染症（特にメチシリン耐性黄色ブドウ球菌〔MRSA〕）に対してより迅速で確実な治癒につながるか？ ... 166
- Q7 リファンピン投与を開始する最も適切なタイミングはいつか？ ... 167
- Q8 PJI に対して施行された一期的（人工関節）再置換術後，どのくらいの期間抗菌薬投与を継続すべきか？ ... 167
- Q9 再置換術後の関節内局所抗菌薬投与は有用か？ もし有用であればその適応は？ ... 167
- Q10 培養陰性の PJI に対する最適な抗菌薬の治療法は？ ... 168
- Q11 再置換術前の関節穿刺は必要か？ ... 168

第12章 一期的再置換術 vs 二期的再置換術 ... 175

- Q1 一期的（人工関節）再置換術の適応と禁忌は？ ... 175
- Q2 二期的（人工関節）再置換術の適応は？ ... 175
- Q3 二期的再置換術 の最適な待機期間はどれくらいか？ ... 176
- Q4 一期的再置換術と二期的再置換術ではコストに差があるか？ ... 176
- Q5 PJI 患者には，再置換術は何回行うべきか？ ... 176

Q6	膝関節固定術の適応は?	176
Q7	感染が慢性化した関節に膝関節固定術を計画する場合,一期的か二期的のどちらで行うべきか?	177
Q8	切断術の適応は?	177

第13章 真菌性あるいは非定型的人工関節周囲感染の治療 ……185

Q1	真菌性あるいは非定型的人工関節周囲感染(PJI)の定義は何か?	185
Q2	どのような場合に真菌微生物がPJIの原因だとみなすべきか?	185
Q3	真菌性PJIを起こしやすい宿主側の因子(合併症や他の因子)は何か?	185
Q4	真菌微生物が対象として考慮される場合,どのような検体が収集されるべきか? どのような追加診断方法を用いるべきか? 診断の最適化のために,それらをいかに用いるべきか?	186
Q5	真菌性PJIにおける最善の外科的治療法は? 洗浄デブリドマン(I&D),一期的再置換術,二期的再置換術,あるいは切除関節形成術のどれか?	187
Q6	真菌性PJI治療における最適(理想的)な抗真菌薬全身投与法は何か? (投与経路と種類と投与量)	187
Q7	真菌性PJIの段階的手術的治療において,セメントスペーサーにはどのような抗真菌薬あるいは抗細菌薬が投与されるべきか? その推奨される投与量は?	187
Q8	真菌性PJIをモニターし,再置換術のタイミングを決定するために推奨される検査は何か?	188
Q9	真菌性PJI治療における全身性抗菌薬(抗真菌薬)の投与期間は?	188

第14章 経口抗菌薬療法 ……195

Q1	適切な外科治療を行いインプラントの温存を試みた急性(早期あるいは晩期)の人工関節周囲感染(PJI)に対して,投与すべき適切な経口抗菌薬,あるいは併用療法は?	195
Q2	デブリドマンによるインプラント温存療法が行われた急性のPJIにおいて,抗菌薬はどれくらいの期間投与するべきか?	195
Q3	外科的治療が適切に行われなかったPJIの治療において,抗菌薬併用療法の役割は?	195

- **Q4** 抗菌薬による抑制療法はどのくらいの期間なされるべきか? ……………………………………………………………………………… 196
- **Q5** 細菌別に,どのような抗菌薬が抑制療法として利用できるか? ……………………………………………………………………………… 196

第15章 晩期人工関節周囲感染の予防 …………… 203

- **Q1** 晩期人工関節周囲感染(PJI)の定義は? ………… 203
- **Q2** 晩期 PJI を診断するには何をすべきか? …………… 203
- **Q3** 予防的に投与する抗凝固剤の種類,投与量および投与期間は,人工関節全置換術(TJA)後の手術部位感染(SSI)の発生に影響するか? ……………………………………………………………………………… 203
- **Q4** TJA 後の患者にルーチンで歯科処置時の予防抗菌薬を投与するべきか? ……………………………………………………………………………… 204
- **Q5** 晩期 PJI のハイリスク患者は,ウイルス性疾患に罹患している間,予防抗菌薬を投与されるべきか? ……………………………… 205
- **Q6** 大腸内視鏡検査などの内視鏡治療の際,晩期 PJI を予防するために,一過性の菌血症を最小化できるか? ……………………… 205
- **Q7** 腸壁からの細菌の転移を減少させるために,薬草サプリメント,プロビオティクス,および代替医療は役に立つか? ……… 205
- **Q8** 無症候性の患者に対する術後のメチシリン耐性黄色ブドウ球菌(MRSA)保菌のモニタリングに意味はあるか? ……………… 205
- **Q9** 晩期 PJI の関節外感染巣を特定する方法は? …………… 206
- **Q10** TJA 後の発熱に対して,いつから精査を行うべきか? ………… 206

"International Consensus Meeting on Periprosthetic Joint Infection" に参加して ……………………………………………………………………………… 219

あとがき ……………………………………………………………………………… 221

索引 ……………………………………………………………………………… 223

1 リスクの軽減と教育

Workgroup 1：Mitigation and Education

Question 1A

- 待機的な人工関節全置換術（TJA）後の，手術部位感染（SSI）あるいは人工関節周囲感染（PJI）発症の重要なリスクファクターにはどのようなものがあるか？

コンセンサス

炎症関節の活動性感染（化膿性関節炎），敗血症の存在，および/または局所皮膚，皮下もしくは深部組織の活動性感染の存在は，全て SSI あるいは PJI 発症の重要なリスクファクターであり，待機的 TJA を行うのは禁忌である．（参考文献 1-9）

投票結果

同意：99％，反対：0％，棄権：1％ （強いコンセンサス）

Question 1B

- 待機的な TJA 後の，SSI あるいは PJI 発症の潜在的リスクファクターにはどのようなものがあるか？

コンセンサス

SSI あるいは PJI のリスクファクターには，過去の手術歴，コントロール不十分な糖尿病（血糖値＞200 mg/dl あるいは HbA1c ＞7％），栄養失調症，病的肥満 （BMI＞40 kg/m^2），活動性肝疾患，慢性腎疾患，過度の喫煙（1 日 1 パック以上），過度のアルコール消費量（1 週間に 40 単位以上），経静脈投与による薬物乱用，最近の入院，リハビリテーション施設入所期間の延長，男性，外傷後関節症，炎症性関節疾患，罹患関節に対する外科治療の既往，重篤な免疫不全などが含まれる．（参考文献 10-60）

投票結果

同意：94％，反対：4％，棄権：2％ （強いコンセンサス）

Question 2

- 待機的人工関節置換術を受ける患者に対する口腔衛生の役割とは何か？

コンセンサス

待機的人工関節置換術を受けるすべての患者に対して口腔内活動性感染の有無についてスクリーニングを行うべきである．手法としては，質問紙法あるいは口腔検査が考えられる．

(参考文献 60-66)

投票結果

同意：80％，反対：18％，棄権：2％（強いコンセンサス）

Question 3A

- メチシリン耐性黄色ブドウ球菌（MRSA）およびメチシリン感受性黄色ブドウ球菌（MSSA）のスクリーニングはどのようなプロセスを経るべきか？

コンセンサス

ワーキング・グループは，人工関節置換術を受ける全ての患者に対して一律にスクリーニングおよび除菌を行うことは推奨しない．一方，黄色ブドウ球菌（MSSA および MRSA）についての術前スクリーニングと検出例に対する除菌は，SSI 発生割合とブドウ球菌およびブドウ球菌以外の細菌による感染の発生を減少させると認識している．(参考文献 67-72)

投票結果

同意：85％，反対：11％，棄権：4％（強いコンセンサス）

Question 3B

- MRSA および MSSA 除菌を目的とした治療法として何が推奨されるか？

コンセンサス

鼻腔内へのムピロシン短期投与が，MRSA および/または MSSA 除菌の方法として，現在最も広く受け入れられている．

(参考文献 67，73-75)

投票結果

同意：80％，反対：11％，棄権：9％（強いコンセンサス）

Question 4

- 医療従事者に対してMRSAやMSSAのスクリーニングを行うべきか？

コンセンサス

行うべきではない．医療従事者に対するルーチンのスクリーニングを正当化するエビデンスはない．MRSAおよびMSSAのスクリーニングは，医療従事者が細菌性感染に関連する症状を呈した場合に備えてとっておかなくてはならない．

(参考文献 76-83)

投票結果

同意：82％，反対：15％，棄権：3％（強いコンセンサス）

Question 5

- 待機的人工関節置換術を受ける患者に対してルーチンの尿検査の役割は？

コンセンサス

待機的人工関節置換術を受ける患者に対するルーチンの尿検査を正当化するエビデンスはない．待機的人工関節置換術前に尿路感染症（UTI）の症状を呈するあるいは既往を有する患者のために，尿検査は温存しておかなければならない．

(参考文献 84-88)

投票結果

同意：74％，反対：24％，棄権：2％（強いコンセンサス）

Question 6

- 待機的なTJAの前に疾患修飾薬は中止すべきか？

コンセンサス

中止すべきである．疾患修飾薬は待機的なTJAの前に中止すべきである．薬物投与を休止するタイミングは個々の薬剤や個々の患者特性に基づくべきである．免疫抑制薬の中止は，治療にあたっている内科医へのコンサルテーションおよび指示に基づいてなされるべきである． (参考文献 89-98)

投票結果

同意：92％，反対：5％，棄権：3％（強いコンセンサス）

薬物	半減期	推奨
非ステロイド性抗炎症薬（NSAIDs）	2〜17時間	術前1週間以内の休止
メトトレキサート	0.7〜5.8時間	術前1週間以内の休止 術後2週間で投薬再開（腎機能障害のある患者は術前2週間の休止）
スルファサラジン	5時間	術前1週間の休止
アザチオプリン	7.6時間	術前1週間の休止
レフルノミド	〜2週間	術前6週間の休止
ヒドロキシクロロキン	1〜2カ月	休止せず，術当日を含めて継続
生物学的製剤		
エタネルセプト	4.3日	術前1.5週間の休薬
インフリキシマブ	8〜10日	術前3週間の休薬
ゴリムマブ	12〜14日	術前1カ月の休薬
トシリズマブ	12〜14日	術前1カ月の休薬
アバタセプト	12〜14日	術前1カ月の休薬
アダリムマブ	12〜14日	術前1カ月の休薬
セトリズマブ	12〜14日	術前1カ月の休薬
リツキシマブ	21日	術前2カ月の休薬
抗痛風薬		
アロプリノール	1〜2時間	術前1週間以内の休薬
コルヒチン	26〜36時間	
プロベネシド	26〜36時間	

Question 7

- 感染性の関節炎に罹患したことのある患者においては，続発性のPJIリスクを最小化するためにどのような対策をとるべきか？

コンセンサス

感染性関節炎既往のある患者は全て，人工関節置換術施行前に血清学的検査による評価と，可能な限り関節穿刺を行うべきである．(参考文献 99-107)

投票結果
同意：84％，反対：14％，棄権：2％（強いコンセンサス）

コンセンサス

過去に人工関節周囲感染に罹患した患者に対し待機的人工関節置換術を施行する最適なタイミングに関してはさらなる研究が必要である．一方で，外科医は術中培養を採取することで，活動性の感染がないという確証を得るべきである．

(参考文献 99-107)

投票結果
同意：85％，反対：14％，棄権：1％（強いコンセンサス）

コンセンサス

人工関節置換術を行っている際に，もし骨セメントを利用するのなら，抗菌薬を添加すべきである．

投票結果
同意：90％，反対：5％，棄権：5％（強いコンセンサス）

コンセンサス

もし，術中培養が陽性と出たら，感染症専門医から得られた情報に基づいて，集中的な抗菌薬の点滴投与が適切に行われるべきである．

投票結果
同意：93％，反対：5％，棄権：2％（強いコンセンサス）

【掲載されている論文】

Mitigation and education.

Aggarwal VK, Tischler EH, Lautenbach C, Williams GR Jr, Abboud JA, Altena M, Bradbury TL, Calhoun JH, Dennis DA, Del Gaizo DJ, Font-Vizcarra L, Huotari K, Kates SL, Koo KH, Mabry TM, Moucha CS, Palacio JC, Peel TN, Poolman RW, Robb WJ 3rd, Salvagno R, Seyler T, Skaliczki G, Vasarhelyi EM, Watters WC 3rd.

J Arthroplasty. 2014 Feb；29（2 Suppl）：19-25. doi：10.1016/j.arth.2013.09.028. Epub 2013 Dec 17.

PMID：24360487

References:

1. Cherney DL, Amstutz HC. Total hip replacement in the previously septic hip. J Bone Joint Surg Am. 1983;65(9):1256-1265.
2. Jupiter JB, Karchmer AW, Lowell JD, Harris WH. Total hip arthroplasty in the treatment of adult hips with current or quiescent sepsis. J Bone Joint Surg Am. 1981;63(2):194-200.
3. Cruess RL, Bickel WS, vonKessler KL. Infections in total hips secondary to a primary source elsewhere. Clin Orthop Relat Res. 1975(106):99-101.
4. del Sel HJ, Charnley J. Total hip replacement following infection in the opposite hip. Clin

Orthop Relat Res. 1979(141):138-142.
5. Fitzgerald RH, Jr., Nolan DR, Ilstrup DM, Van Scoy RE, Washington JA, 2nd, Coventry MB. Deep wound sepsis following total hip arthroplasty. J Bone Joint Surg Am. 1977;59(7):847-855.
6. Hanssen AD, Rand JA. Evaluation and treatment of infection at the site of a total hip or knee arthroplasty. Instr Course Lect. 1999;48:111-122.
7. Schmalzried TP, Amstutz HC, Au MK, Dorey FJ. Etiology of deep sepsis in total hip arthroplasty. The significance of hematogenous and recurrent infections. Clin Orthop Relat Res. 1992(280):200-207.
8. Stinchfield FE, Bigliani LU, Neu HC, Goss TP, Foster CR. Late hematogenous infection of total joint replacement. J Bone Joint Surg Am. 1980;62(8):1345-1350.
9. Thomas BJ, Moreland JR, Amstutz HC. Infection after total joint arthroplasty from distal extremity sepsis. Clin Orthop Relat Res. 1983(181):121-125.
10. Hanssen AD, Osmon DR, Nelson CL. Prevention of deep periprosthetic joint infection. Instr Course Lect. 1997;46:555-567.
11. Peersman G, Laskin R, Davis J, Peterson M. Infection in total knee replacement: a retrospective review of 6489 total knee replacements. Clin Orthop Relat Res. 2001(392):15-23.
12. American Diabetes Association. Standards of medical care in diabetes--2013. Diabetes Care. 2013;36 Suppl 1:S11-66.
13. Jamsen E, Nevalainen P, Kalliovalkama J, Moilanen T. Preoperative hyperglycemia predicts infected total knee replacement. Eur J Intern Med. 2010;21(3):196-201.
14. Marchant MH, Jr., Viens NA, Cook C, Vail TP, Bolognesi MP. The impact of glycemic control and diabetes mellitus on perioperative outcomes after total joint arthroplasty. J Bone Joint Surg Am. 2009;91(7):1621-1629.
15. Pomposelli JJ, Baxter JK, 3rd, Babineau TJ, et al. Early postoperative glucose control predicts nosocomial infection rate in diabetic patients. JPEN J Parenter Enteral Nutr. 1998;22(2):77-81.
16. Adams AL, Paxton EW, Wang JQ, et al. Surgical outcomes of total knee replacement according to diabetes status and glycemic control, 2001 to 2009. J Bone Joint Surg Am. 20 2013;95(6):481-487.
17. Iorio R, Williams KM, Marcantonio AJ, Specht LM, Tilzey JF, Healy WL. Diabetes mellitus, hemoglobin A1C, and the incidence of total joint arthroplasty infection. J Arthroplasty. 2012;27(5):726-729 e721.
18. Del Savio GC, Zelicof SB, Wexler LM, et al. Preoperative nutritional status and outcome of elective total hip replacement. Clin Orthop Relat Res. 1996(326):153-161.
19. Gherini S, Vaughn BK, Lombardi AV, Jr., Mallory TH. Delayed wound healing and nutritional deficiencies after total hip arthroplasty. Clin Orthop Relat Res. 1993(293):188-195.
20. Jaberi FM, Parvizi J, Haytmanek CT, Joshi A, Purtill J. Procrastination of wound drainage and malnutrition affect the outcome of joint arthroplasty. Clin Orthop Relat Res. 2008;466(6):1368-1371.
21. Lavernia CJ, Sierra RJ, Baerga L. Nutritional parameters and short term outcome in arthroplasty. J Am Coll Nutr. 1999;18(3):274-278.
22. Nicholson JA, Dowrick AS, Liew SM. Nutritional status and short-term outcome of hip arthroplasty. J Orthop Surg (Hong Kong). 2012;20(3):331-335.
23. Jensen JE, Jensen TG, Smith TK, Johnston DA, Dudrick SJ. Nutrition in orthopaedic surgery. J Bone Joint Surg Am. 1982;64(9):1263-1272.
24. Fletcher RH, Fairfield KM. Vitamins for chronic disease prevention in adults: clinical applications. JAMA. 19 2002;287(23):3127-3129.
25. Flegal KM, Carroll MD, Kit BK, Ogden CL. Prevalence of obesity and trends in the distribution of body mass index among US adults, 1999-2010. JAMA. 2012;307(5):491-497.
26. Chen J, Cui Y, Li X, et al. Risk factors for deep infection after total knee arthroplasty: a meta-analysis. Arch Orthop Trauma Surg. 2013;133(5):675-687.
27. Dowsey MM, Choong PF. Obese diabetic patients are at substantial risk for deep infection after primary TKA. Clin Orthop Relat Res. 2009;467(6):1577-1581.
28. Everhart JS, Altneu E, Calhoun JH. Medical Comorbidities Are Independent Preoperative Risk Factors for Surgical Infection After Total Joint Arthroplasty. Clin Orthop Relat Res. Mar 22 2013. Epub before print.
29. Malinzak RA, Ritter MA, Berend ME, Meding JB, Olberding EM, Davis KE. Morbidly obese, diabetic, younger, and unilateral joint arthroplasty patients have elevated total joint arthroplasty infection rates. J Arthroplasty. 2009;24(6 Suppl):84-88.
30. Jibodh SR, Gurkan I, Wenz JF. In-hospital outcome and resource use in hip arthroplasty: influence of body mass. Orthopedics. 2004;27(6):594-601.
31. Peersman G, Laskin R, Davis J, Peterson MG, Richart T. Prolonged operative time correlates with increased infection rate after total knee arthroplasty. HSS J. 2006;2(1):70-72.
32. McElroy MJ, Pivec R, Issa K, Harwin SF, Mont MA. The effects of obesity and morbid obesity on outcomes in TKA. J Knee Surg. 2013;26(2):83-88.
33. Freeman JT, Anderson DJ, Hartwig MG, Sexton DJ. Surgical site infections following bariatric surgery in community hospitals: a weighty concern? Obes Surg. 2011;21(7):836-840.

34. Singh JA, Houston TK, Ponce BA, et al. Smoking as a risk factor for short-term outcomes following primary total hip and total knee replacement in veterans. Arthritis Care Res (Hoboken). 2011;63(10):1365-1374.
35. Mills E, Eyawo O, Lockhart I, Kelly S, Wu P, Ebbert JO. Smoking cessation reduces postoperative complications: a systematic review and meta-analysis. Am J Med. 2011;124(2):144-154 e148.
36. Myers K, Hajek P, Hinds C, McRobbie H. Stopping smoking shortly before surgery and postoperative complications: a systematic review and meta-analysis. Arch Intern Med. 2011;171(11):983-989.
37. Sorensen LT. Wound healing and infection in surgery. The clinical impact of smoking and smoking cessation: a systematic review and meta-analysis. Arch Surg. 2012;147(4):373-383.
38. Sorensen LT, Karlsmark T, Gottrup F. Abstinence from smoking reduces incisional wound infection: a randomized controlled trial. Ann Surg. 2003;238(1):1-5.
39. Sadr Azodi O, Bellocco R, Eriksson K, Adami J. The impact of tobacco use and body mass index on the length of stay in hospital and the risk of post-operative complications among patients undergoing total hip replacement. J Bone Joint Surg Br. 2006;88(10):1316-1320.
40. Lindstrom D, Sadr Azodi O, Wladis A, et al. Effects of a perioperative smoking cessation intervention on postoperative complications: a randomized trial. Ann Surg. 2008;248(5):739-745.
41. Harris AH, Reeder R, Ellerbe L, Bradley KA, Rubinsky AD, Giori NJ. Preoperative alcohol screening scores: association with complications in men undergoing total joint arthroplasty. J Bone Joint Surg Am. 2011;93(4):321-327.
42. Bradley KA, Rubinsky AD, Sun H, et al. Alcohol screening and risk of postoperative complications in male VA patients undergoing major non-cardiac surgery. J Gen Intern Med. 2011;26(2):162-169.
43. Tonnesen H, Rosenberg J, Nielsen HJ, et al. Effect of preoperative abstinence on poor postoperative outcome in alcohol misusers: randomised controlled trial. BMJ. 1999;318(7194):1311-1316.
44. Sunday JM, Guille JT, Torg JS. Complications of joint arthroplasty in patients with end-stage renal disease on hemodialysis. Clin Orthop Relat Res. 2002;(397):350-355.
45. Lieberman JR, Fuchs MD, Haas SB, et al. Hip arthroplasty in patients with chronic renal failure. J Arthroplasty. 1995;10(2):191-195.
46. Sakalkale DP, Hozack WJ, Rothman RH. Total hip arthroplasty in patients on long-term renal dialysis. J Arthroplasty. 1999;14(5):571-575.
47. Pour AE, Matar WY, Jafari SM, Purtill JJ, Austin MS, Parvizi J. Total joint arthroplasty in patients with hepatitis C. J Bone Joint Surg Am. 2011;93(15):1448-1454.
48. Hsieh PH, Chen LH, Lee MS, Chen CH, Yang WE, Shih CH. Hip arthroplasty in patients with cirrhosis of the liver. J Bone Joint Surg Br. 2003;85(6):818-821.
49. Cohen SM, Te HS, Levitsky J. Operative risk of total hip and knee arthroplasty in cirrhotic patients. J Arthroplasty. 2005;20(4):460-466.
50. Berbari EF, Osmon DR, Lahr B, et al. The Mayo prosthetic joint infection risk score: implication for surgical site infection reporting and risk stratification. Infect Control Hosp Epidemiol. 2012;33(8):774-781.
51. Guichelaar MM, Schmoll J, Malinchoc M, Hay JE. Fractures and avascular necrosis before and after orthotopic liver transplantation: long-term follow-up and predictive factors. Hepatology. 2007;46(4):1198-1207.
52. Ramsey-Goldman R, Dunn JE, Dunlop DD, et al. Increased risk of fracture in patients receiving solid organ transplants. J Bone Miner Res. 1999;14(3):456-463.
53. Tannenbaum DA, Matthews LS, Grady-Benson JC. Infection around joint replacements in patients who have a renal or liver transplantation. J Bone Joint Surg Am. 1997;79(1):36-43.
54. Lehman CR, Ries MD, Paiement GD, Davidson AB. Infection after total joint arthroplasty in patients with human immunodeficiency virus or intravenous drug use. J Arthroplasty. 2001;16(3):330-335.
55. Habermann B, Eberhardt C, Kurth AA. Total joint replacement in HIV positive patients. J Infect. 2008;57(1):41-46.
56. Hicks JL, Ribbans WJ, Buzzard B, et al. Infected joint replacements in HIV-positive patients with haemophilia. J Bone Joint Surg Br. 2001;83(7):1050-1054.
57. Lee J, Singletary R, Schmader K, Anderson DJ, Bolognesi M, Kaye KS. Surgical site infection in the elderly following orthopaedic surgery. Risk factors and outcomes. J Bone Joint Surg Am. 2006;88(8):1705-1712.
58. Jamsen E, Huhtala H, Puolakka T, Moilanen T. Risk factors for infection after knee arthroplasty. A register-based analysis of 43,149 cases. J Bone Joint Surg Am. 2009;91(1):38-47.
59. Kurtz SM, Ong KL, Lau E, Bozic KJ, Berry D, Parvizi J. Prosthetic joint infection risk after TKA in the Medicare population. Clin Orthop Relat Res. 2010;468(1):52-56.
60. Willis-Owen CA, Konyves A, Martin DK. Factors affecting the incidence of infection in hip and knee replacement: an analysis of 5277 cases. J Bone Joint Surg Br. 2010;92(8):1128-1133.

61. Dye BA, Tan S, Smith V, et al. Trends in oral health status: United States, 1988-1994 and 1999-2004. Vital Health Stat 11. 2007(248):1-92.
62. Bartzokas CA, Johnson R, Jane M, Martin MV, Pearce PK, Saw Y. Relation between mouth and haematogenous infection in total joint replacements. BMJ. 20-27 1994;309(6953):506-508.
63. Barrington JW, Barrington TA. What is the true incidence of dental pathology in the total joint arthroplasty population? J Arthroplasty. 2011;26(6 Suppl):88-91.
64. LaPorte DM, Waldman BJ, Mont MA, Hungerford DS. Infections associated with dental procedures in total hip arthroplasty. J Bone Joint Surg Br. 1999;81(1):56-59.
65. Sandhu SS, Lowry JC, Morton ME, Reuben SF. Antibiotic prophylaxis, dental treatment and arthroplasty: time to explode a myth. J Bone Joint Surg Br. 1997;79(4):521-522.
66. Parvizi J, Della Valle CJ. AAOS Clinical Practice Guideline: diagnosis and treatment of periprosthetic joint infections of the hip and knee. J Am Acad Orthop Surg. 2010;18(12):771-772.
67. Perl TM, Golub JE. New approaches to reduce Staphylococcus aureus nosocomial infection rates: treating S. aureus nasal carriage. Ann Pharmacother. 1998;32(1):S7-16.
68. Kenner J, O'Connor T, Piantanida N, et al. Rates of carriage of methicillin-resistant and methicillin-susceptible Staphylococcus aureus in an outpatient population. Infect Control Hosp Epidemiol. 2003;24(6):439-444.
69. Schwarzkopf R, Takemoto RC, Immerman I, Slover JD, Bosco JA. Prevalence of Staphylococcus aureus colonization in orthopaedic surgeons and their patients: a prospective cohort controlled study. J Bone Joint Surg Am. 2010;92(9):1815-1819.
70. Kalmeijer MD, van Nieuwland-Bollen E, Bogaers-Hofman D, de Baere GA. Nasal carriage of Staphylococcus aureus is a major risk factor for surgical-site infections in orthopedic surgery. Infect Control Hosp Epidemiol. 2000;21(5):319-323.
71. Hacek DM, Robb WJ, Paule SM, Kudrna JC, Stamos VP, Peterson LR. Staphylococcus aureus nasal decolonization in joint replacement surgery reduces infection. Clin Orthop Relat Res. 2008;466(6):1349-1355.
72. Schweizer M, Perencevich E, McDanel J, et al. Effectiveness of a bundled intervention of decolonization and prophylaxis to decrease Gram positive surgical site infections after cardiac or orthopedic surgery: systematic review and meta-analysis. BMJ. 2013;346:f2743.
73. Kallen AJ, Wilson CT, Larson RJ. Perioperative intranasal mupirocin for the prevention of surgical-site infections: systematic review of the literature and meta-analysis. Infect Control Hosp Epidemiol. 2005;26(12):916-922.
74. van Rijen MM, Bonten M, Wenzel RP, Kluytmans JA. Intranasal mupirocin for reduction of Staphylococcus aureus infections in surgical patients with nasal carriage: a systematic review. J Antimicrob Chemother. 2008;61(2):254-261.
75. Johnson AJ, Daley JA, Zywiel MG, Delanois RE, Mont MA. Preoperative chlorhexidine preparation and the incidence of surgical site infections after hip arthroplasty. J Arthroplasty. 2010;25(6 Suppl):98-102.
76. Cox RA, Conquest C. Strategies for the management of healthcare staff colonized with epidemic methicillin-resistant Staphylococcus aureus. J Hosp Infect. 1997;35(2):117-127.
77. Muder RR, Brennen C, Goetz AM. Infection with methicillin-resistant Staphylococcus aureus among hospital employees. Infect Control Hosp Epidemiol. 1993;14(10):576-578.
78. Simmons BP, Munn C, Gelfand M. Toxic shock in a hospital employee due to methicillin-resistant Staphylococcus aureus. Infect Control. 1986;7(7):350.
79. Dutch Working Party for Infection Prevention. MRSA in nursing homes. 2007; www.wip.nl, Accessed 2013.
80. Garner JS. Guideline for isolation precautions in hospitals. The Hospital Infection Control Practices Advisory Committee. Infect Control Hosp Epidemiol. 1996;17(1):53-80.
81. Mitteilung der Kommission für Krankenhaushygiene und Infektionsprävention am RKI. Empfehlung zur prävention und Kontrolle von methicillin-resist-enten Staphylococcus aureus-Stämmen (MRSA) in Krankenhäusern under anderen medizinischen Einrichtungen. Bundesgesundheitsbsl-Gesundheitsforsch-Geseun-dheitsschutz. 1999;42:954-956.
82. Bowler I. Strategies for the management of healthcare staff colonized with epidemic methicillin-resistant Staphylococcus aureus. J Hosp Infect. 1997;36(4):321-322.
83. Lessing MP, Jordens JZ, Bowler IC. When should healthcare workers be screened for methicillin-resistant Staphylococcus aureus? J Hosp Infect. 1996;34(3):205-210.
84. Koulouvaris P, Sculco P, Finerty E, Sculco T, Sharrock NE. Relationship between perioperative urinary tract infection and deep infection after joint arthroplasty. Clin Orthop Relat Res. 2009;467(7):1859-1867.
85. Ollivere BJ, Ellahee N, Logan K, Miller-Jones JC, Allen PW. Asymptomatic urinary tract colonisation predisposes to superficial wound infection in elective orthopaedic surgery. Int Orthop. 2009;33(3):847-850.
86. Lawrence VA, Gafni A, Gross M. The unproven utility of the preoperative urinalysis: economic evaluation. J Clin Epidemiol. 1989;42(12):1185-1192.
87. Nicolle LE, Bradley S, Colgan R, Rice JC, Schaeffer A, Hooton TM. Infectious Diseases Society of America guidelines for the diagnosis and treatment of asymptomatic bacteriuria in

adults. Clin Infect Dis. Mar 1 2005;40(5):643-654.
88. Rajamanickam A, Noor S, Usmani A. Should an asymptomatic patient with an abnormal urinalysis (bacteriuria or pyuria) be treated with antibiotics prior to major joint replacement surgery? Cleve Clin J Med. 2007;74 Suppl 1:S17-18.
89. Bozic KJ, Lau E, Kurtz S, et al. Patient-related risk factors for periprosthetic joint infection and postoperative mortality following total hip arthroplasty in Medicare patients. J Bone Joint Surg Am. 2012;94(9):794-800.
90. Schrama JC, Espehaug B, Hallan G, et al. Risk of revision for infection in primary total hip and knee arthroplasty in patients with rheumatoid arthritis compared with osteoarthritis: a prospective, population-based study on 108,786 hip and knee joint arthroplasties from the Norwegian Arthroplasty Register. Arthritis Care Res (Hoboken). 2010;62(4):473-479.
91. Howe CR, Gardner GC, Kadel NJ. Perioperative medication management for the patient with rheumatoid arthritis. J Am Acad Orthop Surg. 2006;14(9):544-551.
92. Jain A, Maini R, Nanchahal J. Disease modifying treatment and elective surgery in rheumatoid arthritis: the need for more data. Ann Rheum Dis. 2004;63(5):602-603.
93. Giles JT, Bartlett SJ, Gelber AC, et al. Tumor necrosis factor inhibitor therapy and risk of serious postoperative orthopedic infection in rheumatoid arthritis. Arthritis Rheum. 2006;55(2):333-337.
94. Momohara S, Kawakami K, Iwamoto T, et al. Prosthetic joint infection after total hip or knee arthroplasty in rheumatoid arthritis patients treated with nonbiologic and biologic disease-modifying antirheumatic drugs. Mod Rheumatol. 2011;21(5):469-475.
95. Grennan DM, Gray J, Loudon J, Fear S. Methotrexate and early postoperative complications in patients with rheumatoid arthritis undergoing elective orthopaedic surgery. Ann Rheum Dis. 2001;60(3):214-217.
96. Perhala RS, Wilke WS, Clough JD, Segal AM. Local infectious complications following large joint replacement in rheumatoid arthritis patients treated with methotrexate versus those not treated with methotrexate. Arthritis Rheum. 1991;34(2):146-152.
97. Carpenter MT, West SG, Vogelgesang SA, Casey Jones DE. Postoperative joint infections in rheumatoid arthritis patients on methotrexate therapy. Orthopedics. 1996;19(3):207-210.
98. Health Canada Drug Product Database. May 28, 2013; http://hc-sc.gc.ca/dhp-mps/prodpharma/databasdon/index-eng.php, 2013.
99. Le Dantec L, Maury F, Flipo RM, et al. Peripheral pyogenic arthritis. A study of one hundred seventy-nine cases. Rev Rhum Engl Ed. 1996;63(2):103-110.
100. Morgan DS, Fisher D, Merianos A, Currie BJ. An 18 year clinical review of septic arthritis from tropical Australia. Epidemiol Infect. 1996;117(3):423-428.
101. Ryan MJ, Kavanagh R, Wall PG, Hazleman BL. Bacterial joint infections in England and Wales: analysis of bacterial isolates over a four year period. Br J Rheumatol. 1997;36(3):370-373.
102. Li SF, Cassidy C, Chang C, Gharib S, Torres J. Diagnostic utility of laboratory tests in septic arthritis. Emerg Med J. 2007;24(2):75-77.
103. Li SF, Henderson J, Dickman E, Darzynkiewicz R. Laboratory tests in adults with monoarticular arthritis: can they rule out a septic joint? Acad Emerg Med. 2004;11(3):276-280.
104. Margaretten ME, Kohlwes J, Moore D, Bent S. Does this adult patient have septic arthritis? JAMA. 2007;297(13):1478-1488.
105. Parvizi J, Jacovides C, Zmistowski B, Jung KA. Definition of periprosthetic joint infection: is there a consensus? Clin Orthop Relat Res. 2011;469(11):3022-3030.
106. Spangehl MJ, Masri BA, O'Connell JX, Duncan CP. Prospective analysis of preoperative and intraoperative investigations for the diagnosis of infection at the sites of two hundred and two revision total hip arthroplasties. J Bone Joint Surg Am. 1999;81(5):672-683.
107. Atkins BL, Athanasou N, Deeks JJ, et al. Prospective evaluation of criteria for microbiological diagnosis of prosthetic-joint infection at revision arthroplasty. The OSIRIS Collaborative Study Group. J Clin Microbiol. 1998;36(10):2932-2939.

Question 1A

- **What are the significant risk factors for development of surgical site infection (SSI) or periprosthetic joint infection (PJI) after elective total joint arthroplasty (TJA)?**

<u>Consensus:</u> Active infection of the arthritic joint (septic arthritis), presence of septicemia, and/or presence of active local cutaneous, subcutaneous, or deep tissue infection are all significant risk factors predisposing patients to SSI or PJI and are contraindication to undertaking elective TJA.

Delegate Vote

Agree: 99%, Disagree: 0%, Abstain: 1% (Strong Consensus)

Question 1B

- **What are the potential risk factors for development of surgical site infection (SSI) or periprosthetic joint infection (PJI) after elective total joint arthroplasty (TJA)?**

<u>Consensus:</u> The risk factors for SSI or PJI include history of previous surgery, poorly controlled diabetes mellitus (glucose>200 mg/dl or HbA1C>7%), malnutrition, morbid obesity (BMI>40 Kg/m^2), active liver disease, chronic renal disease, excessive smoking (>one pack per day), excessive alcohol consumption (>40 units per week), intravenous drug abuse, recent hospitalization, extended stay in a rehabilitation facility, male gender, diagnosis of post-traumatic arthritis, inflammatory arthropathy, prior surgical procedure in the affected joint, and severe immunodeficiency.

Delegate Vote

Agree: 94%, Disagree: 4%, Abstain: 2% (Strong Consensus)

Question 2

- **What is the role of oral hygiene for patients, undergoing an elective arthroplasty?**

<u>Consensus:</u> All patients undergoing elective arthroplasty should be screened for evidence of active infection. This may be performed by administration of a questionnaire or dental examination.

Delegate Vote
Agree: 80%, Disagree: 18%, Abstain: 2% (Strong Consensus)

Question 3A

- **What should the process be for methicillin-resistant *Staphylococcus aureus* (MRSA) and methicillin-sensitive *Staphylococcus aureus* (MSSA) screening?**

Consensus: While this workgroup does NOT recommend universal screening and decolonization of all patients undergoing joint arthroplasty, it accepts that preoperative screening for *Staphylococcus aureus* (MSSA and MRSA) and decolonization decreases the rate of SSI and the incidence of staphylococcal and nonstaphylococcal infections.

Delegate Vote
Agree: 85%, Disagree: 11%, Abstain: 4% (Strong Consensus)

Question 3B

- **What should the treatment regimen be for methicillin-resistant *Staphylococcus aureus* (MRSA) and methicillin-sensitive *Staphylococcus aureus* (MSSA) decolonization?**

Consensus: Short-term nasal application of mupirocin is the most accepted current method of decolonization for MRSA and/or MSSA.

Delegate Vote
Agree : 80%, Disagree : 11%, Abstain : 9% (Strong Consensus)

Question 4

- **Should healthcare workers be screened for MRSA and MSSA?**

Consensus: NO. Routine MRSA and MSSA screening is not warranted for healthcare workers. MRSA/MSSA screening should be reserved for workers with symptoms associated with bacterial infections.

Delegate Vote
Agree: 82%, Disagree: 15%, Abstain: 3% (Strong Consensus)

Question 5

- **What is the role of routine urine screening in patients undergoing an elective arthroplasty?**

<u>Consensus:</u> Routine urine screening is NOT warranted for patients undergoing elective arthroplasty. Urine screening prior to elective arthroplasty should be reserved for patients with a present history or symptoms of a urinary tract infection (UTI).

Delegate Vote

Agree: 74%, Disagree: 24%, Abstain: 2% (Strong Consensus)

Question 6

- **Should disease-modifying agents be stopped prior to elective TJA?**

<u>Consensus:</u> Yes. Disease-modifying agents should be stopped prior to elective TJA. The timing of drug discontinuation should be based on the specific medication and the individual patient. The cessation of immunosuppressant medications should be performed in consultation and under the direction of the treating physician.

Delegate Vote

Agree: 92%, Disagree: 5%, Abstain: 3% (Strong Consensus)

Question 7

- **In patients with prior septic arthritis what strategies should be undertaken to minimize the risk of subsequent PJI?**

<u>Consensus:</u> ALL patients with prior septic arthritis should undergo evaluation by serology and aspiration of the joint whenever possible, prior to arthroplasty.

Delegate Vote

Agree : 84%, Disagree : 14%, Abstain : 2% (Strong Consensus)

<u>Consensus:</u> While the optimal timing for performing elective arthroplasty in a patient with prior septic arthroplasty needs further research, surgeons should ensure that no evidence of active infection exists by taking intraoperative cultures.

Delegate Vote

Agree: 85%, Disagree: 14%, Abstain: 1% (Strong Consensus)

Consensus: During arthroplasty, if cement is utilized, antibiotics should be added.

Delegate Vote

Agree : 90%, Disagree : 5%, Abstain : 5% (Strong Consensus)

Consensus: If intraoperative cultures are found to be positive, extended intravenous antibiotics should be appropriately administered with input from infectious disease specialists.

Delegate Vote

Agree: 93%, Disagree: 5%, Abstain: 2% (Strong Consensus)

2 周術期の皮膚準備

Workgroup 2 : Perioperative skin preparation

Question 1A

- 術前の皮膚除菌は有用か？

コンセンサス

有用である．術前に皮膚をグルコン酸クロルヘキシジン（CHG）で除菌するべきである．CHG の過敏症があるか，もしくは使用できない場合は，薬用石鹸が適切と思われる．
（参考文献 1-7）

投票結果

同意：90％，反対：8％，棄権：2％（強いコンセンサス）

Question 1B

- 術前皮膚除菌を行う場合は，どのような薬剤を使用し，周術期のどのタイミングで行うべきか？

コンセンサス

人工関節置換術の待機手術では，最低でも手術前日までには全身除菌を開始することを推奨する．入浴後は，何も全身に塗ることなく，清潔な浴衣や寝具を使い就寝することを推奨する．（参考文献 3, 7-13, 37）

投票結果

同意：85％，反対：10％，棄権：5％（強いコンセンサス）

Question 2

- 術前の術野消毒で推奨すべき薬剤はあるか？

コンセンサス

使用できる消毒薬間でその有用性に関する明らかな差は存在しない．アルコールを併用することが有用である可能性を示す根拠はいくつか存在する．（参考文献 10, 14-20）

投票結果
同意:89%,反対:8%,棄権:3%(強いコンセンサス)

Question 3A

- 剃毛の適切な方法は?

コンセンサス

シェービングよりもクリッピングの方が剃毛の方法としては望ましい.除毛を目的とした脱毛効果のあるクリームの有用性については不明である.(参考文献 21-24)

投票結果
同意:92%,反対:3%,棄権:5%(強いコンセンサス)

Question 3B

- 剃毛はいつ行うべきか?

コンセンサス

必要であれば,可能な限り執刀直前が望ましい.

(参考文献 10, 25, 26)

投票結果
同意:94%,反対:4%,棄権:2%(強いコンセンサス)

Question 4

- 皮膚病変のある患者に対して,どのように対応すべきか?

コンセンサス

手術部位付近に活動性の皮膚潰瘍のある患者に対して,人工関節置換術の待機手術は行うべきでない.われわれは,皮膚切開を行う場合は,潰瘍部分をさけて切開するべきというコンセンサスに達した.湿疹や乾癬など特定の皮膚病変を有する患者では,病変部が改善するまでは手術を延期するべきである.

(参考文献 27-30)

投票結果
同意:96%,反対:2%,棄権:2%(強いコンセンサス)

Question 5A

- 術者と助手はどのように手洗いをするべきか？

コンセンサス

術者と手術チームは最初の症例では消毒薬を用いて最低2分間は機械的に手を洗うべきである．その後の手術では，手洗い時間を短縮することは可能である．（参考文献 10, 31-36）

投票結果

同意：71％，反対：24％，棄権：5％（強いコンセンサス）

Question 5B

- 術者と助手は手洗いをする時にどの薬剤を使用すべきか？

コンセンサス

各消毒薬間で手洗いに関する明らかな有用性の差はない．

（参考文献 33, 37, 38）

投票結果

同意：80％，反対：15％，棄権：5％（強いコンセンサス）

【掲載されている論文】

Perioperative skin preparation.

Tokarski AT, Blaha D, Mont MA, Sancheti P, Cardona L, Cotacio GL, Froimson M, Kapadia BH, Kuderna J, López JC, Matar WY, McCarthy J, Morgan-Jones R, Patzakis M, Schwarzkopf R, Shahcheraghi GH, Shang X, Virolainen P, Wongworawat MD, Yates A Jr.

J Arthroplasty. 2014 Feb；29（2 Suppl）：26-8. doi：10.1016/j.arth.2013.09.029. Epub 2013 Dec 15. No abstract available.

PMID：24342277

References:

1. Webster J, Osborne S. Preoperative bathing or showering with skin antiseptics to prevent surgical site infection. Cochrane Database Syst Rev. 2012;9:CD004985.
2. Johnson AJ, Daley JA, Zywiel MG, Delanois RE, Mont MA. Preoperative chlorhexidine preparation and the incidence of surgical site infections after hip arthroplasty. J Arthroplasty. 2010;25(6 Suppl):98-102.
3. Zywiel MG, Daley JA, Delanois RE, Naziri Q, Johnson AJ, Mont MA. Advance pre-operative chlorhexidine reduces the incidence of surgical site infections in knee arthroplasty. Int Orthop. 2011;35(7):1001-1006.
4. Karki S, Cheng AC. Impact of non-rinse skin cleansing with chlorhexidine gluconate on prevention of healthcare-associated infections and colonization with multi-resistant organisms: a systematic review. J Hosp Infect. 2012;82(2):71-84.
5. Mehta S, Hadley S, Hutzler L, Slover J, Phillips M, Bosco JA, 3rd. Impact of preoperative MRSA screening and decolonization on hospital-acquired MRSA burden. Clin Orthop Relat Res.

2013;471(7):2367-2371.
6. Simor AE, Phillips E, McGeer A, et al. Randomized controlled trial of chlorhexidine gluconate for washing, intranasal mupirocin, and rifampin and doxycycline versus no treatment for the eradication of methicillin-resistant Staphylococcus aureus colonization. Clin Infect Dis. 2007;44(2):178-185.
7. Thompson P, Houston S. Decreasing methicillin-resistant Staphylococcus aureus surgical site infections with chlorhexidine and mupirocin. Am J Infect Control. 2013;41(7):629-633.
8. Eiselt D. Presurgical skin preparation with a novel 2% chlorhexidine gluconate cloth reduces rates of surgical site infection in orthopaedic surgical patients. Orthop Nurs. 2009;28(3):141-145.
9. Halpern CH, Mitchell GW, Paul A, et al. Self-administered preoperative antiseptic wash to prevent postoperative infection after deep brain stimulation. Am J Infect Control. 2012;40(5):431-433.
10. Mangram AJ, Horan TC, Pearson ML, Silver LC, Jarvis WR. Guideline for Prevention of Surgical Site Infection, 1999. Centers for Disease Control and Prevention (CDC) Hospital Infection Control Practices Advisory Committee. Am J Infect Control. 1999;27(2):97-132; quiz 133-134; discussion 196.
11. Lilly HA, Lowbury EJ, Wilkins MD. Limits to progressive reduction of resident skin bacteria by disinfection. J Clin Pathol. 1979;32(4):382-385.
12. Lowbury EJ, Lilly HA. Use of 4 per cent chlorhexidine detergent solution (Hibiscrub) and other methods of skin disinfection. Br Med J. Mar 3 1973;1(5852):510-515.
13. Wihlborg O. The effect of washing with chlorhexidine soap on wound infection rate in general surgery. A controlled clinical study. Ann Chir Gynaecol. 1987;76(5):263-265.
14. O'Grady NP, Alexander M, Burns LA, et al. Guidelines for the prevention of intravascular catheter-related infections. Clin Infect Dis. 2011;52(9):e162-193.
15. Darouiche RO, Wall MJ, Jr., Itani KM, et al. Chlorhexidine-Alcohol versus Povidone-Iodine for Surgical-Site Antisepsis. N Engl J Med. 2010;362(1):18-26.
16. Swenson BR, Hedrick TL, Metzger R, Bonatti H, Pruett TL, Sawyer RG. Effects of preoperative skin preparation on postoperative wound infection rates: a prospective study of 3 skin preparation protocols. Infect Control Hosp Epidemiol. 2009;30(10):964-971.
17. Saltzman MD, Nuber GW, Gryzlo SM, Marecek GS, Koh JL. Efficacy of surgical preparation solutions in shoulder surgery. J Bone Joint Surg Am. 2009;91(8):1949-1953.
18. Sistla SC, Prabhu G, Sistla S, Sadasivan J. Minimizing wound contamination in a 'clean' surgery: comparison of chlorhexidine-ethanol and povidone-iodine. Chemotherapy. 2010;56(4):261-267.
19. Dumville JC, McFarlane E, Edwards P, Lipp A, Holmes A. Preoperative skin antiseptics for preventing surgical wound infections after clean surgery. Cochrane Database Syst Rev. 2013;3:CD003949.
20. Apfelbaum JL, Caplan RA, Barker SJ, et al. Practice advisory for the prevention and management of operating room fires: an updated report by the American Society of Anesthesiologists Task Force on Operating Room Fires. Anesthesiology. 2013;118(2):271-290.
21. Tanner J, Norrie P, Melen K. Preoperative hair removal to reduce surgical site infection. Cochrane Database Syst Rev. 2011(11):CD004122.
22. Balthazar ER, Colt JD, Nichols RL. Preoperative hair removal: a random prospective study of shaving versus clipping. South Med J. 1982;75(7):799-801.
23. Ko W, Lazenby WD, Zelano JA, Isom OW, Krieger KH. Effects of shaving methods and intraoperative irrigation on suppurative mediastinitis after bypass operations. Ann Thorac Surg. 1992;53(2):301-305.
24. Sellick JA, Jr., Stelmach M, Mylotte JM. Surveillance of surgical wound infections following open heart surgery. Infect Control Hosp Epidemiol. 1991;12(10):591-596.
25. Alexander JW, Fischer JE, Boyajian M, Palmquist J, Morris MJ. The influence of hair-removal methods on wound infections. Arch Surg. 1983;118(3):347-352.
26. Seropian R, Reynolds BM. Wound infections after preoperative depilatory versus razor preparation. Am J Surg. 1971;121(3):251-254.
27. Penington A. Ulceration and antihypertensive use are risk factors for infection after skin lesion excision. ANZ J Surg. 2010;80(9):642-645.
28. Menon TJ, Wroblewski BM. Charnley low-friction arthroplasty in patients with psoriasis. Clin Orthop Relat Res. 1983(176):127-128.
29. Stern SH, Insall JN, Windsor RE, Inglis AE, Dines DM. Total knee arthroplasty in patients with psoriasis. Clin Orthop Relat Res. 1989(248):108-110; discussion 111.
30. Aly R, Maibach HE, Mandel A. Bacterial flora in psoriasis. Br J Dermatol. 1976;95(6):603-606.
31. Kappstein I, Schulgen G, Waninger J, Daschner F. [Microbiological and economic studies of abbreviated procedures for surgical hand disinfection]. Chirurg. 1993;64(5):400-405.
32. Pereira LJ, Lee GM, Wade KJ. The effect of surgical handwashing routines on the microbial counts of operating room nurses. Am J Infect Control. 1990;18(6):354-364.
33. Tanner J, Swarbrook S, Stuart J. Surgical hand antisepsis to reduce surgical site infection. Cochrane Database Syst Rev. 2008(1):CD004288.

34. Wheelock SM, Lookinland S. Effect of surgical hand scrub time on subsequent bacterial growth. AORN J. 1997;65(6):1087-1092; 1094-1088.
35. Pereira LJ, Lee GM, Wade KJ. An evaluation of five protocols for surgical handwashing in relation to skin condition and microbial counts. J Hosp Infect. 1997;36(1):49-65.
36. Recommended practices for surgical hand antisepsis/hand scrubs. AORN J. 2004;79(2):416-418, 421-416, 429-431.
37. Parienti JJ, Thibon P, Heller R, et al. Hand-rubbing with an aqueous alcoholic solution vs traditional surgical hand-scrubbing and 30-day surgical site infection rates: a randomized equivalence study. JAMA. 2002;288(6):722-727.
38. Weight CJ, Lee MC, Palmer JS. Avagard hand antisepsis vs. traditional scrub in 3600 pediatric urologic procedures. Urology. 2010;76(1):15-17.

Question 1A

- **Is there a role for preoperative skin cleansing with an antiseptic?**

<u>Consensus:</u> Yes. Preoperative cleansing of the skin with chlorhexidine gluconate (CHG) should be implemented. In the presence of a sensitivity to CHG, or when it is unavailable, it is our consensus that antiseptic soap is appropriate.

Delegate Vote
Agree: 90%, Disagree: 8%, Abstain: 2% (Strong Consensus)

Question 1B

- **What type and when should preoperative skin cleansing with an antiseptic be implemented?**

<u>Consensus:</u> We recommend that whole-body skin cleansing should start at least the night prior to elective arthroplasty. It is a consensus that after bathing patients are advised to sleep in clean garments and bedding without the application of any topical products.

Delegate Vote
Agree: 85%, Disagree: 10%, Abstain: 5% (Strong Consensus)

Question 2

- **Which agent, if any, is the optimal agent for surgical skin preparation?**

<u>Consensus:</u> There is no clear difference between various skin preparation agents. There is some evidence that combinations of antiseptic agents with alcohol may be important for skin antisepsis.

Delegate Vote
Agree: 89%, Disagree: 8%, Abstain: 3% (Strong Consensus)

Question 3A

- **What is the proper method of hair removal?**

<u>Consensus:</u> Clipping, as opposed to shaving, is the preferred method for hair removal. We cannot advise for or against the use of depilatory cream for removal of hair.

Delegate Vote
Agree: 92%, Disagree: 3%, Abstain: 5% (Strong Consensus)

Question 3B

- **When should hair removal be performed?**

Consensus: If necessary, hair removal should be performed as close to the time of the surgical procedure as possible.

Delegate Vote
Agree: 94%, Disagree: 4%, Abstain: 2% (Strong Consensus)

Question 4

- **What special considerations should be given to a patient with skin lesions?**

Consensus: Elective arthroplasty should NOT be performed in patients with active ulceration of the skin in the vicinity of the surgical site. It is our consensus that incisions should not be placed through active skin lesions. For certain lesions, such as those due to eczema and psoriasis, surgery should be delayed in these patients until their lesions have been optimized.

Delegate Vote
Agree: 96%, Disagree: 2%, Abstain: 2% (Strong Consensus)

Question 5A

- **How should the surgeon and assistants wash their hands?**

Consensus: The surgeon and operating room personnel should mechanically wash their hands with an antiseptic agent for a minimum of 2 minutes for the first case. A shorter period may be appropriate for subsequent cases.

Delegate Vote
Agree: 71%, Disagree: 24%, Abstain: 5% (Strong Consensus)

Question 5B

- **With what agent should the surgeon and assistants wash their hands?**

Consensus: There is no clear difference among various antiseptic agents for hand washing.

Delegate Vote

Agree: 80%, Disagree: 15%, Abstain: 5% (Strong Consensus)

3 周術期抗菌薬投与

Workgroup 3：Perioperative antibiotics

Question 1

- 抗菌薬の術前投与として適切なタイミングはいつか？

コンセンサス

術前の抗菌薬は，執刀開始前1時間以内に投与するべきである．ただし，バンコマイシンやフルオロキノロンは開始前2時間以内でよい．さらに，サーベイランスを行うことは現場のコンプライアンスを確実なものとするために非常に重要である．

(参考文献 1-14)

投票結果

同意：97％，反対：2％，棄権：1％（強いコンセンサス）

Question 2

- 予防抗菌薬投与で通常使用すべき適切な抗菌薬はあるか？

コンセンサス

第1世代，もしくは第2世代セファロスポリン（セファゾリンもしくはセフロキシム）が通常の予防抗菌薬として推奨される．イソキサゾリルペニシリンも代替薬としては適切である．

(参考文献 6, 15-23)

投票結果

同意：89％，反対：8％，棄権：3％（強いコンセンサス）

Question 3

- 心臓の人工弁などの人工物が体内に存在する患者に対して，どの予防抗菌薬を使用すべきか？

コンセンサス

予防抗菌薬では，通常行う人工関節の待機手術と同様の抗菌薬を使用するべきである． (参考文献 23-28)

投票結果
同意:94%,反対:3%,棄権:3%(強いコンセンサス)

Question 4
- セファロスポリンが投与できないとき,どのような抗菌薬を予防抗菌薬として使用すべきか?

コンセンサス

テイコプラニンやバンコマイシンは,通常使用する抗菌薬が投与できない場合の代替薬として妥当である.(参考文献 29-35)

投票結果
同意:73%,反対:22%,棄権:5%(強いコンセンサス)

Question 5A
- アナフィラキシー型のペニシリンアレルギー患者では,どの抗菌薬を投与するべきか?

コンセンサス

アナフィラキシー型のペニシリンアレルギー患者では,バンコマイシンやクリンダマイシンを予防的に投与するべきである.テイコプラニンが使用可能な国ではテイコプラニンも候補である.

投票結果
同意:88%,反対:10%,棄権:2%(強いコンセンサス)

Question 5B
- アナフィラキシー型でないペニシリンアレルギーの場合,予防抗菌薬として使用すべき抗菌薬は何か?

コンセンサス

ペニシリンに対してアナフィラキシー型でない反応を示した患者では,第2世代セファロスポリンが安全に使用できる.これは交差反応性が限定的であるからである.本当にペニシリンアレルギーであるかどうかを調べるためには,ペニシリンの皮内テストが有用である場合がある.(参考文献 3, 8, 36-50)

投票結果
同意:87%,反対:9%,棄権:4%(強いコンセンサス)

Question 6

- バンコマイシンの予防的投与の適応は？

コンセンサス

バンコマイシンは，メチシリン耐性黄色ブドウ球菌（MRSA）保菌者もしくはアナフィラキシー型のペニシリンアレルギー患者に対して用いることを検討すべきである．

下記のハイリスク患者に対しては，スクリーニングを行うことを検討すべきである
—MRSA 割合の高い地域にいる患者
—施設にいる患者（施設に入所中の患者，透析患者，ICU 入院中の患者）
—医療従事者

（参考文献 6, 51, 52）

投票結果

同意：93％，反対：7％，棄権：0％（強いコンセンサス）

Question 7

- バンコマイシンのルーチン使用を正当化できる医学的根拠は存在するか？

コンセンサス

存在しない．バンコマイシンの術前予防投与をルーチンで行うことは推奨できない．（参考文献 1, 8, 53-78）

投票結果

同意：93％，反対：6％，棄権：1％（強いコンセンサス）

Question 8

- 抗菌薬の併用療法をルーチンで行うことは推奨できるか？（セファロスポリンとアミノグリコシド，もしくはセファロスポリンとバンコマイシン）

コンセンサス

併用療法をルーチンで行うことは推奨できない．

（参考文献 78-83）

投票結果

同意：85％，反対：14％，棄権：1％（強いコンセンサス）

Question 9

- 尿検査で異常所見を呈した患者,および/あるいは尿路カテーテルが留置されている患者では,どのような抗菌薬を予防的に投与すべきか？

コンセンサス

尿路症状を訴える患者では,人工関節全置換術（TJA）を施行する前に尿検査を行うことが勧められる.非症候性の細菌尿患者では,通常どおりの予防抗菌薬投与で安全に TJA を行うことができる.急性尿路感染症（UTI）の患者では,待機的な人工関節置換術を行う前に治療が行われるべきである.
(参考文献 84-95)

投票結果
同意：82%,反対：12%,棄権：6%（強いコンセンサス）

Question 10

- 他の関節の感染治療を受けた患者では,術前に予防抗菌薬として使用する抗菌薬を変えるべきか？

コンセンサス

化膿性関節炎,もしくは人工関節周囲感染（PJI）の既往がある患者では,罹患関節の原因菌もカバーする抗菌薬を術前に投与すべきである.このような患者でセメントを使用する場合は,抗菌薬含有セメントの使用を推奨する.(参考文献 96-98)

投票結果
同意：84%,反対：10%,棄権：6%（強いコンセンサス）

Question 11

- 尿路カテーテル,あるいは術後ドレーンが留置されている間,術後の予防抗菌薬投与は継続するべきか？

コンセンサス

継続するべきではない.術後尿路カテーテルやドレーンが留置されている間も抗菌薬投与を継続するべきとする医学的根拠はない.尿路カテーテルやドレーンは安全に抜去できるタイミングで可及的早期に抜去するべきである.

(参考文献 2,87,88,99-113)

投票結果
同意：90％，反対：7％，棄権：3％（強いコンセンサス）

Question 12

- 手術部位感染（SSI）や PJI 予防のために最適な術後予防抗菌薬投与期間は？

コンセンサス

予防抗菌薬投与は術後 24 時間以降は継続されるべきではない．（参考文献　1, 22, 24, 114-121）

投票結果
同意：87％，反対：10％，棄権：3％（強いコンセンサス）

Question 13

- 感染の疑いがある患者では，培養結果が出るまでどの抗菌薬を投与するべきか？

コンセンサス

感染を疑う患者では，培養結果が出るまでの経験的抗菌薬投与は，それぞれの地域の微生物学的疫学調査に基づき選択するべきである．培養結果は，その後の抗菌薬選択に有用な情報となる．（参考文献　23, 122-131）

投票結果
同意：96％，反対：1％，棄権：3％（強いコンセンサス）

Question 14

- （二期的再置換術の）第二期の手術を行う場合は，どの抗菌薬が予防抗菌薬投与として適切か？

コンセンサス

第二期の手術を行う場合，予防的に投与する抗菌薬は，原因菌に対しても感受性のある抗菌薬を使用するべきである．セメントを使用する人工関節置換術では，抗菌薬含有骨セメントを使用するべきである．（参考文献　126, 132-136）

投票結果
同意：66％，反対：31％，棄権：3％（強いコンセンサス）

Question 15

- 長時間手術では,抗菌薬の術中追加投与はどのタイミングで行うべきか?

コンセンサス

使用する抗菌薬の半減期の2倍を目安に追加投与を行うべきである.抗菌薬の追加投与に関する一般的ガイドラインの情報を追加した.われわれは,出血量>2000 ccや補液量>2000 ccの症例では追加投与を行うことを推奨する.これらは独立した指標であり,いずれかの条件を満たした場合には,速やかに追加投与を検討することを推奨する. (参考文献 1-3, 10, 74, 75, 137-148)

投票結果

同意:94%,反対:5%,棄権:1%(強いコンセンサス)

Question 16

- 予防抗菌薬投与は体重により投与量を調整するべきか?

コンセンサス

予防抗菌薬は体重により異なった薬物動態を呈するため,体重によって調整するべきである. (参考文献 2, 18, 61, 149-159)

投票結果

同意:95%,反対:4%,棄権:1%(強いコンセンサス)

抗菌薬	実体重	推奨投与量	周術期投与間隔	適応
セファゾリン	60 kg 未満	1,000 mg	4時間毎	初回の予防抗菌薬投与
	60〜120 kg	2,000 mg	4時間毎	
	120 kg 超	3,000 mg	4時間毎	
セフロキシム	調整不要	1,500 mg	4時間毎	初回の予防抗菌薬投与
バンコマイシン	体重による調整が推奨される	15 mg/kg(最大 2,000 mg)	術前,術後12時間,術後24時間にそれぞれ1回投与する.	MRSA保菌者および/あるいはβラクタムアレルギー患者に対する予防抗菌薬投与

クリンダマイシン	調整不要	900 mg	3 時間毎	βラクタムアレルギー患者に対する予防抗菌薬投与
テイコプラニン	調整不要	400 mg	該当データなし	MRSA 保菌者および/あるいはβラクタムアレルギー患者に対する予防抗菌薬投与

Question 17A

- MRSA 保菌者では，予防抗菌薬としてどの抗菌薬が推奨されるか？

コンセンサス

MRSA 保菌者では，バンコマイシンかテイコプラニンが予防抗菌薬投与として推奨される．

投票結果

同意：86％，反対：12％，棄権：2％（強いコンセンサス）

Question 17B

- MRSA の既往のある患者では，再度スクリーニングを行うべきか？ また，このような患者では，どのような抗菌薬を予防的に投与するべきか？

コンセンサス

MRSA の既往がある患者も術前に再度スクリーニングは行うべきである．もし，MRSA 陰性であった場合は，通常どおりの予防抗菌薬投与を行うことを推奨する．

(参考文献 1, 52, 59, 70, 79, 160, 161)

投票結果

同意：76％，反対：23％，棄権：1％（強いコンセンサス）

Question 18

- 腫瘍，もしくは腫瘍以外でメガプロステーシスを使用する大規模な整形外科的再建の場合，どの抗菌薬が推奨されるか？

コンセンサス

さらなる重大な医学的根拠が示されるまでは，大規模な再建であっても通常どおり予防抗菌薬投与を行うことを推奨する．

(参考文献 162-174, 176)

投票結果

同意：93%，反対：6%，棄権：1%（強いコンセンサス）

Question 19

- 塊状他家骨移植（bulk allograft）で再建を行った患者では，予防的に投与する抗菌薬は変更するべきか？

コンセンサス

塊状他家骨移植で再建を行う場合でも，通常どおりの予防抗菌薬投与を行うべきである．(参考文献 175-184)

投票結果

同意：93%，反対：5%，棄権：2%（強いコンセンサス）

Question 20

- コントロール不良な糖尿病患者，免疫不全疾患や自己免疫性疾患の患者では，予防抗菌薬投与は異なった抗菌薬を選択するべきか？

コンセンサス

異なった抗菌薬を選択する必要はない．これらの患者でも通常どおりの抗菌薬が推奨される．(参考文献 185-209)

投票結果

同意：90%，反対：9%，棄権：1%（強いコンセンサス）

Question 21A

- 術前の予防抗菌薬は，初回人工関節置換手術と再置換手術では異なった抗菌薬を使用するべきか？

コンセンサス

異なった抗菌薬を使用する必要はない．予防抗菌薬投与は初回手術と非感染性の再置換手術では，同じ抗菌薬を使用するべきである．

投票結果

同意：89%，反対：10%，棄権：1%（強いコンセンサス）

Question 21B

- 術前の予防抗菌薬は股関節と膝関節では異なる抗菌薬を使用するべきか？

コンセンサス

周術期の予防抗菌薬は，股関節と膝関節で同じ抗菌薬を使用するべきである．（参考文献 201-213, 219）

投票結果

同意：99％，反対：1％，棄権：0％（強いコンセンサス）

Question 22

- カルバペネム耐性腸球菌や多剤耐性アシネトバクター保菌患者では，どの抗菌薬が予防抗菌薬投与として最も適しているか？

コンセンサス

多剤耐性菌に感染，もしくは保菌している者に対して，予防抗菌薬の選択を拡張するだけの十分な医学的根拠はない．
（参考文献 214-221）

投票結果

同意：76％，反対：8％，棄権：16％（強いコンセンサス）

【掲載されている論文】

Perioperative antibiotics.

Hansen E, Belden K, Silibovsky R, Vogt M, Arnold WV, Bicanic G, Bini SA, Catani F, Chen J, Ghazavi MT, Godefroy KM, Holham P, Hosseinzadeh H, Kim KI, Kirketerp-Møller K, Lidgren L, Lin JH, Lonner JH, Moore CC, Papagelopoulos P, Poultsides L, Randall RL, Roslund B, Saleh K, Salmon JV, Schwarz EM, Stuyck J, Dahl AW, Yamada K.

J Arthroplasty. 2014 Feb；29（2 Suppl）：29-48. doi：10.1016/j.arth.2013.09.030. Epub 2013 Dec 16. No abstract available.

PMID：24355256

References:

1. Recommendations for the Use of Intravenous Antibiotic Prophylaxis in Primary Total Joint Arthroplasty. http://www.aaos.org/about/papers/advistmt/1027.asp. Accessed 2013.
2. Prokuski L. Prophylactic antibiotics in orthopaedic surgery. J Am Acad Orthop Surg. 2008;16(5):283-293.
3. Bratzler DW, Houck PM. Antimicrobial prophylaxis for surgery: an advisory statement from the National Surgical Infection Prevention Project. Clin Infect Dis. 2004;38(12):1706-1715.
4. van Kasteren ME, Mannien J, Ott A, Kullberg BJ, de Boer AS, Gyssens IC. Antibiotic prophylaxis and the risk of surgical site infections following total hip arthroplasty: timely administration is the most important factor. Clin Infect Dis. 2007;44(7):921-927.
5. Classen DC, Evans RS, Pestotnik SL, Horn SD, Menlove RL, Burke JP. The timing of prophylactic administration of antibiotics and the risk of surgical-wound infection. N Engl J Med. 1992;326(5):281-286.
6. Bratzler DW, Houck PM. Antimicrobial prophylaxis for surgery: an advisory statement from the National Surgical Infection Prevention Project. Am J Surg. 2005;189(4):395-404.
7. Galandiuk S, Polk HC, Jr., Jagelman DG, Fazio VW. Re-emphasis of priorities in surgical antibiotic prophylaxis. Surg Gynecol Obstet. 1989;169(3):219-222.
8. Hawn MT, Richman JS, Vick CC, et al. Timing of surgical antibiotic prophylaxis and the risk of surgical site infection. JAMA Surg. 2013;148(7):649-657.
9. Weber WP, Marti WR, Zwahlen M, et al. The timing of surgical antimicrobial prophylaxis. Ann Surg. 2008;247(6):918-926.
10. Steinberg JP, Braun BI, Hellinger WC, et al. Timing of antimicrobial prophylaxis and the risk of surgical site infections: results from the Trial to Reduce Antimicrobial Prophylaxis Errors. Ann Surg. 2009;250(1):10-16.
11. Johnson DP. Antibiotic prophylaxis with cefuroxime in arthroplasty of the knee. J Bone Joint Surg Br. 1987;69(5):787-789.
12. Friedman RJ, Friedrich LV, White RL, Kays MB, Brundage DM, Graham J. Antibiotic prophylaxis and tourniquet inflation in total knee arthroplasty. Clin Orthop Relat Res. 1990;(260):17-23.
13. Soriano A, Bori G, Garcia-Ramiro S, et al. Timing of antibiotic prophylaxis for primary total knee arthroplasty performed during ischemia. Clin Infect Dis. 2008;46(7):1009-1014.
14. A WD, Robertsson O, Stefansdottir A, Gustafson P, Lidgren L. Timing of preoperative antibiotics for knee arthroplasties: Improving the routines in Sweden. Patient Saf Surg.5:22.
15. Neu HC. Cephalosporin antibiotics as applied in surgery of bones and joints. Clin Orthop Relat Res. 1984;(190):50-64.
16. Oishi CS, Carrion WV, Hoaglund FT. Use of parenteral prophylactic antibiotics in clean orthopaedic surgery. A review of the literature. Clin Orthop Relat Res. 1993;(296):249-255.
17. Schurman DJ, Hirshman HP, Kajiyama G, Moser K, Burton DS. Cefazolin concentrations in bone and synovial fluid. J Bone Joint Surg Am. 1978;60(3):359-362.
18. Forse RA, Karam B, MacLean LD, Christou NV. Antibiotic prophylaxis for surgery in morbidly obese patients. Surgery. 1989;106(4):750-756; discussion 756-757.
19. Sodhi M, Axtell SS, Callahan J, Shekar R. Is it safe to use carbapenems in patients with a history of allergy to penicillin? J Antimicrob Chemother. 2004;54(6):1155-1157.
20. Hill C, Flamant R, Mazas F, Evrard J. Prophylactic cefazolin versus placebo in total hip replacement. Report of a multicentre double-blind randomised trial. Lancet. 1981;1(8224):795-796.
21. Tyllianakis ME, Karageorgos A, Marangos MN, Saridis AG, Lambiris EE. Antibiotic prophylaxis in primary hip and knee arthroplasty: comparison between cefuroxime and two specific antistaphylococcal agents. J Arthroplasty. 2010;25(7):1078-1082.
22. Mauerhan DR, Nelson CL, Smith DL, et al. Prophylaxis against infection in total joint arthroplasty. One day of cefuroxime compared with three days of cefazolin. J Bone Joint Surg Am. 1994;76(1):39-45.
23. Stefansdottir A, Johansson D, Knutson K, Lidgren L, Robertsson O. Microbiology of the infected knee arthroplasty: report from the Swedish Knee Arthroplasty Register on 426 surgically revised cases. Scand J Infect Dis. 2009;41(11-12):831-840.
24. Enzler MJ, Berbari E, Osmon DR. Antimicrobial prophylaxis in adults. Mayo Clin Proc. 2011;86(7):686-701.
25. Wilson W, Taubert KA, Gewitz M, et al. Prevention of infective endocarditis: guidelines from the American Heart Association: a guideline from the American Heart Association Rheumatic Fever, Endocarditis, and Kawasaki Disease Committee, Council on Cardiovascular Disease in the Young, and the Council on Clinical Cardiology, Council on Cardiovascular Surgery and Anesthesia, and the Quality of Care and Outcomes Research Interdisciplinary Working Group. Circulation. 2007;116(15):1736-1754.
26. Eagle KA, Guyton RA, Davidoff R, et al. ACC/AHA 2004 guideline update for coronary artery bypass graft surgery: a report of the American College of Cardiology/American Heart Association Task Force on Practice Guidelines (Committee to Update the 1999 Guidelines for Coronary Artery Bypass Graft Surgery). Circulation. 2004;110(14):e340-437.

27. Edwards FH, Engelman RM, Houck P, Shahian DM, Bridges CR. The Society of Thoracic Surgeons Practice Guideline Series: Antibiotic Prophylaxis in Cardiac Surgery, Part I: Duration. Ann Thorac Surg. 2006;81(1):397-404.
28. Haydon TP, Presneill JJ, Robertson MS. Antibiotic prophylaxis for cardiac surgery in Australia. Med J Aust. 2010;192(3):141-143.
29. Mollan RA, Haddock M, Webb CH. Teicoplanin vs cephamandole for antimicrobial prophylaxis in prosthetic joint implant surgery: (preliminary results). Eur J Surg Suppl. 1992(567):19-21.
30. Lazzarini L, Pellizzer G, Stecca C, Viola R, de Lalla F. Postoperative infections following total knee replacement: an epidemiological study. J Chemother. 2001;13(2):182-187.
31. Periti P, Pannuti F, Della Cuna GR, et al. Combination chemotherapy with cyclophosphamide, fluorouracil, and either epirubicin or mitoxantrone: a comparative randomized multicenter study in metastatic breast carcinoma. Cancer Invest. 1991;9(3):249-255.
32. Periti P, Stringa G, Mini E. Comparative multicenter trial of teicoplanin versus cefazolin for antimicrobial prophylaxis in prosthetic joint implant surgery. Italian Study Group for Antimicrobial Prophylaxis in Orthopedic Surgery. Eur J Clin Microbiol Infect Dis. 1999;18(2):113-119.
33. Brogden RN, Peters DH. Teicoplanin. A reappraisal of its antimicrobial activity, pharmacokinetic properties and therapeutic efficacy. Drugs. 1994;47(5):823-854.
34. Wood MJ. The comparative efficacy and safety of teicoplanin and vancomycin. J Antimicrob Chemother. 1996;37(2):209-222.
35. Wilson AP. Antibiotic prophylaxis in cardiac surgery. J Antimicrob Chemother. 1988;21(5):522-524.
36. Darley ES, MacGowan AP. Antibiotic treatment of gram-positive bone and joint infections. J Antimicrob Chemother. 2004;53(6):928-935.
37. Dash CH. Penicillin allergy and the cephalosporins. J Antimicrob Chemother. 1975;1(3 Suppl):107-118.
38. Petz LD. Immunologic cross-reactivity between penicillins and cephalosporins: a review. J Infect Dis. 1978;137 Suppl:S74-S79.
39. Kelkar PS, Li JT. Cephalosporin allergy. N Engl J Med. 2001;345(11):804-809.
40. Saxon A, Beall GN, Rohr AS, Adelman DC. Immediate hypersensitivity reactions to beta-lactam antibiotics. Ann Intern Med. 1987;107(2):204-215.
41. Pichichero ME. Use of selected cephalosporins in penicillin-allergic patients: a paradigm shift. Diagn Microbiol Infect Dis. 2007;57(3 Suppl):13S-18S.
42. Pichichero ME, Casey JR. Safe use of selected cephalosporins in penicillin-allergic patients: a meta-analysis. Otolaryngol Head Neck Surg. 2007;136(3):340-347.
43. Audicana M, Bernaola G, Urrutia I, et al. Allergic reactions to betalactams: studies in a group of patients allergic to penicillin and evaluation of cross-reactivity with cephalosporin. Allergy. 1994;49(2):108-113.
44. Solensky R, Earl HS, Gruchalla RS. Lack of penicillin resensitization in patients with a history of penicillin allergy after receiving repeated penicillin courses. Arch Intern Med. 2002;162(7):822-826.
45. Campagna JD, Bond MC, Schabelman E, Hayes BD. The use of cephalosporins in penicillin-allergic patients: a literature review. J Emerg Med. 2012;42(5):612-620.
46. DePestel DD, Benninger MS, Danziger L, et al. Cephalosporin use in treatment of patients with penicillin allergies. J Am Pharm Assoc (2003). 2008;48(4):530-540.
47. Platt R. Adverse effects of third-generation cephalosporins. J Antimicrob Chemother. 1982;10 Suppl C:135-140.
48. Goodman EJ, Morgan MJ, Johnson PA, Nichols BA, Denk N, Gold BB. Cephalosporins can be given to penicillin-allergic patients who do not exhibit an anaphylactic response. J Clin Anesth. 2001;13(8):561-564.
49. Apter AJ, Kinman JL, Bilker WB, et al. Is there cross-reactivity between penicillins and cephalosporins? Am J Med. 2006;119(4):354 e311-359.
50. Park MA, Koch CA, Klemawesch P, Joshi A, Li JT. Increased adverse drug reactions to cephalosporins in penicillin allergy patients with positive penicillin skin test. Int Arch Allergy Immunol. 2010;153(3):268-273.
51. Advisory statement. Recommendations for the use of intravenous antibiotic prophylaxis in primary total joint arthroplasty. http://www.aaos.org/about/papers/advistmt/1027.asp, Accessed 2013.
52. Muto CA, Jernigan JA, Ostrowsky BE, et al. SHEA guideline for preventing nosocomial transmission of multidrug-resistant strains of Staphylococcus aureus and enterococcus. Infect Control Hosp Epidemiol. 2003;24(5):362-386.
53. Cantoni L, Glauser MP, Bille J. Comparative efficacy of daptomycin, vancomycin, and cloxacillin for the treatment of Staphylococcus aureus endocarditis in rats and role of test conditions in this determination. Antimicrob Agents Chemother. 1990;34(12):2348-2353.
54. Patel M, Kumar RA, Stamm AM, Hoesley CJ, Moser SA, Waites KB. USA300 genotype community-associated methicillin-resistant Staphylococcus aureus as a cause of surgical site

infections. J Clin Microbiol. 2007;45(10):3431-3433.
55. Manian FA, Griesnauer S. Community-associated methicillin-resistant Staphylococcus aureus (MRSA) is replacing traditional health care-associated MRSA strains in surgical-site infections among inpatients. Clin Infect Dis. 2008;47(3):434-435.
56. Recommendations for preventing the spread of vancomycin resistance. Recommendations of the Hospital Infection Control Practices Advisory Committee (HICPAC). MMWR Recomm Rep. 1995;44(RR-12):1-13.
57. Hiramatsu K, Aritaka N, Hanaki H, et al. Dissemination in Japanese hospitals of strains of Staphylococcus aureus heterogeneously resistant to vancomycin. Lancet. 1997;350(9092):1670-1673.
58. Michel M, Gutmann L. Methicillin-resistant Staphylococcus aureus and vancomycin-resistant enterococci: therapeutic realities and possibilities. Lancet. 1997;349(9069):1901-1906.
59. Fulkerson E, Valle CJ, Wise B, Walsh M, Preston C, Di Cesare PE. Antibiotic susceptibility of bacteria infecting total joint arthroplasty sites. J Bone Joint Surg Am. 2006;88(6):1231-1237.
60. UK Health protection agency. Surgical Site Infection surveillance service. Protocol for surveillance of surgical site infection. . http://www.hpa.org/uk/we/HPAwebFile/HPAweb_C/1194947388966, Accessed 2013.
61. Meehan J, Jamali AA, Nguyen H. Prophylactic antibiotics in hip and knee arthroplasty. J Bone Joint Surg Am. 2009;91(10):2480-2490.
62. Wiesel BB, Esterhai JL. Prophylaxis of musculoskeletal infections. In: J C, JT M, eds. Musculosketal Infections. New York: Marcel Dekker; 2003:115-129.
63. Merrer J, Desbouchages L, Serazin V, Razafimamonjy J, Pauthier F, Leneveu M. Comparison of routine prophylaxis with vancomycin or cefazolin for femoral neck fracture surgery: microbiological and clinical outcomes. Infect Control Hosp Epidemiol. 2006;27(12):1366-1371.
64. Cranny G, Elliott R, Weatherly H, et al. A systematic review and economic model of switching from non-glycopeptide to glycopeptide antibiotic prophylaxis for surgery. Health Technol Assess. 2008;12(1):iii-iv, xi-xii, 1-147.
65. Bolon MK, Morlote M, Weber SG, Koplan B, Carmeli Y, Wright SB. Glycopeptides are no more effective than beta-lactam agents for prevention of surgical site infection after cardiac surgery: a meta-analysis. Clin Infect Dis. 2004;38(10):1357-1363.
66. Mangram AJ, Horan TC, Pearson ML, Silver LC, Jarvis WR. Guideline for prevention of surgical site infection, 1999. Hospital Infection Control Practices Advisory Committee. Infect Control Hosp Epidemiol. 1999;20(4):250-278; quiz 279-280.
67. Tacconelli E, Cataldo MA, Albanese A, et al. Vancomycin versus cefazolin prophylaxis for cerebrospinal shunt placement in a hospital with a high prevalence of meticillin-resistant Staphylococcus aureus. J Hosp Infect. 2008;69(4):337-344.
68. Finkelstein R, Rabino G, Mashiah T, et al. Vancomycin versus cefazolin prophylaxis for cardiac surgery in the setting of a high prevalence of methicillin-resistant staphylococcal infections. J Thorac Cardiovasc Surg. 2002;123(2):326-332.
69. Garey KW, Lai D, Dao-Tran TK, Gentry LO, Hwang LY, Davis BR. Interrupted time series analysis of vancomycin compared to cefuroxime for surgical prophylaxis in patients undergoing cardiac surgery. Antimicrob Agents Chemother. 2008;52(2):446-451.
70. Spelman D, Harrington G, Russo P, Wesselingh S. Clinical, microbiological, and economic benefit of a change in antibiotic prophylaxis for cardiac surgery. Infect Control Hosp Epidemiol. 2002;23(7):402-404.
71. Smith EB, Wynne R, Joshi A, Liu H, Good RP. Is it time to include vancomycin for routine perioperative antibiotic prophylaxis in total joint arthroplasty patients? J Arthroplasty. 2012;27(8 Suppl):55-60.
72. Bull AL, Worth LJ, Richards MJ. Impact of vancomycin surgical antibiotic prophylaxis on the development of methicillin-sensitive staphylococcus aureus surgical site infections: report from Australian Surveillance Data (VICNISS). Ann Surg. 2012;256(6):1089-1092.
73. Miller LG, McKinnell JA, Vollmer ME, Spellberg B. Impact of methicillin-resistant Staphylococcus aureus prevalence among S. aureus isolates on surgical site infection risk after coronary artery bypass surgery. Infect Control Hosp Epidemiol. 2011;32(4):342-350.
74. Zanetti G, Giardina R, Platt R. Intraoperative redosing of cefazolin and risk for surgical site infection in cardiac surgery. Emerg Infect Dis. 2001;7(5):828-831.
75. Zanetti G, Goldie SJ, Platt R. Clinical consequences and cost of limiting use of vancomycin for perioperative prophylaxis: example of coronary artery bypass surgery. Emerg Infect Dis. 2001;7(5):820-827.
76. Muralidhar B, Anwar SM, Handa AI, Peto TE, Bowler IC. Prevalence of MRSA in emergency and elective patients admitted to a vascular surgical unit: implications for antibiotic prophylaxis. Eur J Vasc Endovasc Surg. 2006;32(4):402-407.
77. Gemmell CG, Edwards DI, Fraise AP, Gould FK, Ridgway GL, Warren RE. Guidelines for the prophylaxis and treatment of methicillin-resistant Staphylococcus aureus (MRSA) infections in the UK. J Antimicrob Chemother. 2006;57(4):589-608.
78. Elliott RA, Weatherly HL, Hawkins NS, et al. An economic model for the prevention of

MRSA infections after surgery: non-glycopeptide or glycopeptide antibiotic prophylaxis? Eur J Health Econ. 2010;11(1):57-66.
79. Walsh EE, Greene L, Kirshner R. Sustained reduction in methicillin-resistant Staphylococcus aureus wound infections after cardiothoracic surgery. Arch Intern Med. 2011;171(1):68-73.
80. Dhadwal K, Al-Ruzzeh S, Athanasiou T, et al. Comparison of clinical and economic outcomes of two antibiotic prophylaxis regimens for sternal wound infection in high-risk patients following coronary artery bypass grafting surgery: a prospective randomised double-blind controlled trial. Heart. 2007;93(9):1126-1133.
81. Patrick S, James C, Ali A, Lawson D, Mary E, Modak A. Vascular surgical antibiotic prophylaxis study (VSAPS). Vasc Endovascular Surg. 2010;44(7):521-528.
82. Sewick A, Makani A, Wu C, O'Donnell J, Baldwin KD, Lee GC. Does dual antibiotic prophylaxis better prevent surgical site infections in total joint arthroplasty? Clin Orthop Relat Res. 2012;470(10):2702-2707.
83. Ritter MA, Barzilauskas CD, Faris PM, Keating EM. Vancomycin prophylaxis and elective total joint arthroplasty. Orthopedics. 1989;12(10):1333-1336.
84. Cruess RL, Bickel WS, vonKessler KL. Infections in total hips secondary to a primary source elsewhere. Clin Orthop Relat Res. 1975(106):99-101.
85. Hall AJ. Late infection about a total knee prosthesis. Report of a case secondary to urinary tract infection. J Bone Joint Surg Br. 1974;56(1):144-147.
86. David TS, Vrahas MS. Perioperative lower urinary tract infections and deep sepsis in patients undergoing total joint arthroplasty. J Am Acad Orthop Surg. 2000;8(1):66-74.
87. Ritter MA, Fechtman RW. Urinary tract sequelae: possible influence on joint infections following total joint replacement. Orthopedics. 1987;10(3):467-469.
88. Wymenga AB, van Horn JR, Theeuwes A, Muytjens HL, Slooff TJ. Perioperative factors associated with septic arthritis after arthroplasty. Prospective multicenter study of 362 knee and 2,651 hip operations. Acta Orthop Scand. 1992;63(6):665-671.
89. Glynn MK, Sheehan JM. The significance of asymptomatic bacteriuria in patients undergoing hip/knee arthroplasty. Clin Orthop Relat Res. 1984(185):151-154.
90. Waterhouse N, Beaumont AR, Murray K, Staniforth P, Stone MH. Urinary retention after total hip replacement. A prospective study. J Bone Joint Surg Br. 1987;69(1):64-66.
91. Walton JK, Robinson RG. An analysis of a male population having total hip replacement with regard to urological assessment and post-operative urinary retention. Br J Urol. 1982;54(5):519-521.
92. Drekonja DM, Rector TS, Cutting A, Johnson JR. Urinary tract infection in male veterans: treatment patterns and outcomes. JAMA Intern Med. 2013;173(1):62-68.
93. Irvine R, Johnson BL, Jr., Amstutz HC. The relationship of genitourinary tract procedures and deep sepsis after total hip replacements. Surg Gynecol Obstet. 1974;139(5):701-706.
94. Garibaldi RA, Burke JP, Dickman ML, Smith CB. Factors predisposing to bacteriuria during indwelling urethral catheterization. N Engl J Med. 1974;291(5):215-219.
95. Kunin CM, McCormack RC. Prevention of catheter-induced urinary-tract infections by sterile closed drainage. N Engl J Med. 1966;274(21):1155-1161.
96. Jerry GJ, Jr., Rand JA, Ilstrup D. Old sepsis prior to total knee arthroplasty. Clin Orthop Relat Res. 1988(236):135-140.
97. Lee GC, Pagnano MW, Hanssen AD. Total knee arthroplasty after prior bone or joint sepsis about the knee. Clin Orthop Relat Res. 2002(404):226-231.
98. Larson AN, Hanssen AD, Cass JR. Does prior infection alter the outcome of TKA after tibial plateau fracture? Clin Orthop Relat Res. 2009;467(7):1793-1799.
99. Michelson JD, Lotke PA, Steinberg ME. Urinary-bladder management after total joint-replacement surgery. N Engl J Med. 1988;319(6):321-326.
100. Martinez OV, Civetta JM, Anderson K, Roger S, Murtha M, Malinin TI. Bacteriuria in the catheterized surgical intensive care patient. Crit Care Med. 1986;14(3):188-191.
101. Schaeffer AJ. Catheter-associated bacteriuria. Urol Clin North Am. 1986;13(4):735-747.
102. Skelly JM, Guyatt GH, Kalbfleisch R, Singer J, Winter L. Management of urinary retention after surgical repair of hip fracture. CMAJ. 1992;146(7):1185-1189.
103. Donovan TL, Gordon RO, Nagel DA. Urinary infections in total hip arthroplasty. Influences of prophylactic cephalosporins and catheterization. J Bone Joint Surg Am. 1976;58(8):1134-1137.
104. Fitzgerald RH, Jr., Nolan DR, Ilstrup DM, Van Scoy RE, Washington JA, 2nd, Coventry MB. Deep wound sepsis following total hip arthroplasty. J Bone Joint Surg Am. 1977;59(7):847-855.
105. Surin VV, Sundholm K, Backman L. Infection after total hip replacement. With special reference to a discharge from the wound. J Bone Joint Surg Br. 1983;65(4):412-418.
106. Felippe WA, Werneck GL, Santoro-Lopes G. Surgical site infection among women discharged with a drain in situ after breast cancer surgery. World J Surg. 2007;31(12):2293-2299; discussion 2300-2291.
107. Lanier ST, Wang ED, Chen JJ, et al. The effect of acellular dermal matrix use on complication rates in tissue expander/implant breast reconstruction. Ann Plast Surg.

2010;64(5):674-678.
108. Sorensen AI, Sorensen TS. Bacterial growth on suction drain tips. Prospective study of 489 clean orthopedic operations. Acta Orthop Scand. 1991;62(5):451-454.
109. van den Brand IC, Castelein RM. Total joint arthroplasty and incidence of postoperative bacteriuria with an indwelling catheter or intermittent catheterization with one-dose antibiotic prophylaxis: a prospective randomized trial. J Arthroplasty. 2001;16(7):850-855.
110. Oishi CS, Williams VJ, Hanson PB, Schneider JE, Colwell CW, Jr., Walker RH. Perioperative bladder management after primary total hip arthroplasty. J Arthroplasty. 1995;10(6):732-736.
111. Koulouvaris P, Sculco P, Finerty E, Sculco T, Sharrock NE. Relationship between perioperative urinary tract infection and deep infection after joint arthroplasty. Clin Orthop Relat Res. 2009;467(7):1859-1867.
112. Brahmbhatt RD, Huebner M, Scow JS, et al. National practice patterns in preoperative and postoperative antibiotic prophylaxis in breast procedures requiring drains: survey of the American Society of Breast Surgeons. Ann Surg Oncol. 2012;19(10):3205-3211.
113. Phillips BT, Wang ED, Mirrer J, et al. Current practice among plastic surgeons of antibiotic prophylaxis and closed-suction drains in breast reconstruction: experience, evidence, and implications for postoperative care. Ann Plast Surg. 2011;66(5):460-465.
114. Turano A. New clinical data on the prophylaxis of infections in abdominal, gynecologic, and urologic surgery. Multicenter Study Group. Am J Surg. 1992;164(4A Suppl):16S-20S.
115. Niederhauser U, Vogt M, Vogt P, Genoni M, Kunzli A, Turina MI. Cardiac surgery in a high-risk group of patients: is prolonged postoperative antibiotic prophylaxis effective? J Thorac Cardiovasc Surg. 1997;114(2):162-168.
116. Wymenga AB, Hekster YA, Theeuwes A, Muytjens HL, van Horn JR, Slooff TJ. Antibiotic use after cefuroxime prophylaxis in hip and knee joint replacement. Clin Pharmacol Ther. 1991;50(2):215-220.
117. McDonald M, Grabsch E, Marshall C, Forbes A. Single- versus multiple-dose antimicrobial prophylaxis for major surgery: a systematic review. Aust N Z J Surg. 1998;68(6):388-396.
118. Heydemann JS, Nelson CL. Short-term preventive antibiotics. Clin Orthop Relat Res. 1986(205):184-187.
119. Stone HH, Haney BB, Kolb LD, Geheber CE, Hooper CA. Prophylactic and preventive antibiotic therapy: timing, duration and economics. Ann Surg. 1979;189(6):691-699.
120. Williams DN, Gustilo RB. The use of preventive antibiotics in orthopaedic surgery. Clin Orthop Relat Res. 1984(190):83-88.
121. Tang WM, Chiu KY, Ng TP, Yau WP, Ching PT, Seto WH. Efficacy of a single dose of cefazolin as a prophylactic antibiotic in primary arthroplasty. J Arthroplasty. 2003;18(6):714-718.
122. Sharma D, Douglas J, Coulter C, Weinrauch P, Crawford R. Microbiology of infected arthroplasty: implications for empiric peri-operative antibiotics. J Orthop Surg (Hong Kong). 2008;16(3):339-342.
123. Nickinson RS, Board TN, Gambhir AK, Porter ML, Kay PR. The microbiology of the infected knee arthroplasty. Int Orthop. 2010;34(4):505-510.
124. Bengston S, Knutson K, Lidgren L. Treatment of infected knee arthroplasty. Clin Orthop Relat Res. 1989(245):173-178.
125. Peersman G, Laskin R, Davis J, Peterson M. Infection in total knee replacement: a retrospective review of 6489 total knee replacements. Clin Orthop Relat Res. 2001(392):15-23.
126. Mont MA, Waldman BJ, Hungerford DS. Evaluation of preoperative cultures before second-stage reimplantation of a total knee prosthesis complicated by infection. A comparison-group study. J Bone Joint Surg Am. 2000;82-A(11):1552-1557.
127. Rafiq I, Gambhir AK, Wroblewski BM, Kay PR. The microbiology of infected hip arthroplasty. Int Orthop. 2006;30(6):532-535.
128. Al-Maiyah M, Hill D, Bajwa A, et al. Bacterial contaminants and antibiotic prophylaxis in total hip arthroplasty. J Bone Joint Surg Br. 2005;87(9):1256-1258.
129. Phillips JE, Crane TP, Noy M, Elliott TS, Grimer RJ. The incidence of deep prosthetic infections in a specialist orthopaedic hospital: a 15-year prospective survey. J Bone Joint Surg Br. 2006;88(7):943-948.
130. Tsukayama DT, Estrada R, Gustilo RB. Infection after total hip arthroplasty. A study of the treatment of one hundred and six infections. J Bone Joint Surg Am. 1996;78(4):512-523.
131. Moran E, Masters S, Berendt AR, McLardy-Smith P, Byren I, Atkins BL. Guiding empirical antibiotic therapy in orthopaedics: The microbiology of prosthetic joint infection managed by debridement, irrigation and prosthesis retention. J Infect. 2007;55(1):1-7.
132. Azzam K, McHale K, Austin M, Purtill JJ, Parvizi J. Outcome of a second two-stage reimplantation for periprosthetic knee infection. Clin Orthop Relat Res. 2009;467(7):1706-1714.
133. Kalra KP, Lin KK, Bozic KJ, Ries MD. Repeat 2-stage revision for recurrent infection of total hip arthroplasty. J Arthroplasty. 2010;25(6):880-884.
134. Jamsen E, Stogiannidis I, Malmivaara A, Pajamaki J, Puolakka T, Konttinen YT. Outcome of prosthesis exchange for infected knee arthroplasty: the effect of treatment approach. Acta Orthop. 2009;80(1):67-77.

135. Kubista B, Hartzler RU, Wood CM, Osmon DR, Hanssen AD, Lewallen DG. Reinfection after two-stage revision for periprosthetic infection of total knee arthroplasty. Int Orthop. 2012;36(1):65-71.
136. Mortazavi SM, O'Neil JT, Zmistowski B, Parvizi J, Purtill JJ. Repeat 2-stage exchange for infected total hip arthroplasty: a viable option? J Arthroplasty. 2012;27(6):923-926 e921.
137. Fletcher N, Sofianos D, Berkes MB, Obremskey WT. Prevention of perioperative infection. J Bone Joint Surg Am. 2007;89(7):1605-1618.
138. Dellinger EP, Gross PA, Barrett TL, et al. Quality standard for antimicrobial prophylaxis in surgical procedures. The Infectious Diseases Society of America. Infect Control Hosp Epidemiol. 1994;15(3):182-188.
139. Scher KS. Studies on the duration of antibiotic administration for surgical prophylaxis. Am Surg. 1997;63(1):59-62.
140. Shapiro M, Munoz A, Tager IB, Schoenbaum SC, Polk BF. Risk factors for infection at the operative site after abdominal or vaginal hysterectomy. N Engl J Med. 1982;307(27):1661-1666.
141. Polk HC, Jr., Trachtenberg L, Finn MP. Antibiotic activity in surgical incisions. The basis of prophylaxis in selected operations. JAMA. 19 1980;244(12):1353-1354.
142. Ohge H, Takesue Y, Yokoyama T, et al. An additional dose of cefazolin for intraoperative prophylaxis. Surg Today. 1999;29(12):1233-1236.
143. Morita S, Nishisho I, Nomura T, et al. The significance of the intraoperative repeated dosing of antimicrobials for preventing surgical wound infection in colorectal surgery. Surg Today. 2005;35(9):732-738.
144. Swoboda SM, Merz C, Kostuik J, Trentler B, Lipsett PA. Does intraoperative blood loss affect antibiotic serum and tissue concentrations? Arch Surg. 1996;131(11):1165-1171; discussion 1171-1162.
145. Markantonis SL, Kostopanagiotou G, Panidis D, Smirniotis V, Voros D. Effects of blood loss and fluid volume replacement on serum and tissue gentamicin concentrations during colorectal surgery. Clin Ther. 2004;26(2):271-281.
146. Klekamp JW, DiPersio D, Haas DW. No influence of large volume blood loss on serum vancomycin concentrations during orthopedic procedures. Acta Orthop Scand. 1999;70(1):47-50.
147. Meter JJ, Polly DW, Jr., Brueckner RP, Tenuta JJ, Asplund L, Hopkinson WJ. Effect of intraoperative blood loss on the serum level of cefazolin in patients managed with total hip arthroplasty. A prospective, controlled study. J Bone Joint Surg Am. 1996;78(8):1201-1205.
148. Polly DW, Jr., Meter JJ, Brueckner R, Asplund L, van Dam BE. The effect of intraoperative blood loss on serum cefazolin level in patients undergoing instrumented spinal fusion. A prospective, controlled study. Spine (Phila Pa 1976). 1996;21(20):2363-2367.
149. The Sanford guide to antimicrobial therapy. 30th ed; 2000.
150. Wurtz R, Itokazu G, Rodvold K. Antimicrobial dosing in obese patients. Clin Infect Dis. 1997;25(1):112-118.
151. Leader WG, Tsubaki T, Chandler MH. Creatinine-clearance estimates for predicting gentamicin pharmacokinetic values in obese patients. Am J Hosp Pharm. 1994;51(17):2125-2130.
152. Begg EJ, Barclay ML, Duffull SB. A suggested approach to once-daily aminoglycoside dosing. Br J Clin Pharmacol. 1995;39(6):605-609.
153. Janson B, Thursky K. Dosing of antibiotics in obesity. Curr Opin Infect Dis. 2012;25(6):634-649.
154. Truong J, Levkovich BJ, Padiglione AA. Simple approach to improving vancomycin dosing in intensive care: a standardised loading dose results in earlier therapeutic levels. Intern Med J. 2012;42(1):23-29.
155. Ho VP, Nicolau DP, Dakin GF, et al. Cefazolin dosing for surgical prophylaxis in morbidly obese patients. Surg Infect (Larchmt). 2012;13(1):33-37.
156. Rybak MJ, Lomaestro BM, Rotschafer JC, et al. Vancomycin therapeutic guidelines: a summary of consensus recommendations from the infectious diseases Society of America, the American Society of Health-System Pharmacists, and the Society of Infectious Diseases Pharmacists. Clin Infect Dis. 2009;49(3):325-327.
157. Traynor AM, Nafziger AN, Bertino JS, Jr. Aminoglycoside dosing weight correction factors for patients of various body sizes. Antimicrob Agents Chemother. 1995;39(2):545-548.
158. van Kralingen S, Taks M, Diepstraten J, et al. Pharmacokinetics and protein binding of cefazolin in morbidly obese patients. Eur J Clin Pharmacol. 2011;67(10):985-992.
159. Edmiston CE, Krepel C, Kelly H, et al. Perioperative antibiotic prophylaxis in the gastric bypass patient: do we achieve therapeutic levels? Surgery. 2004;136(4):738-747.
160. Liu C. The bundled approach to MRSA surgical site infection prevention: is the whole greater than the sum of its parts?: comment on "Sustained reduction in methicillin-resistant Staphylococcus aureus wound infections after cardiothoracic surgery". Arch Intern Med. 2011;171(1):73-74.
161. Pofahl WE, Goettler CE, Ramsey KM, Cochran MK, Nobles DL, Rotondo MF. Active surveillance screening of MRSA and eradication of the carrier state decreases surgical-site

infections caused by MRSA. J Am Coll Surg. 2009;208(5):981-986; discussion 986-988.
162. Wirganowicz PZ, Eckardt JJ, Dorey FJ, Eilber FR, Kabo JM. Etiology and results of tumor endoprosthesis revision surgery in 64 patients. Clin Orthop Relat Res. 1999(358):64-74.
163. Safran MR, Kody MH, Namba RS, et al. 151 endoprosthetic reconstructions for patients with primary tumors involving bone. Contemp Orthop. 1994;29(1):15-25.
164. Malawer MM, Chou LB. Prosthetic survival and clinical results with use of large-segment replacements in the treatment of high-grade bone sarcomas. J Bone Joint Surg Am. 1995;77(8):1154-1165.
165. Capanna R, Morris HG, Campanacci D, Del Ben M, Campanacci M. Modular uncemented prosthetic reconstruction after resection of tumours of the distal femur. J Bone Joint Surg Br. 1994;76(2):178-186.
166. Mittermayer F, Krepler P, Dominkus M, et al. Long-term followup of uncemented tumor endoprostheses for the lower extremity. Clin Orthop Relat Res. 2001(388):167-177.
167. Ghert M, Deheshi B, Holt G, et al. Prophylactic antibiotic regimens in tumour surgery (PARITY): protocol for a multicentre randomised controlled study. BMJ Open. 2012;2(6).
168. Jansen B, Rinck M, Wolbring P, Strohmeier A, Jahns T. In vitro evaluation of the antimicrobial efficacy and biocompatibility of a silver-coated central venous catheter. J Biomater Appl. 1994;9(1):55-70.
169. Karchmer TB, Giannetta ET, Muto CA, Strain BA, Farr BM. A randomized crossover study of silver-coated urinary catheters in hospitalized patients. Arch Intern Med. 2000;160(21):3294-3298.
170. Tsuchiya H, Shirai T, Nishida H. New implant technology:iodine-coating for infection control. Paper presented at: 26th European Musculoskeletal Oncology Society Meeting, 2013; Gothenburg, Sweden.
171. Tsuchiya H, Shirai T, Nishida H, et al. Innovative antimicrobial coating of titanium implants with iodine. J Orthop Sci. 2012;17(5):595-604.
172. Gosheger G, Hardes J, Ahrens H, et al. Silver-coated megaendoprostheses in a rabbit model--an analysis of the infection rate and toxicological side effects. Biomaterials. 2004;25(24):5547-5556.
173. Hardes J, von Eiff C, Streitbuerger A, et al. Reduction of periprosthetic infection with silver-coated megaprostheses in patients with bone sarcoma. J Surg Oncol. 2010;101(5):389-395.
174. Gosheger G, Goetze C, Hardes J, Joosten U, Winkelmann W, von Eiff C. The influence of the alloy of megaprostheses on infection rate. J Arthroplasty. 2008;23(6):916-920.
175. Witso E, Persen L, Benum P, Aamodt A, Husby OS, Bergh K. High local concentrations without systemic adverse effects after impaction of netilmicin-impregnated bone. Acta Orthop Scand. 2004;75(3):339-346.
176. Buttaro MA, Gimenez MI, Greco G, Barcan L, Piccaluga F. High active local levels of vancomycin without nephrotoxicity released from impacted bone allografts in 20 revision hip arthroplasties. Acta Orthop. 2005;76(3):336-340.
177. Buttaro MA, Pusso R, Piccaluga F. Vancomycin-supplemented impacted bone allografts in infected hip arthroplasty. Two-stage revision results. J Bone Joint Surg Br. 2005;87(3):314-319.
178. Michalak KA, Khoo PP, Yates PJ, Day RE, Wood DJ. Iontophoresed segmental allografts in revision arthroplasty for infection. J Bone Joint Surg Br. 2006;88(11):1430-1437.
179. Khoo PP, Michalak KA, Yates PJ, Megson SM, Day RE, Wood DJ. Iontophoresis of antibiotics into segmental allografts. J Bone Joint Surg Br. 2006;88(9):1149-1157.
180. Winkler H, Stoiber A, Kaudela K, Winter F, Menschik F. One stage uncemented revision of infected total hip replacement using cancellous allograft bone impregnated with antibiotics. J Bone Joint Surg Br. 2008;90(12):1580-1584.
181. Buttaro MA, Guala AJ, Comba F, Suarez F, Piccaluga F. Incidence of deep infection in aseptic revision THA using vancomycin-impregnated impacted bone allograft. Hip Int. 2010;20(4):535-541.
182. Witso E, Persen L, Loseth K, Bergh K. Adsorption and release of antibiotics from morselized cancellous bone. In vitro studies of 8 antibiotics. Acta Orthop Scand. 1999;70(3):298-304.
183. Buttaro MA, Gonzalez Della Valle AM, Pineiro L, Mocetti E, Morandi AA, Piccaluga F. Incorporation of vancomycin-supplemented bone incorporation of vancomycin-supplemented bone allografts: radiographical, histopathological and immunohistochemical study in pigs. Acta Orthop Scand. 2003;74(5):505-513.
184. Witso E, Persen L, Loseth K, Benum P, Bergh K. Cancellous bone as an antibiotic carrier. Acta Orthop Scand. 2000;71(1):80-84.
185. Berbari EF, Hanssen AD, Duffy MC, et al. Risk factors for prosthetic joint infection: case-control study. Clin Infect Dis. 1998;27(5):1247-1254.
186. Yang K, Yeo SJ, Lee BP, Lo NN. Total knee arthroplasty in diabetic patients: a study of 109 consecutive cases. J Arthroplasty. 2001;16(1):102-106.
187. Meding JB, Reddleman K, Keating ME, et al. Total knee replacement in patients with diabetes mellitus. Clin Orthop Relat Res. 2003(416):208-216.

188. Pedersen AB, Mehnert F, Johnsen SP, Sorensen HT. Risk of revision of a total hip replacement in patients with diabetes mellitus: a population-based follow up study. J Bone Joint Surg Br. 2010;92(7):929-934.
189. Adams AL, Paxton EW, Wang JQ, et al. Surgical outcomes of total knee replacement according to diabetes status and glycemic control, 2001 to 2009. J Bone Joint Surg Am. 20 2013;95(6):481-487.
190. Haverkamp D, Klinkenbijl MN, Somford MP, Albers GH, van der Vis HM. Obesity in total hip arthroplasty--does it really matter? A meta-analysis. Acta Orthop. 2011;82(4):417-422.
191. Namba RS, Paxton L, Fithian DC, Stone ML. Obesity and perioperative morbidity in total hip and total knee arthroplasty patients. J Arthroplasty. 2005;20(7 Suppl 3):46-50.
192. Dowsey MM, Choong PF. Early outcomes and complications following joint arthroplasty in obese patients: a review of the published reports. ANZ J Surg. 2008;78(6):439-444.
193. Parvizi J, Sullivan TA, Pagnano MW, Trousdale RT, Bolander ME. Total joint arthroplasty in human immunodeficiency virus-positive patients: an alarming rate of early failure. J Arthroplasty. 2003;18(3):259-264.
194. Ragni MV, Crossett LS, Herndon JH. Postoperative infection following orthopaedic surgery in human immunodeficiency virus-infected hemophiliacs with CD4 counts < or = 200/mm3. J Arthroplasty. 1995;10(6):716-721.
195. Habermann B, Eberhardt C, Kurth AA. Total joint replacement in HIV positive patients. J Infect. 2008;57(1):41-46.
196. Wang TI, Chen CF, Chen WM, et al. Joint replacement in human immunodeficiency virus-infected patients. J Chin Med Assoc. 2012;75(11):595-599.
197. Unger AS, Kessler CM, Lewis RJ. Total knee arthroplasty in human immunodeficiency virus-infected hemophiliacs. J Arthroplasty. 1995;10(4):448-452.
198. Silva M, Luck JV, Jr. Long-term results of primary total knee replacement in patients with hemophilia. J Bone Joint Surg Am. 2005;87(1):85-91.
199. Rodriguez-Merchan EC. Total knee replacement in haemophilic arthropathy. J Bone Joint Surg Br. 2007;89(2):186-188.
200. Shaarani SR, Collins D, O'Byrne JM. The need for guidelines in asplenic patients undergoing total joint arthroplasty: a case report. Case Rep Orthop. 2012;2012:147042.
201. McCleery MA, Leach WJ, Norwood T. Rates of infection and revision in patients with renal disease undergoing total knee replacement in Scotland. J Bone Joint Surg Br. 2010;92(11):1535-1539.
202. Lieberman JR, Fuchs MD, Haas SB, et al. Hip arthroplasty in patients with chronic renal failure. J Arthroplasty. 1995;10(2):191-195.
203. Sakalkale DP, Hozack WJ, Rothman RH. Total hip arthroplasty in patients on long-term renal dialysis. J Arthroplasty. 1999;14(5):571-575.
204. Li WC, Shih CH, Ueng SW, Shih HN, Lee MS, Hsieh PH. Uncemented total hip arthroplasty in chronic hemodialysis patients. Acta Orthop. 2010;81(2):178-182.
205. Nagoya S, Nagao M, Takada J, Kuwabara H, Kaya M, Yamashita T. Efficacy of cementless total hip arthroplasty in patients on long-term hemodialysis. J Arthroplasty. 2005;20(1):66-71.
206. Pour AE, Matar WY, Jafari SM, Purtill JJ, Austin MS, Parvizi J. Total joint arthroplasty in patients with hepatitis C. J Bone Joint Surg Am. 2011;93(15):1448-1454.
207. Orozco F, Post ZD, Baxi O, Miller A, Ong A. Fibrosis in Hepatitis C Patients Predicts Complications After Elective Total Joint Arthroplasty. J Arthroplasty. May 3 2013.
208. Vergidis P, Lesnick TG, Kremers WK, Razonable RR. Prosthetic joint infection in solid organ transplant recipients: a retrospective case-control study. Transpl Infect Dis. 2012;14(4):380-386.
209. Tannenbaum DA, Matthews LS, Grady-Benson JC. Infection around joint replacements in patients who have a renal or liver transplantation. J Bone Joint Surg Am. 1997;79(1):36-43.
210. Mortazavi SM, Molligan J, Austin MS, Purtill JJ, Hozack WJ, Parvizi J. Failure following revision total knee arthroplasty: infection is the major cause. Int Orthop. 2011;35(8):1157-1164.
211. Poss R, Thornhill TS, Ewald FC, Thomas WH, Batte NJ, Sledge CB. Factors influencing the incidence and outcome of infection following total joint arthroplasty. Clin Orthop Relat Res. 1984(182):117-126.
212. Sierra RJ, Cooney WPt, Pagnano MW, Trousdale RT, Rand JA. Reoperations after 3200 revision TKAs: rates, etiology, and lessons learned. Clin Orthop Relat Res. 2004(425):200-206.
213. Liu C, Kakis A, Nichols A, Ries MD, Vail TP, Bozic KJ. Targeted Use of Vancomycin as Perioperative Prophylaxis Reduces Periprosthetic Joint Infection in Revision TKA. Clin Orthop Relat Res. May 4 2013. Epub before print.
214. Nordmann P, Cuzon G, Naas T. The real threat of Klebsiella pneumoniae carbapenemase-producing bacteria. Lancet Infect Dis. 2009;9(4):228-236.
215. Queenan AM, Bush K. Carbapenemases: the versatile beta-lactamases. Clin Microbiol Rev. 2007;20(3):440-458, table of contents.
216. Schwaber MJ, Carmeli Y. Carbapenem-resistant Enterobacteriaceae: a potential threat. JAMA. 2008;300(24):2911-2913.
217. Bratu S, Landman D, Haag R, et al. Rapid spread of carbapenem-resistant Klebsiella

pneumoniae in New York City: a new threat to our antibiotic armamentarium. Arch Intern Med. 2005;165(12):1430-1435.

218. Marchaim D, Navon-Venezia S, Schwaber MJ, Carmeli Y. Isolation of imipenem-resistant Enterobacter species: emergence of KPC-2 carbapenemase, molecular characterization, epidemiology, and outcomes. Antimicrob Agents Chemother. 2008;52(4):1413-1418.

219. Cuzon G, Naas T, Demachy MC, Nordmann P. Plasmid-mediated carbapenem-hydrolyzing beta-lactamase KPC-2 in Klebsiella pneumoniae isolate from Greece. Antimicrob Agents Chemother. 2008;52(2):796-797.

220. de Smet AM, Kluytmans JA, Cooper BS, et al. Decontamination of the digestive tract and oropharynx in ICU patients. N Engl J Med. 2009;360(1):20-31.

221. Perez F, Pultz MJ, Endimiani A, Bonomo RA, Donskey CJ. Effect of antibiotic treatment on establishment and elimination of intestinal colonization by KPC-producing Klebsiella pneumoniae in mice. Antimicrob Agents Chemother. 2011;55(6):2585-2589.

Question 1

- **What is the optimal timing of the preoperative dose of antibiotics?**

<u>Consensus:</u> The preoperative dose of antibiotics should be administered within one hour of surgical incision; this can be extended to two hours for vancomycin and fluoroquinolones. Furthermore, surveillance measures are critical in ensuring clinician compliance with this objective.

Delegate Vote

Agree: 97%, Disagree: 2%, Abstain: 1% (Strong Consensus)

Question 2

- **Is there an optimal antibiotic that should be administered for routine perioperative surgical prophylaxis?**

<u>Consensus:</u> A first or second generation cephalosporin (cefazolin or cefuroxime) should be administered for routine perioperative surgical prophylaxis. Isoxazolyl penicillin is used as an appropriate alternative.

Delegate Vote

Agree: 89%, Disagree: 8%, Abstain: 3% (Strong Consensus)

Question 3

- **What is the choice of antibiotic in patients who have pre-existing prostheses such as heart valves?**

<u>Consensus:</u> The choice of antibiotics for patients with pre-existing prostheses such as heart valves is the same as that for routine elective arthroplasty.

Delegate Vote

Agree: 94%, Disagree: 3%, Abstain: 3% (Strong Consensus)

Question 4

- **What alternatives are available for routine prophylaxis when cephalosporins are not an option?**

<u>Consensus:</u> Curently teicoplanin and vancomycin are reasonable alternatives when routine antibiotic prophylaxis cannot be adminis-

tered.

Delegate Vote
Agree: 73%, Disagree: 22%, Abstain: 5% (Strong Consensus)

Question 5A

- **What antibiotic should be administered in a patient with a known anaphylactic penicillin allergy?**

Consensus: In a patient with a known anaphylactic reaction to penicillin, vancomycin or clindamycin should be administered as prophylaxis. Teicoplanin is an option in countries where it is available.

Delegate Vote
Agree: 88%, Disagree: 10%, Abstain: 2% (Strong Consensus)

Question 5B

- **What antibiotic should be administered in a patient with a known nonanaphylactic penicillin allergy?**

Consensus: In a patient with a reported non-anaphylactic reaction to penicillin, a second generation cephalosporin can be used safely as there is limited cross-reactivity. Penicillin skin testing may be helpful in certain situations to clarify whether the patient has a true penicillin allergy.

Delegate Vote
Agree: 87%, Disagree: 9%, Abstain: 4% (Strong Consensus)

Question 6

- **What are the indications for administration of vancomycin?**

Consensus: Vancomycin should be considered for patients who are current MRSA carriers or have anaphylactic allergy to penicillins.

Consideration should be given to screening high risk patients such as:

—Patients in regions with a high prevalence of MRSA.

—Institutionalized patients (nursing home residents, dialysis-dependent patients, and those who have been in the intensive care unit).

—Healthcare workers.

Delegate Vote

Agree: 93%, Disagree: 7%, Abstain: 0% (Strong Consensus)

Question 7

- **Is there evidence to support the routine use of vancomycin for preoperative prophylaxis?**

<u>Consensus:</u> No. Routine use of vancomycin for preoperative prophylaxis is not recommended.

Delegate Vote

Agree: 93%, Disagree: 6%, Abstain: 1% (Strong Consensus)

Question 8

- **Is there a role for routine prophylactic use of dual antibiotics (cephalosporins and aminoglycosides or cephalosporins and vancomycin)?**

<u>Consensus:</u> Routine prophylactic use of dual antibiotics is not recommended.

Delegate Vote

Agree: 85%, Disagree: 14%, Abstain: 1% (Strong Consensus)

Question 9

- **What should be the antibiotic of choice for patients with abnormal urinary screening and/or an indwelling urinary catheter?**

<u>Consensus:</u> The presence of urinary tract symptoms should trigger urinary screening prior to TJA. Asymptomatic patients with bacteriuria may safely undergo TJA provided that routine prophylactic antibiotics are administered. Patients with acute urinary tract infections (UTI) need to be treated prior to elective arthroplasty

Delegate Vote

Agree: 82%, Disagree: 12%, Abstain: 6% (Strong Consensus)

Question 10

- **Should the preoperative antibiotic choice be different in patients who have previously been treated for another joint infection?**

Consensus: The type of preoperative antibiotic administered to a patient with prior septic arthritis or PJI should cover the previous infecting organism of the same joint. In these patients, we recommend the use of antibiotic-impregnated cement, if a cemented component is utilized.

Delegate Vote
Agree: 84%, Disagree: 10%, Abstain: 6% (Strong Consensus)

Question 11

- **Should postoperative antibiotics be continued while a urinary catheter or surgical drain remains in place?**

Consensus: No. There is no evidence to support the support the continued use of postoperative antibiotics when urinary catheter or surgical drains are in place. Urinary catheters and surgical drains should be removed as soon as safely possible.

Delegate Vote
Agree: 90%, Disagree: 7%, Abstain: 3% (Strong Consensus)

Question 12

- **What is the evidence for the optimal duration of postoperative antibiotics in decreasing SSI or PJI?**

Consensus: Postoperative antibiotics should not be administered for greater than 24 hours after surgery.

Delegate Vote
Agree: 87%, Disagree: 10%, Abstain: 3% (Strong Consensus)

Question 13

- **Until culture results are finalized, what antibiotic should be administered to a patient with a presumed infection?**

Consensus: In a patient with a presumed infection when culture results are pending, empiric antibiotic coverage should depend on the local microbiological epidemiology. Culture data should assist in the tailoring of antibiotic regimens.

Delegate Vote
Agree: 96%, Disagree: 1%, Abstain: 3% (Strong Consensus)

Question 14

- **What is the appropriate preoperative antibiotic for a second-stage procedure?**

Consensus: The appropriate preoperative antibiotic for the second stage should include coverage of the prior organism (s). Cemented arthroplasty components should be inserted with antibiotic-laden bone cement.

Delegate Vote

Agree: 66%, Disagree: 31%, Abstain: 3% (Strong Consensus)

Question 15

- **For surgeries of longer duration, when should an additional dose of antibiotic be administered intraoperatively?**

Consensus: An additional dose of antibiotic should be administered intraoperatively after two half-lives of the prophylactic agent. The general guidelines for frequency of intraoperative antibiotic administration are provided. We recommend that re-dosing of antibiotics be considered in cases of large blood volume loss (>2000 cc) and fluid resuscitation (>2000 cc). As these are independent variables, re-dosing should be considered as soon as the first of these parameters are met.

Delegate Vote

Agree: 94%, Disagree: 5%, Abstain: 1% (Strong Consensus)

Question 16

- **Should preoperative antibiotic doses be weight-adjusted?**

Consensus: Preoperative antibiotics have different pharmacokinetics based on patient weight and should be weight-adjusted.

Delegate Vote

Agree: 95%, Disagree: 4%, Abstain: 1% (Strong Consensus)

Question 17A

- **What type of perioperative antibiotic prophylaxis is recommended for current MRSA carriers?**

Consensus: For current MRSA carriers, vancomycin or teicoplanin is the recommended perioperative antibiotic prophylaxis.

Delegate Vote

Agree: 86%, Disagree: 12%, Abstain: 2% (Strong Consensus)

Question 17B

- **Should patients with prior history of MRSA be re-screened? What should the choice of perioperative prophylactic antibiotics be in these patients?**

Consensus: Patients with prior history of MRSA should be re-screened preoperatively. If patients are found to be negative for MRSA, we recommend routine perioperative antibiotic prophylaxis.

Delegate Vote

Agree: 76%, Disagree: 23%, Abstain: 1% (Strong Consensus)

Question 18

- **What is the recommended prophylaxis in patients undergoing major orthopaedic reconstructions for either tumor or non-neoplastic conditions using megaprosthesis?**

Consensus: Until the emergence of further evidence, we recommend the use of routine antibiotic prophylaxis for patients undergoing major reconstruction.

Delegate Vote

Agree: 93%, Disagree: 6%, Abstain: 1% (Strong Consensus)

Question 19

- **Should antibiotic prophylaxis be different in patients who have reconstruction by bulk allograft?**

Consensus: We recommend the use of routine antibiotic prophylaxis in patients who have reconstruction by bulk allograft.

Delegate Vote

Agree: 93%, Disagree: 5%, Abstain: 2% (Strong Consensus)

Question 20

- **Do patients with poorly controlled diabetes, immunosuppression, or autoimmune disease require a different perioperative**

antibiotic prophylaxis?

Consensus: No. Routine antibiotic prophylaxis is recommended in these patients.

Delegate Vote

Agree: 90%, Disagree: 9%, Abstain: 1% (Strong Consensus)

Question 21A

- **Should preoperative antibiotics be different for primary and revision TJA?**

Consensus: No. Perioperative antibiotic prophylaxis should be the same for primary and uninfected revision arthroplasty.

Delegate Vote

Agree: 89%, Disagree: 10%, Abstain: 1% (Strong Consensus)

Question 21B

- **Should preoperative antibiotics be different for hips and knees?**

Consensus: Perioperative antibiotic prophylaxis should be the same for hips and knees.

Delegate Vote

Agree: 99%, Disagree: 1%, Abstain: 0% (Strong Consensus)

Question 22

- **What is the best antibiotic prophylaxis to choose in patients with colonization by carbapenem resistant enterobacteriaceae or multi-drug resistant (MDR) —*Acinetobacter* spp?**

Consensus: There is insufficient data to recommend expanded antibiotic prophylaxis in patients known to be colonized or recently infected with MDR pathogens.

Delegate Vote

Agree: 76%, Disagree: 8%, Abstain: 16% (Strong Consensus)

4 手術環境

Workgroup 4：Operative Environment

Question 1

- 手術創内の細菌量は，手術部位感染（SSI）のしやすさと直接相関するか？

コンセンサス

SSI のしやすさと創内の細菌量は直接的に相関する．そのため，手術部位の微粒子や汚染細菌量を減らすための対策を支持する．（参考文献 1-3）

投票結果

同意：97％，反対：2％，棄権：1％（強いコンセンサス）

Question 2

- 手術室環境内の汚染細菌量は，SSI のしやすさと直接相関するか？

コンセンサス

手術室の浮遊細菌が，手術室環境で最も大きな汚染源である．また，これら汚染物質の一番の源は，人間であると考える．われわれの提言の目的は，手術室内の汚染細菌量をいかにして減らすかであり，特に落下細菌に注目した．（参考文献 1-8）

投票結果

同意：93％，反対：5％，棄権：2％（強いコンセンサス）

Question 3

- 待機的人工関節置換術を行う場合の手術室は，層流換気を備えている（バイオクリーンルームである）必要があるか？

コンセンサス

人工関節置換手術は，層流換気のない手術室で行っても良い．バイオクリーンルームやその他手術室内の浮遊微粒子を減少させる効果が期待される対策は，微粒子の蓄積量減少効果が

期待できる．バイオクリーンルームを使うことで SSI が減ることは証明されておらず，むしろいくつかの研究では SSI 割合増加と関連していた．層流換気は保守規定を忠実かつ厳密に守って使用すべき複雑な技術である．本領域では，さらなる研究が必要である．(参考文献 9-17)

投票結果
同意：85％，反対：7％，棄権：8％（強いコンセンサス）

Question 4
- 人工関節全置換術（TJA）で全身排気スーツを必ず着用するべきとする十分な医学的根拠はあるか？

コンセンサス
現在，TJA を行う際にルーチンで全身排気スーツを使用することを支持する決定的な根拠はない．(参考文献 13, 14, 18, 19)

投票結果
同意：84％，反対：11％，棄権：5％（強いコンセンサス）

Question 5
- 手術室の人の出入りでは，どのような対策をとるべきか？

コンセンサス
手術室への人の出入りは，最小限にとどめることを推奨する．(参考文献 15, 17, 20-22)

投票結果
同意：100％，反対：0％，棄権：0％（満場一致）

Question 6
- 手術室のライトは，目線より上の物を触れないようにするためにフットペダルで操作できるようにするべきか？

コンセンサス
まず全員が，ライトハンドルは汚染の原因になり得るということを十分に認識するべきである．また，ライトハンドルの操作は可能な限り控えることを推奨する．将来的には，汚染を最小限にするために，ライトをコントロールするための他の方法を開発するべきである．(参考文献 23, 24)

投票結果
同意：91%，反対：4%，棄権：5%（強いコンセンサス）

Question 7
- 紫外線照射（ultraviolet（UV）light）はTJA後の感染予防に有用か？

コンセンサス
紫外線照射は感染割合を軽減できると思うが，同時に手術室スタッフへのリスクも伴う．われわれは，UVの利点は手術室への人の出入りが抑制されることではないかと考える．

(参考文献 5, 25-30)

投票結果
同意：74%，反対：13%，棄権：13%（強いコンセンサス）

Question 8
- （夜間や週末の）使用されていない手術室で，殺菌用や滅菌用UVライトは手術室環境の清潔度に違いをもたらすか？

コンセンサス
UVは手術室の細菌量を減らすことが期待できる．しかし，本設定での研究は行われていない．従来どおりの清掃法に追加することはよいが，従来どおりの清掃法の代わりになるものではない．仕事開始時に不注意につけっぱなしにされるなど，手術室スタッフに対し潜在的なリスクがある．

投票結果
同意：84%，反対：3%，棄権：13%（強いコンセンサス）

Question 9
- 患者や手術室スタッフは手術室内空気汚染を助長しないようにマスクを使用するべきか？

コンセンサス
手術室マスクをしっかりと全スタッフが着用することでSSI割合が軽減するという決定的な医学的根拠はないものの，手術室マスクをしっかり使用することで空気汚染細菌数の減少が期待できると信じている．マスクを着用しない方がむしろ良いとする医学的根拠が示されるまで，手術室にいる間は全員が手術

室マスクを着用することは患者安全上の問題である．患者がマスクを装着することが気道確保の利点に勝るということを支持する十分な証拠はない．(参考文献 31-35)
投票結果
同意：85％，反対：7％，棄権：8％（強いコンセンサス）

Question 10
- 手術室スタッフはどのような術衣を使用するべきか？

コンセンサス
手術室に入る際には，全員，清潔な術衣と使い捨ての帽子を着用することを推奨する．病院の外で着用した術衣は，人工関節置換術の際は着用するべきではない．(参考文献 28, 36-42)
投票結果
同意：98％，反対：1％，棄権：1％（強いコンセンサス）

Question 11
- 手術室での電子機器（携帯電話，ノート型パソコン，タブレットや音楽関係の器具）の使用に対してどのような規制を設けるべきか？

コンセンサス
携帯用電子機器は細菌に汚染されている可能性がある．また，会話量が増えることは，手術室環境の汚染度の増悪と関連することが知られている．そのため，携帯電子機器の使用は，患者管理にどうしても必要な用途に制限することを推奨する．
(参考文献 43-51)
投票結果
同意：84％，反対：14％，棄権：2％（強いコンセンサス）

Question 12
- 手術時間の延長は人工関節周囲感染(PJI)リスクを助長するか？

コンセンサス
SSI 割合は手術時間と直接相関すると考えている．手術は，より多くの時間をかけなければならないほど複雑なものがある．手術時間の短縮は非常に重要であり，施設や執刀チーム全員の協力が必要である．手術時間短縮のため，手術手技を妥協

することなく全員で一丸となって協力し努力することを推奨する．（参考文献 9, 52-70）

投票結果

同意：96％，反対：3％，棄権：1％（強いコンセンサス）

Question 13

- 待機的 TJA の前に既感染，不潔や汚染手術が入らないようにするべきか？

コンセンサス

汚染手術後に清潔手術を行うことが，感染のリスクになるかどうかは興味のあるところである．汚染手術後に清潔手術を行った場合に，感染割合が上昇したという研究はない．汚染手術後は，追加手術を行う前に施設ごとの基準に従った清掃を徹底的に行うことを推奨する．（参考文献 71-73）

投票結果

同意：89％，反対：8％，棄権：3％（強いコンセンサス）

Question 14

- 感染性合併症を予防するために患者体温管理は重要か？

コンセンサス

整形外科手術以外の領域で患者体温管理の重要性が指摘されている．われわれは，一般外科の文献にある一般的な推奨事項を支持するが，本領域はさらなる研究が必要である．
（参考文献 74, 75）

投票結果

同意：92％，反対：1％，棄権：7％（強いコンセンサス）

Question 15

- 温風式加温（FAW）ブランケットは SSI リスクを助長するか？

コンセンサス

温風式加温ブランケットを使用することの理論的な問題点はあるが，実際に FAW ブランケットを使用することで SSI 割合が上昇したとする文献はない．さらなる研究が必要であるが，現在実践している方法を変更する必要はない．（参考文献 76-84）

投票結果
同意:89%,反対:5%,棄権:6%(強いコンセンサス)

Question 16
- 手術室スタッフは患者周囲におかれている医療機器などを触った際に,都度手指をアルコール製剤で消毒する必要があるか?

コンセンサス
現行の患者管理のための手指衛生の推奨事項を支持する.
(参考文献 85-96)

投票結果
同意:86%,反対:8%,棄権:6%(強いコンセンサス)

Question 17
- 患者への診察,手技や手術台への移動などを行う際に遵守すべき手指衛生や手袋使用法のガイドラインは何か?

コンセンサス
標準予防策(standard precautions)の原則に従った現行の患者管理方法を推奨する. (参考文献 86, 92, 93, 97-99)

投票結果
同意:92%,反対:1%,棄権:7%(強いコンセンサス)

Question 18
- TJA では汚染予防のため3重手袋を着用するべきか?

コンセンサス
2重手袋を推奨する.3重にすることは理論的に有用である.
(参考文献 100-104)

投票結果
同意:89%,反対:7%,棄権:4%(強いコンセンサス)

Question 19
- 手術中はどの程度の頻度で手袋を交換するべきか?

コンセンサス
90分,あるいはそれよりも短い間隔で手袋を交換することが有用である.また,手袋が破れた場合は交換するべきである.透過性はメタクリレートセメントの影響を受けるため,セメン

トを使用した後に手袋は交換するべきである.
(参考文献 100, 105-108)
投票結果
同意：89%，反対：6%，棄権：5%（強いコンセンサス）

Question 20
- 器械台はいつ広げるべきか？

コンセンサス
器械台の展開は，手術開始になるべく近いタイミングで行うことを推奨する．器械台を展開した際は，執刀開始が遅れないようにするべきである．(参考文献 109, 110)

投票結果
同意：98%，反対：1%，棄権：1%（強いコンセンサス）

Question 21
- 器械台は使用していない間は滅菌ドレープやタオルで覆うべきか？

コンセンサス
手術器具を使用していない間は，器械台を覆うことが有用である．また，より大きなカバーは汚染野から清潔野を通って移動させる場合に不利である．本手技のタイミングや方法についてはさらなる研究が必要である．(参考文献 109, 111, 112)

投票結果
同意：90%，反対：4%，棄権：6%（強いコンセンサス）

Question 22
- 皮膚を切開後，さらに深層の切開のためにメス刃は交換するべきか？

コンセンサス
皮膚切開時にメス刃は高い確率で汚染されるため，皮膚切開後にメス刃を交換することを推奨する．(参考文献 23, 113-116)

投票結果
同意：88%，反対：8%，棄権：4%（強いコンセンサス）

Question 23

- 電気メスの先端は TJA 中に交換するべきか？ もし交換するとしたら，どのような頻度で交換するべきか？

コンセンサス

医学的根拠が不足しており，さらなる研究が必要である．

投票結果

同意：95%，反対：0%，棄権：5%（強いコンセンサス）

Question 24

- 吸引の先は，手術中定期的に交換するべきか？ もし交換するとしたら，どのような頻度で行うべきか？ また，吸引の先は大腿骨の髄腔内に入れるべきか？

コンセンサス

汚染割合増加を指摘する数々の報告を考慮し，吸引の先を 60 分毎に交換することを推奨する．吸引の先は大腿骨の髄腔内に入れても良いが，液体を吸引するために必要な時間だけにとどめるべきであり，吸引後は留置するべきではない．これは，大量の汚染した空気や微粒子を吸い込み，術野を汚染する可能性があるからである．（参考文献 23, 117-123）

投票結果

同意：85%，反対：8%，棄権：7%（強いコンセンサス）

Question 25

- 膿盆は汚染源として知られているが，使用するべきか？

コンセンサス

液体を満たしたまま，手術中に野ざらしになっている膿盆は使用すべきでない．（参考文献 15, 124-126）

投票結果

同意：88%，反対：3%，棄権：9%（強いコンセンサス）

Question 26

- 使い捨ての手術器具やカッティングガイドは，術野汚染リスクや PJI リスクを改善するか？

コンセンサス

使い捨て器具は，理論的に有用である可能性があるが，デー

タが不足しており特定のコメントはできない．
(参考文献 127, 128)
投票結果
同意：95％，反対：2％，棄権：3％（強いコンセンサス）

Question 27
- 粘着ドレープは有用か？ 有用であるならば，どのようなタイプのドレープを使用するべきか（ヨード含有か，非含有か）？

コンセンサス
ヨード含有粘着ドレープが皮膚細菌量を減少させるという報告があるが，SSI 自体との関連は明らかでない．皮膚バリアに関する特定のコメントはできないが，さらなる研究を行うことを勧める．(参考文献 129-144)

投票結果
同意：89％，反対：7％，棄権：4％（強いコンセンサス）

Question 28
- 術中，創縁や皮下脂肪にタオルや他の滅菌材料を当て，確実に創縁にクリップすることで，術野汚染や SSI は減少するか？

コンセンサス
滅菌ドレープを用いて皮膚創縁をカバーする従来どおりの方法もあるが，臨床の現場では様々なやり方があり，特に勧告は行わない．(参考文献 145-148)

投票結果
同意：94％，反対：2％，棄権：4％（強いコンセンサス）

Question 29
- どのようなドレープを使用すべきか（再利用可能なものか使い捨てか）？

コンセンサス
ドレープを液体が通過することは汚染と同等であると考えており，不浸透性のドレープを推奨する．使い捨てのものと布のドレープについての比較データは無く，さらなる研究が必要であること以外に勧告は行わない．(参考文献 149-156)

投票結果
同意：90％，反対：6％，棄権：4％（強いコンセンサス）

Question 30
- 術野の消毒前後に使用される粘着型 U 型ドレープは術野から非消毒エリアを効果的に遮るか？

コンセンサス
"会陰部との交通を絶つためのU-ドレープ(U-drapes to isolate the perineum)" は従来実践に供されてきたが，データがないため勧告は行わない．

投票結果
同意：83％，反対：11％，棄権：6％（強いコンセンサス）

Question 31
- 洗浄は有効か？ どのような洗浄方法が良いか（高パルス，低パルス，もしくはバルブ）？

コンセンサス
理論的に，洗浄により汚染物質を希釈でき，大量に洗浄すればするほど希釈されることは分かっている．洗浄方法ごとに利点と欠点があり，優劣はつけがたく，いずれか一つを推奨することはできない．（参考文献 91，157-182）

投票結果
同意：91％，反対：4％，棄権：5％（強いコンセンサス）

Question 32
- どのような洗浄液を使用すべきか？ 抗菌薬を洗浄液に加えるべきか？

コンセンサス
第31項で述べたように，洗浄をすることは物理的に有利であることについては認識している．しかし，いずれの洗浄液もその有用性について相反する科学的根拠があり，洗浄液のタイプに関する勧告はできない．（参考文献 157，160，165，183-211）

投票結果
同意：90％，反対：7％，棄権：3％（強いコンセンサス）

Question 33

- 感染予防のための創内に自己血製剤を術中投与することに意味はあるか?

コンセンサス

データがないので,自己血製剤を感染予防のために創内で使用することについて,特に勧告は行わない. (参考文献 212-219)

投票結果

同意:94%,反対:2%,棄権:4% (強いコンセンサス)

Question 34

- ステープル,あるいは縫合糸の種類は感染イベントに影響するか? もしするならば,感染を予防するうえで最良の閉鎖法は何か?

コンセンサス

決定的なデータはなく,多種多様の術式があることから,感染予防のため特定の縫合糸やステープルを推奨することはしない. (参考文献 220-224)

投票結果

同意:92%,反対:3%,棄権:5% (強いコンセンサス)

Question 35

- 手術用安全チェックリストを使用したり,タイムアウトを行うことは人工関節患者の SSI 割合に影響を及ぼすか?

コンセンサス

手術用チェックリストのプロトコールは,患者安全にとって有益であること,そしてとりわけ適切な予防抗菌薬の使用につながることから,その使用を推奨する. (参考文献 225-232)

投票結果

同意:97%,反対:1%,棄権:2% (強いコンセンサス)

【掲載されている論文】

Operative environment.

Alijanipour P, Karam J, Llinás A, Vince KG, Zalavras C, Austin M, Garrigues G, Heller S, Huddleston J, Klatt B, Krebs V, Lohmann C, McPherson EJ, Molloy R, Oliashirazi A, Schwaber M, Sheehan E, Smith E, Sterling R, Stocks G, Vaidya S.

J Arthroplasty. 2014 Feb：29（2 Suppl）：49-64. doi：10.1016/j.arth.2013.09.031.

Epub 2013 Dec 15. No abstract available.

PMID：24342274

References:

1. Lidwell OM, Lowbury EJ, Whyte W, Blowers R, Stanley SJ, Lowe D. Airborne contamination of wounds in joint replacement operations: the relationship to sepsis rates. J Hosp Infect. 1983;4(2):111-131.
2. McPherson EJ, Peters CL. Chapter 20 Musculoskeletal Infection. Orthopedic Knowledge Update 10; 2011:239-258.
3. Whyte W, Hodgson R, Tinkler J. The importance of airborne bacterial contamination of wounds. J Hosp Infect. 1982;3(2):123-135.
4. Edmiston CE, Jr., Seabrook GR, Cambria RA, et al. Molecular epidemiology of microbial contamination in the operating room environment: Is there a risk for infection? Surgery. 2005;138(4):573-579; discussion 579-582.
5. Taylor GJ, Bannister GC, Leeming JP. Wound disinfection with ultraviolet radiation. J Hosp Infect. 1995;30(2):85-93.
6. Seal DV, Clark RP. Electronic particle counting for evaluating the quality of air in operating theatres: a potential basis for standards? J Appl Bacteriol. 1990;68(3):225-230.
7. Stocks GW, Self SD, Thompson B, Adame XA, O'Connor DP. Predicting bacterial populations based on airborne particulates: a study performed in nonlaminar flow operating rooms during joint arthroplasty surgery. Am J Infect Control. 2010;38(3):199-204.
8. Friberg B, Friberg S, Burman LG. Correlation between surface and air counts of particles carrying aerobic bacteria in operating rooms with turbulent ventilation: an experimental study. J Hosp Infect. 1999;42(1):61-68.
9. Charnley J. Postoperative infection after total hip replacement with special reference to air contamination in the operating room. Clin Orthop Relat Res. 1972;87:167-187.
10. Lidwell OM, Lowbury EJ, Whyte W, Blowers R, Stanley SJ, Lowe D. Effect of ultraclean air in operating rooms on deep sepsis in the joint after total hip or knee replacement: a randomised study. Br Med J (Clin Res Ed). 1982;285(6334):10-14.
11. Breier AC, Brandt C, Sohr D, Geffers C, Gastmeier P. Laminar airflow ceiling size: no impact on infection rates following hip and knee prosthesis. Infect Control Hosp Epidemiol. 2011;32(11):1097-1102.
12. Gastmeier P, Breier AC, Brandt C. Influence of laminar airflow on prosthetic joint infections: a systematic review. J Hosp Infect. 2012;81(2):73-78.
13. Hooper GJ, Rothwell AG, Frampton C, Wyatt MC. Does the use of laminar flow and space suits reduce early deep infection after total hip and knee replacement?: the ten-year results of the New Zealand Joint Registry. J Bone Joint Surg Br. 2011;93(1):85-90.
14. Miner AL, Losina E, Katz JN, Fossel AH, Platt R. Deep infection after total knee replacement: impact of laminar airflow systems and body exhaust suits in the modern operating room. Infect Control Hosp Epidemiol. 2007;28(2):222-226.
15. Andersson BM, Lidgren L, Schalen C, Steen A. Contamination of irrigation solutions in an operating theatre. Infect Control. 1984;5(7):339-341.
16. Brandt C, Hott U, Sohr D, Daschner F, Gastmeier P, Ruden H. Operating room ventilation with laminar airflow shows no protective effect on the surgical site infection rate in orthopedic and abdominal surgery. Ann Surg. 2008;248(5):695-700.
17. Ritter MA, Eitzen H, French ML, Hart JB. The operating room environment as affected by people and the surgical face mask. Clin Orthop Relat Res. 1975(111):147-150.
18. Salvati EA, Robinson RP, Zeno SM, Koslin BL, Brause BD, Wilson PD, Jr. Infection rates after 3175 total hip and total knee replacements performed with and without a horizontal unidirectional filtered air-flow system. J Bone Joint Surg Am. 1982;64(4):525-535.
19. Taylor GJ, Bannister GC. Infection and interposition between ultraclean air source and wound. J Bone Joint Surg Br. 1993;75(3):503-504.
20. Quraishi ZA, Blais FX, Sottile WS, Adler LM. Movement of personnel and wound contamination. AORN J. 1983;38(1):146-147, 150-146.
21. Panahi P, Stroh M, Casper DS, Parvizi J, Austin MS. Operating room traffic is a major concern during total joint arthroplasty. Clin Orthop Relat Res. 2012;470(10):2690-2694.
22. Lynch RJ, Englesbe MJ, Sturm L, et al. Measurement of foot traffic in the operating room: implications for infection control. Am J Med Qual. 2009;24(1):45-52.
23. Davis N, Curry A, Gambhir AK, et al. Intraoperative bacterial contamination in operations for joint replacement. J Bone Joint Surg Br. 1999;81(5):886-889.
24. Hussein JR, Villar RN, Gray AJ, Farrington M. Use of light handles in the laminar flow operating theatre--is it a cause of bacterial concern? Ann R Coll Surg Engl. 2001;83(5):353-354.

25. Berg M, Bergman BR, Hoborn J. Ultraviolet radiation compared to an ultra-clean air enclosure. Comparison of air bacteria counts in operating rooms. J Bone Joint Surg Br. 1991;73(5):811-815.
26. Carlsson AS, Nilsson B, Walder MH, Osterberg K. Ultraviolet radiation and air contamination during total hip replacement. J Hosp Infect. 1986;7(2):176-184.
27. Lowell JD, Kundsin RB, Schwartz CM, Pozin D. Ultraviolet radiation and reduction of deep wound infection following hip and knee arthroplasty. Ann N Y Acad Sci. 1980;353:285-293.
28. Mangram AJ, Horan TC, Pearson ML, Silver LC, Jarvis WR. Guideline for Prevention of Surgical Site Infection, 1999. Centers for Disease Control and Prevention (CDC) Hospital Infection Control Practices Advisory Committee. Am J Infect Control. 1999;27(2):97-132; quiz 133-134; discussion 196.
29. Moggio M, Goldner JL, McCollum DE, Beissinger SF. Wound infections in patients undergoing total hip arthroplasty. Ultraviolet light for the control of airborne bacteria. Arch Surg. 1979;114(7):815-823.
30. Ritter MA, Olberding EM, Malinzak RA. Ultraviolet lighting during orthopaedic surgery and the rate of infection. J Bone Joint Surg Am. 2007;89(9):1935-1940.
31. Belkin NL. The surgical mask has its first performance standard--a century after it was introduced. Bull Am Coll Surg. 2009;94(12):22-25.
32. Lipp A, Edwards P. Disposable surgical face masks: a systematic review. Can Oper Room Nurs J. 2005;23(3):20-21, 24-25, 33-28.
33. Romney MG. Surgical face masks in the operating theatre: re-examining the evidence. J Hosp Infect. 2001;47(4):251-256.
34. Sellden E. Is routine use of a face mask necessary in the operating room? Anesthesiology. 2010;113(6):1447.
35. Webster J, Croger S, Lister C, Doidge M, Terry MJ, Jones I. Use of face masks by non-scrubbed operating room staff: a randomized controlled trial. ANZ J Surg. 2010;80(3):169-173.
36. Berger SA, Kramer M, Nagar H, Finkelstein A, Frimmerman A, Miller HI. Effect of surgical mask position on bacterial contamination of the operative field. J Hosp Infect. 1993;23(1):51-54.
37. Chamberlain GV, Houang E. Trial of the use of masks in the gynaecological operating theatre. Ann R Coll Surg Engl. 1984;66(6):432-433.
38. Laslett LJ, Sabin A. Wearing of caps and masks not necessary during cardiac catheterization. Cathet Cardiovasc Diagn. 1989;17(3):158-160.
39. Mitchell NJ, Hunt S. Surgical face masks in modern operating rooms--a costly and unnecessary ritual? J Hosp Infect. 1991;18(3):239-242.
40. Orr NW, Bailey S. Masks in surgery. J Hosp Infect. 1992;20(1):57.
41. Tunevall TG. Postoperative wound infections and surgical face masks: a controlled study. World J Surg. 1991;15(3):383-387; discussion 387-388.
42. Tunevall TG, Jorbeck H. Influence of wearing masks on the density of airborne bacteria in the vicinity of the surgical wound. Eur J Surg. 1992;158(5):263-266.
43. Brady RR, Chitnis S, Stewart RW, Graham C, Yalamarthi S, Morris K. NHS connecting for health: healthcare professionals, mobile technology, and infection control. Telemed J E Health. 2012;18(4):289-291.
44. Jeske HC, Tiefenthaler W, Hohlrieder M, Hinterberger G, Benzer A. Bacterial contamination of anaesthetists' hands by personal mobile phone and fixed phone use in the operating theatre. Anaesthesia. 2007;62(9):904-906.
45. Lee YJ, Yoo CG, Lee CT, et al. Contamination rates between smart cell phones and non-smart cell phones of healthcare workers. J Hosp Med. 2013;8(3):144-147.
46. Sadat-Ali M, Al-Omran AK, Azam Q, et al. Bacterial flora on cell phones of health care providers in a teaching institution. Am J Infect Control. 2010;38(5):404-405.
47. Singh A, Purohit B. Mobile phones in hospital settings: a serious threat to infection. Occup Health Saf. 2012;81(3):42-44.
48. Ulger F, Esen S, Dilek A, Yanik K, Gunaydin M, Leblebicioglu H. Are we aware how contaminated our mobile phones with nosocomial pathogens? Ann Clin Microbiol Antimicrob. 2009;8:7.
49. Ustun C, Cihangiroglu M. Health care workers' mobile phones: a potential cause of microbial cross-contamination between hospitals and community. J Occup Environ Hyg. 2012;9(9):538-542.
50. Singh D, Kaur H, Gardner WG, Treen LB. Bacterial contamination of hospital pagers. Infect Control Hosp Epidemiol. 2002;23(5):274-276.
51. Hassoun A, Vellozzi EM, Smith MA. Colonization of personal digital assistants carried by healthcare professionals. Infect Control Hosp Epidemiol. 2004;25(11):1000-1001.
52. Carroll K, Dowsey M, Choong P, Peel T. Risk factors for superficial wound complications in hip and knee arthroplasty. Clin Microbiol Infect. 2013.
53. Cordero-Ampuero J, de Dios M. What are the risk factors for infection in hemiarthroplasties and total hip arthroplasties? Clin Orthop Relat Res. 2010;468(12):3268-3277.

54. Huotari K, Agthe N, Lyytikainen O. Validation of surgical site infection surveillance in orthopedic procedures. Am J Infect Control. 2007;35(4):216-221.
55. Masgala A, Chronopoulos E, Nikolopoulos G, et al. Risk factors affecting the incidence of infection after orthopaedic surgery: the role of chemoprophylaxis. Cent Eur J Public Health. 2012;20(4):252-256.
56. Namba RS, Inacio MC, Paxton EW. Risk factors associated with deep surgical site infections after primary total knee arthroplasty: an analysis of 56,216 knees. J Bone Joint Surg Am. 2013;95(9):775-782.
57. Pedersen AB, Svendsson JE, Johnsen SP, Riis A, Overgaard S. Risk factors for revision due to infection after primary total hip arthroplasty. A population-based study of 80,756 primary procedures in the Danish Hip Arthroplasty Registry. Acta Orthop. 2010;81(5):542-547.
58. Peersman G, Laskin R, Davis J, Peterson MG, Richart T. Prolonged operative time correlates with increased infection rate after total knee arthroplasty. HSS J. 2006;2(1):70-72.
59. Pulido L, Ghanem E, Joshi A, Purtill JJ, Parvizi J. Periprosthetic joint infection: the incidence, timing, and predisposing factors. Clin Orthop Relat Res. 2008;466(7):1710-1715.
60. Ridgeway S, Wilson J, Charlet A, Kafatos G, Pearson A, Coello R. Infection of the surgical site after arthroplasty of the hip. J Bone Joint Surg Br. 2005;87(6):844-850.
61. Skramm I, Saltyte Benth J, Bukholm G. Decreasing time trend in SSI incidence for orthopaedic procedures: surveillance matters! J Hosp Infect. 2012;82(4):243-247.
62. Smabrekke A, Espehaug B, Havelin LI, Furnes O. Operating time and survival of primary total hip replacements: an analysis of 31,745 primary cemented and uncemented total hip replacements from local hospitals reported to the Norwegian Arthroplasty Register 1987-2001. Acta Orthop Scand. 2004;75(5):524-532.
63. Urquhart DM, Hanna FS, Brennan SL, et al. Incidence and risk factors for deep surgical site infection after primary total hip arthroplasty: a systematic review. J Arthroplasty. 2010;25(8):1216-1222 e1211-1213.
64. van Kasteren ME, Mannien J, Ott A, Kullberg BJ, de Boer AS, Gyssens IC. Antibiotic prophylaxis and the risk of surgical site infections following total hip arthroplasty: timely administration is the most important factor. Clin Infect Dis. Apr 1 2007;44(7):921-927.
65. Willis-Owen CA, Konyves A, Martin DK. Factors affecting the incidence of infection in hip and knee replacement: an analysis of 5277 cases. J Bone Joint Surg Br. 2010;92(8):1128-1133.
66. Culver DH, Horan TC, Gaynes RP, et al. Surgical wound infection rates by wound class, operative procedure, and patient risk index. National Nosocomial Infections Surveillance System. Am J Med. Sep 16 1991;91(3B):152S-157S.
67. Wymenga AB, van Horn JR, Theeuwes A, Muytjens HL, Slooff TJ. Perioperative factors associated with septic arthritis after arthroplasty. Prospective multicenter study of 362 knee and 2,651 hip operations. Acta Orthop Scand. Dec 1992;63(6):665-671.
68. de Boer AS, Geubbels EL, Wille J, Mintjes-de Groot AJ. Risk assessment for surgical site infections following total hip and total knee prostheses. J Chemother. 2001;13 Spec No 1(1):42-47.
69. Jaffer AK, Barsoum WK, Krebs V, Hurbanek JG, Morra N, Brotman DJ. Duration of anesthesia and venous thromboembolism after hip and knee arthroplasty. Mayo Clin Proc. 2005;80(6):732-738.
70. Strum DP, Sampson AR, May JH, Vargas LG. Surgeon and type of anesthesia predict variability in surgical procedure times. Anesthesiology. 2000;92(5):1454-1466.
71. Kramer A, Schwebke I, Kampf G. How long do nosocomial pathogens persist on inanimate surfaces? A systematic review. BMC Infect Dis. 2006;6:130.
72. Abolghasemian M, Sternheim A, Shakib A, Safir OA, Backstein D. Is arthroplasty immediately after an infected case a risk factor for infection? Clin Orthop Relat Res. 2013;471(7):2253-2258.
73. Namdari S, Voleti PB, Baldwin KD, Lee GC. Primary total joint arthroplasty performed in operating rooms following cases of known infection. Orthopedics. 2011;34(9):e541-545.
74. Kurz A, Sessler DI, Lenhardt R. Perioperative normothermia to reduce the incidence of surgical-wound infection and shorten hospitalization. Study of Wound Infection and Temperature Group. N Engl J Med. May 9 1996;334(19):1209-1215.
75. Melling AC, Ali B, Scott EM, Leaper DJ. Effects of preoperative warming on the incidence of wound infection after clean surgery: a randomised controlled trial. Lancet. Sep 15 2001;358(9285):876-880.
76. McGovern PD, Albrecht M, Belani KG, et al. Forced-air warming and ultra-clean ventilation do not mix: an investigation of theatre ventilation, patient warming and joint replacement infection in orthopaedics. J Bone Joint Surg Br. 2011;93(11):1537-1544.
77. Legg AJ, Cannon T, Hamer AJ. Do forced air patient-warming devices disrupt unidirectional downward airflow? J Bone Joint Surg Br. 2012;94(2):254-256.
78. Sessler DI, Olmsted RN, Kuelpmann R. Forced-air warming does not worsen air quality in laminar flow operating rooms. Anesth Analg. 2011;113(6):1416-1421.
79. Memarzadeh F. Active warming systems to maintain perioperative normothermia in hip replacement surgery. J Hosp Infect. 2010;75(4):332-333.
80. Moretti B, Larocca AM, Napoli C, et al. Active warming systems to maintain perioperative

normothermia in hip replacement surgery: a therapeutic aid or a vector of infection? J Hosp Infect. 2009;73(1):58-63.
81. Tumia N, Ashcroft GP. Convection warmers--a possible source of contamination in laminar airflow operating theatres? J Hosp Infect. 2002;52(3):171-174.
82. Sharp RJ, Chesworth T, Fern ED. Do warming blankets increase bacterial counts in the operating field in a laminar-flow theatre? J Bone Joint Surg Br. 2002;84(4):486-488.
83. Zink RS, Iaizzo PA. Convective warming therapy does not increase the risk of wound contamination in the operating room. Anesth Analg. 1993;76(1):50-53.
84. Albrecht M, Gauthier RL, Belani K, Litchy M, Leaper D. Forced-air warming blowers: An evaluation of filtration adequacy and airborne contamination emissions in the operating room. Am J Infect Control. 2011;39(4):321-328.
85. World Health Organization. Clean care is safer care. http://who.int/gpsc/5may/background/5moments/en. Accessed July 30, 2013.
86. Pittet D, Allegranzi B, Sax H, et al. Evidence-based model for hand transmission during patient care and the role of improved practices. Lancet Infect Dis. 2006;6(10):641-652.
87. Chou DT, Achan P, Ramachandran M. The World Health Organization '5 moments of hand hygiene': the scientific foundation. J Bone Joint Surg Br. 2012;94(4):441-445.
88. Larson EL, Hughes CA, Pyrek JD, Sparks SM, Cagatay EU, Bartkus JM. Changes in bacterial flora associated with skin damage on hands of health care personnel. Am J Infect Control. Oct 1998;26(5):513-521.
89. Noble WC. Dispersal of skin microorganisms. Br J Dermatol. Oct 1975;93(4):477-485.
90. Bonten MJ, Hayden MK, Nathan C, et al. Epidemiology of colonisation of patients and environment with vancomycin-resistant enterococci. Lancet. 1996;348(9042):1615-1619.
91. Boyce JM, Potter-Bynoe G, Chenevert C, King T. Environmental contamination due to methicillin-resistant Staphylococcus aureus: possible infection control implications. Infect Control Hosp Epidemiol. 1997;18(9):622-627.
92. Hayden MK, Blom DW, Lyle EA, Moore CG, Weinstein RA. Risk of hand or glove contamination after contact with patients colonized with vancomycin-resistant enterococcus or the colonized patients' environment. Infect Control Hosp Epidemiol. 2008;29(2):149-154.
93. Bhalla A, Pultz NJ, Gries DM, et al. Acquisition of nosocomial pathogens on hands after contact with environmental surfaces near hospitalized patients. Infect Control Hosp Epidemiol. 2004;25(2):164-167.
94. Boyce JM, Opal SM, Chow JW, et al. Outbreak of multidrug-resistant Enterococcus faecium with transferable vanB class vancomycin resistance. J Clin Microbiol. 1994;32(5):1148-1153.
95. McFarland LV, Mulligan ME, Kwok RY, Stamm WE. Nosocomial acquisition of Clostridium difficile infection. N Engl J Med. Jan 26 1989;320(4):204-210.
96. Hilburn J, Hammond BS, Fendler EJ, Groziak PA. Use of alcohol hand sanitizer as an infection control strategy in an acute care facility. Am J Infect Control. 2003;31(2):109-116.
97. Centers for Disease Control and Prevention. 2007 Guideline for isolation precautions: preventing transmission of infecitous agents in healthcare settings. http://www.cdc.gov/hicpac/2007ip/2007ip_table4.html. Accessed July 30, 2013.
98. Lucet JC, Rigaud MP, Mentre F, et al. Hand contamination before and after different hand hygiene techniques: a randomized clinical trial. J Hosp Infect. 2002;50(4):276-280.
99. McBryde ES, Bradley LC, Whitby M, McElwain DL. An investigation of contact transmission of methicillin-resistant Staphylococcus aureus. J Hosp Infect. 2004;58(2):104-108.
100. Carter AH, Casper DS, Parvizi J, Austin MS. A prospective analysis of glove perforation in primary and revision total hip and total knee arthroplasty. J Arthroplasty. 2012;27(7):1271-1275.
101. Demircay E, Unay K, Bilgili MG, Alataca G. Glove perforation in hip and knee arthroplasty. J Orthop Sci. 2010;15(6):790-794.
102. Hester RA, Nelson CL, Harrison S. Control of contamination of the operative team in total joint arthroplasty. J Arthroplasty. 1992;7(3):267-269.
103. Sebold EJ, Jordan LR. Intraoperative glove perforation. A comparative analysis. Clin Orthop Relat Res. Dec 1993(297):242-244.
104. Sutton PM, Greene T, Howell FR. The protective effect of a cut-resistant glove liner. A prospective, randomised trial. J Bone Joint Surg Br. 1998;80(3):411-413.
105. Al-Maiyah M, Bajwa A, Mackenney P, et al. Glove perforation and contamination in primary total hip arthroplasty. J Bone Joint Surg Br. 2005;87(4):556-559.
106. Kaya I, Ugras A, Sungur I, Yilmaz M, Korkmaz M, Cetinus E. Glove perforation time and frequency in total hip arthroplasty procedures. Acta Orthop Traumatol Turc. 2012;46(1):57-60.
107. Dawson-Bowling S, Smith J, Butt D, Cottam H, Umasankar S, Armitage A. Should outer surgical gloves be changed intraoperatively before orthopaedic prosthesis implantation? J Hosp Infect. 2011;78(2):156-157.
108. Beldame J, Lagrave B, Lievain L, Lefebvre B, Frebourg N, Dujardin F. Surgical glove bacterial contamination and perforation during total hip arthroplasty implantation: when gloves should be changed. Orthop Traumatol Surg Res. 2012;98(4):432-440.
109. Dalstrom DJ, Venkatarayappa I, Manternach AL, Palcic MS, Heyse BA, Prayson MJ.

Time-dependent contamination of opened sterile operating-room trays. J Bone Joint Surg Am. 2008;90(5):1022-1025.
110. Brown AR, Taylor GJ, Gregg PJ. Air contamination during skin preparation and draping in joint replacement surgery. J Bone Joint Surg Br. 1996;78(1):92-94.
111. Chosky SA, Modha D, Taylor GJ. Optimisation of ultraclean air. The role of instrument preparation. J Bone Joint Surg Br. 1996;78(5):835-837.
112. Recommended practices for maintaining a sterile field. AORN J. 2006;83(2):402-404, 407-410, 413-406.
113. Fairclough JA, Mackie IG, Mintowt-Czyz W, Phillips GE. The contaminated skin-knife. A surgical myth. J Bone Joint Surg Br. 1983;65(2):210.
114. Grabe N, Falstie-Jensen S, Fredberg U, Schroder H, Sorensen I. The contaminated skin-knife--fact or fiction. J Hosp Infect. 1985;6(3):252-256.
115. Ritter RA, French ML, Eitzen HE. Bacterial contamination of the surgical knife. Clin Orthop Relat Res. 1975(108):158-160.
116. Schindler OS, Spencer RF, Smith MD. Should we use a separate knife for the skin? J Bone Joint Surg Br. 2006;88(3):382-385.
117. Givissis P, Karataglis D, Antonarakos P, Symeonidis PD, Christodoulou A. Suction during orthopaedic surgery. How safe is the suction tip? Acta Orthop Belg. 2008;74(4):531-533.
118. Greenough CG. An investigation into contamination of operative suction. J Bone Joint Surg Br. 1986;68(1):151-153.
119. Insull PJ, Hudson J. Suction tip: a potential source of infection in clean orthopaedic procedures. ANZ J Surg. 2012;82(3):185-186.
120. Meals RA, Knoke L. The surgical suction top--a contaminated instrument. J Bone Joint Surg Am. 1978;60(3):409-410.
121. Mulcahy DM, Johnson AJ, McCormack D, McElwain JP. Intraoperative suction catheter tip contamination. J R Coll Surg Edinb. Dec 1994;39(6):371-373.
122. Robinson AH, Drew S, Anderson J, Bentley G, Ridgway GL. Suction tip contamination in the ultraclean-air operating theatre. Ann R Coll Surg Engl. 1993;75(4):254-256.
123. Strange-Vognsen HH, Klareskov B. Bacteriologic contamination of suction tips during hip arthroplasty. Acta Orthop Scand. Aug 1988;59(4):410-411.
124. Baird RA, Nickel FR, Thrupp LD, Rucker S, Hawkins B. Splash basin contamination in orthopaedic surgery. Clin Orthop Relat Res. Jul-Aug 1984(187):129-133.
125. Anto B, McCabe J, Kelly S, Morris S, Rynn L, Corbett-Feeney G. Splash basin bacterial contamination during elective arthroplasty. J Infect. 2006;52(3):231-232.
126. Glait SA, Schwarzkopf R, Gould S, Bosco J, Slover J. Is repetitive intraoperative splash basin use a source of bacterial contamination in total joint replacement? Orthopedics. 2011;34(9):e546-549.
127. Mont MA, Johnson AJ, Issa K, et al. Single-Use Instrumentation, Cutting Blocks, and Trials Decrease Contamination during Total Knee Arthroplasty: A Prospective Comparison of Navigated and Nonnavigated Cases. J Knee Surg. 2013;26(4):285-290.
128. Barrack RL, Ruh EL, Williams BM, Ford AD, Foreman K, Nunley RM. Patient specific cutting blocks are currently of no proven value. J Bone Joint Surg Br. 2012;94(11 Suppl A):95-99.
129. Gilliam DL, Nelson CL. Comparison of a one-step iodophor skin preparation versus traditional preparation in total joint surgery. Clin Orthop Relat Res. 1990(250):258-260.
130. Jacobson C, Osmon DR, Hanssen A, et al. Prevention of wound contamination using DuraPrep solution plus Ioban 2 drapes. Clin Orthop Relat Res. 2005;439:32-37.
131. Johnston DH, Fairclough JA, Brown EM, Morris R. Rate of bacterial recolonization of the skin after preparation: four methods compared. Br J Surg. 1987;74(1):64.
132. Kuhme T, Isaksson B, Dahlin LG. Wound contamination in cardiac surgery. A systematic quantitative and qualitative study of the bacterial growth in sternal wounds in cardiac surgery patients. APMIS. 2007;115(9):1001-1007.
133. Lewis DA, Leaper DJ, Speller DC. Prevention of bacterial colonization of wounds at operation: comparison of iodine-impregnated ('Ioban') drapes with conventional methods. J Hosp Infect. Dec 1984;5(4):431-437.
134. Bady S, Wongworawat MD. Effectiveness of antimicrobial incise drapes versus cyanoacrylate barrier preparations for surgical sites. Clin Orthop Relat Res. 2009;467(7):1674-1677.
135. Falk-Brynhildsen K, Friberg O, Soderquist B, Nilsson UG. Bacterial colonization of the skin following aseptic preoperative preparation and impact of the use of plastic adhesive drapes. Biol Res Nurs. 2013;15(2):242-248.
136. French ML, Eitzen HE, Ritter MA. The plastic surgical adhesive drape: an evaluation of its efficacy as a microbial barrier. Ann Surg. 1976;184(1):46-50.
137. Chiu KY, Lau SK, Fung B, Ng KH, Chow SP. Plastic adhesive drapes and wound infection after hip fracture surgery. Aust N Z J Surg. Oct 1993;63(10):798-801.
138. Dewan PA, Van Rij AM, Robinson RG, Skeggs GB, Fergus M. The use of an iodophor-impregnated plastic incise drape in abdominal surgery--a controlled clinical trial. Aust N Z J Surg. 1987;57(11):859-863.

139. Fairclough JA, Johnson D, Mackie I. The prevention of wound contamination by skin organisms by the pre-operative application of an iodophor impregnated plastic adhesive drape. J Int Med Res. 1986;14(2):105-109.
140. Webster J, Alghamdi A. Use of plastic adhesive drapes during surgery for preventing surgical site infection. Cochrane Database Syst Rev. 2013;1:CD006353.
141. Grove GL, Eyberg CI. Comparison of two preoperative skin antiseptic preparations and resultant surgical incise drape adhesion to skin in healthy volunteers. J Bone Joint Surg Am. 2012;94(13):1187-1192.
142. Alexander JW, Aerni S, Plettner JP. Development of a safe and effective one-minute preoperative skin preparation. Arch Surg. Dec 1985;120(12):1357-1361.
143. Erdmann S, Hertl M, Merk HF. Allergic contact dermatitis from povidone-iodine. Contact Dermatitis. 1999;40(6):331-332.
144. Zokaie S, White IR, McFadden JD. Allergic contact dermatitis caused by iodophor-impregnated surgical incise drape. Contact Dermatitis. 2011;65(5):309.
145. Gheorghe A, Calvert M, Pinkney TD, et al. Systematic review of the clinical effectiveness of wound-edge protection devices in reducing surgical site infection in patients undergoing open abdominal surgery. Ann Surg. 2012;255(6):1017-1029.
146. Edwards JP, Ho AL, Tee MC, Dixon E, Ball CG. Wound protectors reduce surgical site infection: a meta-analysis of randomized controlled trials. Ann Surg. 2012;256(1):53-59.
147. Mihaljevic AL, Michalski CW, Erkan M, et al. Standard abdominal wound edge protection with surgical dressings vs coverage with a sterile circular polyethylene drape for prevention of surgical site infections (BaFO): study protocol for a randomized controlled trial. Trials. 2012;13:57.
148. Pinkney TD, Bartlett DC, Hawkins W, et al. Reduction of surgical site infection using a novel intervention (ROSSINI): study protocol for a randomised controlled trial. Trials. 2011;12:217
149. Blom AW, Gozzard C, Heal J, Bowker K, Estela CM. Bacterial strike-through of re-usable surgical drapes: the effect of different wetting agents. J Hosp Infect. 2002;52(1):52-55.
150. Laufman H, Siegal JD, Edberg SC. Moist bacterial strike-through of surgical materials: confirmatory tests. Ann Surg. 1979;189(1):68-74.
151. Blom A, Estela C, Bowker K, MacGowan A, Hardy JR. The passage of bacteria through surgical drapes. Ann R Coll Surg Engl. 2000;82(6):405-407.
152. Ha'eri GB, Wiley AM. Wound contamination through drapes and gowns: a study using tracer particles. Clin Orthop Relat Res. Jan-Feb 1981(154):181-184.
153. Macxintosh CA, Lidwell OM. The evaluation of fabrics in relation to their use as protective garments in nursing and surgery. III. Wet penetration and contact transfer of particles through clothing. J Hyg (Lond). Dec 1980;85(3):393-403.
154. Blom AW, Barnett A, Ajitsaria P, Noel A, Estela CM. Resistance of disposable drapes to bacterial penetration. J Orthop Surg (Hong Kong). 2007;15(3):267-269.
155. Bellchambers J, Harris JM, Cullinan P, Gaya H, Pepper JR. A prospective study of wound infection in coronary artery surgery. Eur J Cardiothorac Surg. 1999;15(1):45-50.
156. Garibaldi RA, Maglio S, Lerer T, Becker D, Lyons R. Comparison of nonwoven and woven gown and drape fabric to prevent intraoperative wound contamination and postoperative infection. Am J Surg. 1986;152(5):505-509.
157. Anglen JO, Gainor BJ, Simpson WA, Christensen G. The use of detergent irrigation for musculoskeletal wounds. Int Orthop. 2003;27(1):40-46.
158. Niki Y, Matsumoto H, Otani T, Tomatsu T, Toyama Y. How much sterile saline should be used for efficient lavage during total knee arthroplasty? Effects of pulse lavage irrigation on removal of bone and cement debris. J Arthroplasty. 2007;22(1):95-99.
159. Bhandari M, Schemitsch EH, Adili A, Lachowski RJ, Shaughnessy SG. High and low pressure pulsatile lavage of contaminated tibial fractures: an in vitro study of bacterial adherence and bone damage. J Orthop Trauma. 1999;13(8):526-533.
160. Brown LL, Shelton HT, Bornside GH, Cohn I, Jr. Evaluation of wound irrigation by pulsatile jet and conventional methods. Ann Surg. Feb 1978;187(2):170-173.
161. Gross A, Cutright DE, Bhaskar SN. Effectiveness of pulsating water jet lavage in treatment of contaminated crushed wounds. Am J Surg. 1972;124(3):373-377.
162. Kalteis T, Lehn N, Schroder HJ, et al. Contaminant seeding in bone by different irrigation methods: an experimental study. J Orthop Trauma. 2005;19(9):591-596.
163. Moussa FW, Gainor BJ, Anglen JO, Christensen G, Simpson WA. Disinfecting agents for removing adherent bacteria from orthopaedic hardware. Clin Orthop Relat Res. Aug 1996(329):255-262.
164. Rodeheaver GT, Pettry D, Thacker JG, Edgerton MT, Edlich RF. Wound cleansing by high pressure irrigation. Surg Gynecol Obstet. 1975;141(3):357-362.
165. Bratzler DW, Dellinger EP, Olsen KM, et al. Clinical practice guidelines for antimicrobial prophylaxis in surgery. Am J Health Syst Pharm. Feb 1 2013;70(3):195-283.
166. Cervantes-Sanchez CR, Gutierrez-Vega R, Vazquez-Carpizo JA, Clark P, Athie-Gutierrez C. Syringe pressure irrigation of subdermic tissue after appendectomy to decrease the incidence of postoperative wound infection. World J Surg. 2000;24(1):38-41; discussion 41-32.

167. Eklund AE, Tunevall TG. Prevention of postoperative wound infection after appendectomy by local application of tinidazole: a double-blind study. World J Surg. 1987;11(2):263-266.
168. Hassinger SM, Harding G, Wongworawat MD. High-pressure pulsatile lavage propagates bacteria into soft tissue. Clin Orthop Relat Res. 2005;439:27-31.
169. Ackland DC, Yap V, Ackland ML, Williams JF, Hardidge A, de Steiger R. Pulse-lavage brushing followed by hydrogen peroxide-gauze packing for bone-bed preparation in cemented total hip arthroplasty: a bovine model. J Orthop Surg (Hong Kong). 2009;17(3):296-300.
170. Clarius M, Seeger JB, Jaeger S, Mohr G, Bitsch RG. The importance of pulsed lavage on interface temperature and ligament tension force in cemented unicompartmental knee arthroplasty. Clin Biomech (Bristol, Avon). 2012;27(4):372-376.
171. Kalteis T, Pforringer D, Herold T, Handel M, Renkawitz T, Plitz W. An experimental comparison of different devices for pulsatile high-pressure lavage and their relevance to cement intrusion into cancellous bone. Arch Orthop Trauma Surg. 2007;127(10):873-877.
172. Maistrelli GL, Antonelli L, Fornasier V, Mahomed N. Cement penetration with pulsed lavage versus syringe irrigation in total knee arthroplasty. Clin Orthop Relat Res. 1995(312):261-265.
173. Miskovsky C, Whiteside LA, White SE. The cemented unicondylar knee arthroplasty. An in vitro comparison of three cement techniques. Clin Orthop Relat Res. 1992(284):215-220.
174. Seeger JB, Jaeger S, Bitsch RG, Mohr G, Rohner E, Clarius M. The effect of bone lavage on femoral cement penetration and interface temperature during Oxford unicompartmental knee arthroplasty with cement. J Bone Joint Surg Am. Jan 2 2013;95(1):48-53.
175. Clarius M, Hauck C, Seeger JB, James A, Murray DW, Aldinger PR. Pulsed lavage reduces the incidence of radiolucent lines under the tibial tray of Oxford unicompartmental knee arthroplasty: pulsed lavage versus syringe lavage. Int Orthop. 2009;33(6):1585-1590.
176. Polzin B, Ellis T, Dirschl DR. Effects of varying pulsatile lavage pressure on cancellous bone structure and fracture healing. J Orthop Trauma. 2006;20(4):261-266.
177. Dirschl DR, Duff GP, Dahners LE, Edin M, Rahn BA, Miclau T. High pressure pulsatile lavage irrigation of intraarticular fractures: effects on fracture healing. J Orthop Trauma. Sep-Oct 1998;12(7):460-463.
178. Draeger RW, Dahners LE. Traumatic wound debridement: a comparison of irrigation methods. J Orthop Trauma. 2006;20(2):83-88.
179. Bhandari M, Adili A, Lachowski RJ. High pressure pulsatile lavage of contaminated human tibiae: an in vitro study. J Orthop Trauma. Sep-Oct 1998;12(7):479-484.
180. Svoboda SJ, Bice TG, Gooden HA, Brooks DE, Thomas DB, Wenke JC. Comparison of bulb syringe and pulsed lavage irrigation with use of a bioluminescent musculoskeletal wound model. J Bone Joint Surg Am. 2006;88(10):2167-2174.
181. Hargrove R, Ridgeway S, Russell R, Norris M, Packham I, Levy B. Does pulse lavage reduce hip hemiarthroplasty infection rates? J Hosp Infect. 2006;62(4):446-449.
182. Munoz-Mahamud E, Garcia S, Bori G, et al. Comparison of a low-pressure and a high-pressure pulsatile lavage during debridement for orthopaedic implant infection. Arch Orthop Trauma Surg. 2011;131(9):1233-1238.
183. Howell JM, Dhindsa HS, Stair TO, Edwards BA. Effect of scrubbing and irrigation on staphylococcal and streptococcal counts in contaminated lacerations. Antimicrob Agents Chemother. Dec 1993;37(12):2754-2755.
184. McHugh SM, Collins CJ, Corrigan MA, Hill AD, Humphreys H. The role of topical antibiotics used as prophylaxis in surgical site infection prevention. J Antimicrob Chemother. 2011;66(4):693-701.
185. Farnell MB, Worthington-Self S, Mucha P, Jr., Ilstrup DM, McIlrath DC. Closure of abdominal incisions with subcutaneous catheters. A prospective randomized trial. Arch Surg. 1986;121(6):641-648.
186. Greig J, Morran C, Gunn R, Mason B, Sleigh D, McArdle C. Wound sepsis after colorectal surgery: the effect of cefotetan lavage. Chemioterapia. 1987;6(2 Suppl):595-596.
187. Rambo WM. Irrigation of the peritoneal cavity with cephalothin. Am J Surg. Feb 1972;123(2):192-195.
188. Schein M, Gecelter G, Freinkel W, Gerding H, Becker PJ. Peritoneal lavage in abdominal sepsis. A controlled clinical study. Arch Surg. 1990;125(9):1132-1135.
189. Sherman JO, Luck SR, Borger JA. Irrigation of the peritoneal cavity for appendicitis in children: a double-blind study. J Pediatr Surg. 1976;11(3):371-374.
190. Conroy BP, Anglen JO, Simpson WA, et al. Comparison of castile soap, benzalkonium chloride, and bacitracin as irrigation solutions for complex contaminated orthopaedic wounds. J Orthop Trauma. Jun-1999;13(5):332-337.
191. Anglen J, Apostoles PS, Christensen G, Gainor B, Lane J. Removal of surface bacteria by irrigation. J Orthop Res. 1996;14(2):251-254.
192. Anglen JO, Apostoles S, Christensen G, Gainor B. The efficacy of various irrigation solutions in removing slime-producing Staphylococcus. J Orthop Trauma. Oct 1994;8(5):390-396.

193. Anglen JO. Comparison of soap and antibiotic solutions for irrigation of lower-limb open fracture wounds. A prospective, randomized study. J Bone Joint Surg Am. 2005;87(7):1415-1422.
194. Sindelar WF, Mason GR. Irrigation of subcutaneous tissue with povidone-iodine solution for prevention of surgical wound infections. Surg Gynecol Obstet. Feb 1979;148(2):227-231.
195. Brown NM, Cipriano CA, Moric M, Sporer SM, Della Valle CJ. Dilute betadine lavage before closure for the prevention of acute postoperative deep periprosthetic joint infection. J Arthroplasty. 2012;27(1):27-30.
196. Cheng MT, Chang MC, Wang ST, Yu WK, Liu CL, Chen TH. Efficacy of dilute betadine solution irrigation in the prevention of postoperative infection of spinal surgery. Spine (Phila Pa 1976). Aug 1 2005;30(15):1689-1693.
197. Chundamala J, Wright JG. The efficacy and risks of using povidone-iodine irrigation to prevent surgical site infection: an evidence-based review. Can J Surg. 2007;50(6):473-481.
198. Kataoka M, Tsumura H, Kaku N, Torisu T. Toxic effects of povidone-iodine on synovial cell and articular cartilage. Clin Rheumatol. 2006;25(5):632-638.
199. Schaumburger J, Beckmann J, Springorum HR, et al. [Toxicity of antiseptics on chondrocytes in vitro]. Z Orthop Unfall. 2010;148(1):39-43.
200. Kaysinger KK, Nicholson NC, Ramp WK, Kellam JF. Toxic effects of wound irrigation solutions on cultured tibiae and osteoblasts. J Orthop Trauma. 1995;9(4):303-311.
201. Goldenheim PD. An appraisal of povidone-iodine and wound healing. Postgrad Med J. 1993;69 Suppl 3:S97-105.
202. Berkelman RL, Lewin S, Allen JR, et al. Pseudobacteremia attributed to contamination of povidone-iodine with Pseudomonas cepacia. Ann Intern Med. 1981;95(1):32-36.
203. Panlilio AL, Beck-Sague CM, Siegel JD, et al. Infections and pseudoinfections due to povidone-iodine solution contaminated with Pseudomonas cepacia. Clin Infect Dis. 1992;14(5):1078-1083.
204. Howells RJ, Salmon JM, McCullough KG. The effect of irrigating solutions on the strength of the cement-bone interface. Aust N Z J Surg. 1992;62(3):215-218.
205. Dimick JB, Lipsett PA, Kostuik JP. Spine update: antimicrobial prophylaxis in spine surgery: basic principles and recent advances. Spine (Phila Pa 1976). Oct 1 2000;25(19):2544-2548.
206. Lipsky BA, Hoey C. Topical antimicrobial therapy for treating chronic wounds. Clin Infect Dis. Nov 15 2009;49(10):1541-1549.
207. Antevil JL, Muldoon MP, Battaglia M, Green R. Intraoperative anaphylactic shock associated with bacitracin irrigation during revision total knee arthroplasty. A case report. J Bone Joint Surg Am. 2003;85-A(2):339-342.
208. Dirschl DR, Wilson FC. Topical antibiotic irrigation in the prophylaxis of operative wound infections in orthopedic surgery. Orthop Clin North Am. 1991;22(3):419-426.
209. Gelman ML, Frazier CH, Chandler HP. Acute renal failure after total hip replacement. J Bone Joint Surg Am. 1979;61(5):657-660.
210. Savitz SI, Savitz MH, Goldstein HB, Mouracade CT, Malangone S. Topical irrigation with polymyxin and bacitracin for spinal surgery. Surg Neurol. 1998;50(3):208-212.
211. Petty W, Spanier S, Shuster JJ. Prevention of infection after total joint replacement. Experiments with a canine model. J Bone Joint Surg Am. 1988;70(4):536-539.
212. Everts PA, Devilee RJ, Brown Mahoney C, et al. Platelet gel and fibrin sealant reduce allogeneic blood transfusions in total knee arthroplasty. Acta Anaesthesiol Scand. 2006;50(5):593-599.
213. Levy O, Martinowitz U, Oran A, Tauber C, Horoszowski H. The use of fibrin tissue adhesive to reduce blood loss and the need for blood transfusion after total knee arthroplasty. A prospective, randomized, multicenter study. J Bone Joint Surg Am. 1999;81(11):1580-1588.
214. Wang GJ, Hungerford DS, Savory CG, et al. Use of fibrin sealant to reduce bloody drainage and hemoglobin loss after total knee arthroplasty: a brief note on a randomized prospective trial. J Bone Joint Surg Am. 2001;83-A(10):1503-1505.
215. Wang GJ, Goldthwaite CA, Jr., Burks S, Crawford R, Spotnitz WD. Fibrin sealant reduces perioperative blood loss in total hip replacement. J Long Term Eff Med Implants. 2003;13(5):399-411.
216. Lassen MR, Solgaard S, Kjersgaard AG, et al. A pilot study of the effects of Vivostat patient-derived fibrin sealant in reducing blood loss in primary hip arthroplasty. Clin Appl Thromb Hemost. 2006;12(3):352-357.
217. Mawatari M, Higo T, Tsutsumi Y, Shigematsu M, Hotokebuchi T. Effectiveness of autologous fibrin tissue adhesive in reducing postoperative blood loss during total hip arthroplasty: a prospective randomised study of 100 cases. J Orthop Surg (Hong Kong). 2006;14(2):117-121.
218. Molloy DO, Archbold HA, Ogonda L, McConway J, Wilson RK, Beverland DE. Comparison of topical fibrin spray and tranexamic acid on blood loss after total knee replacement: a prospective, randomised controlled trial. J Bone Joint Surg Br. 2007;89(3):306-309.
219. Carless PA, Henry DA, Anthony DM. Fibrin sealant use for minimising peri-operative

allogeneic blood transfusion. Cochrane Database Syst Rev. 2003(2):CD004171.
220. Eggers MD, Fang L, Lionberger DR. A comparison of wound closure techniques for total knee arthroplasty. J Arthroplasty. 2011;26(8):1251-1258 e1251-1254.
221. Khan RJ, Fick D, Yao F, et al. A comparison of three methods of wound closure following arthroplasty: a prospective, randomised, controlled trial. J Bone Joint Surg Br. 2006;88(2):238-242.
222. Livesey C, Wylde V, Descamps S, et al. Skin closure after total hip replacement: a randomised controlled trial of skin adhesive versus surgical staples. J Bone Joint Surg Br. 2009;91(6):725-729.
223. Coulthard P, Esposito M, Worthington HV, van der Elst M, van Waes OJ, Darcey J. Tissue adhesives for closure of surgical incisions. Cochrane Database Syst Rev. 2010(5):CD004287.
224. Smith TO, Sexton D, Mann C, Donell S. Sutures versus staples for skin closure in orthopaedic surgery: meta-analysis. BMJ. 2010;340:c1199.
225. Lingard L, Regehr G, Orser B, et al. Evaluation of a preoperative checklist and team briefing among surgeons, nurses, and anesthesiologists to reduce failures in communication. Arch Surg. 2008;143(1):12-17; discussion 18.
226. de Vries EN, Prins HA, Crolla RM, et al. Effect of a comprehensive surgical safety system on patient outcomes. N Engl J Med. Nov 11 2010;363(20):1928-1937.
227. Lingard L, Regehr G, Cartmill C, et al. Evaluation of a preoperative team briefing: a new communication routine results in improved clinical practice. BMJ Qual Saf. 2011;20(6):475-482.
228. Rosenberg AD, Wambold D, Kraemer L, et al. Ensuring appropriate timing of antimicrobial prophylaxis. J Bone Joint Surg Am. 2008;90(2):226-232.
229. Haynes AB, Weiser TG, Berry WR, et al. A surgical safety checklist to reduce morbidity and mortality in a global population. N Engl J Med. Jan 29 2009;360(5):491-499.
230. Andersson AE, Bergh I, Karlsson J, Eriksson BI, Nilsson K. The application of evidence-based measures to reduce surgical site infections during orthopedic surgery - report of a single-center experience in Sweden. Patient Saf Surg. 2012;6(1):11.
231. Burden AR, Torjman MC, Dy GE, et al. Prevention of central venous catheter-related bloodstream infections: is it time to add simulation training to the prevention bundle? J Clin Anesth. 2012;24(7):555-560.
232. Schulman J, Stricof R, Stevens TP, et al. Statewide NICU central-line-associated bloodstream infection rates decline after bundles and checklists. Pediatrics. 2011;127(3):436-444.

Question 1

- **Do numbers of bacteria arriving in the surgical wound correlate directly with the probability of surgical site infection (SSI)?**

<u>Consensus:</u> We recognize that the probability of SSI correlates directly with the quantity of bacteria that reach the wound. Accordingly we support strategies to lower particulate and bacterial counts at surgical wounds.

Delegate Vote

Agree: 97%, Disagree: 2%, Abstain: 1% (Strong Consensus)

Question 2

- **Do numbers of bacteria in the operating room (OR) environment correlate directly with the probability of SSI?**

<u>Consensus:</u> We recognize that airborne particulate bacteria are a major source of contamination in the OR environment and that bacteria shed by personnel are the predominant source of these particles. The focus of our recommendations is to reduce the volume of bacteria in the OR with particular attention to airborne particles.

Delegate Vote

Agree: 93%, Disagree: 5%, Abstain: 2% (Strong Consensus)

Question 3

- **Should the OR in which an elective arthroplasty is performed be fitted with laminar air flow (LAF)?**

<u>Consensus:</u> We believe that arthroplasty surgery may be performed in operating theaters without laminar flow. Laminar flow rooms and other strategies that may reduce particulates in operating rooms would be expected to reduce particulate load. Studies have not shown lower SSI in laminar flow rooms and some cases are associated with increased rates of SSI. These are complex technologies that must function in strict adherence to maintenance protocols. We recommend further investigation in this field.

Delegate Vote

Agree: 85%, Disagree: 7%, Abstain: 8% (Strong Consensus)

Question 4

- **Is there enough evidence to enforce the universal use of body exhaust suits during total joint arthroplasty (TJA) ?**

<u>Consensus:</u> There is currently no conclusive evidence to support the routine use of space suits in performing TJA.

Delegate Vote

Agree: 84%, Disagree: 11%, Abstain: 5% (Strong Consensus)

Question 5

- **What strategies should be implemented regarding OR traffic?**

<u>Consensus:</u> We recommend that OR traffic should be kept to a minimum.

Delegate Vote

Agree: 100%, Disagree: 0%, Abstain: 0% (Unanimous Consensus)

Question 6

- **Should operating lights be controlled with a foot pedal as opposed to reaching above eye level?**

<u>Consensus:</u> We recommend a general awareness that light handles can be a source of contamination and to minimize handling of lights as much as possible. Other strategies for light control need to be developed in the future to minimize contamination.

Delegate Vote

Agree: 91%, Disagree: 4%, Abstain: 5% (Strong Consensus)

Question 7

- **Is there a role for ultraviolet (UV) light use in the prevention of infection after TJA?**

<u>Consensus:</u> We agree that UV light environments can lower infection rates, but recognize that this can pose a risk to OR personnel. We recognize that the benefit of UV might be the inhibition of operating traffic.

Delegate Vote

Agree: 74%, Disagree: 13%, Abstain: 13% (Strong Consensus)

Question 8

- **Do UV decontamination/sterilization lights or portable units in unoccupied ORs (nights and weekends) make a difference in the sterility of the OR environment?**

Consensus: UV would be expected to lower bacterial load in ORs, but the technology has not been studied in this application. It might be considered an adjunct but not a replacement for conventional cleaning. There are potential risks to staff by UV technology inadvertently left on at the start of the work day.

Delegate Vote

Agree: 84%, Disagree: 3%, Abstain: 13% (Strong Consensus)

Question 9

- **Should the patient and OR personnel wear a mask to avoid contamination of the OR air?**

Consensus: Despite the absence of conclusive studies that show a reduction in SSI when surgical masks are worn properly and uniformly by all staff, we believe there is reason to expect particulate airborne bacteria counts to be reduced by disciplined use of surgical masks. Until evidence appears that shows an advantage to NOT wearing a mask, we believe that it is in the interest of patient safety that all personnel wear surgical masks at all time that they are in the OR. There is insufficient evidence to support the use of masks by patients that outweighs the benefit of airway access.

Delegate Vote

Agree: 85%, Disagree: 7%, Abstain: 8% (Strong Consensus)

Question 10

- **What garments are required for OR personnel?**

Consensus: We recommend that all personnel wear clean theater attire including a disposable head covering, when entering an OR. Garments worn outside of the hospital should not be worn during TJA.

Delegate Vote

Agree: 98%, Disagree: 1%, Abstain: 1% (Strong Consensus)

Question 11

- **What restrictions should be placed on the use of portable electronic devices (such as mobile phones, laptops, tablets, or music devices) in the OR?**

<u>Consensus:</u> We recognize that portable electronic devices may be contaminated with bacteria. We also recognize that increased levels of talking are associated with higher levels of bacteria in the OR environment. Accordingly we recommend that portable electronic device usage be limited to that which is necessary for patient care.

Delegate Vote

Agree: 84%, Disagree: 14%, Abstain: 2% (Strong Consensus)

Question 12

- **Does prolonged surgical time predispose to an increased risk of PJI?**

<u>Consensus:</u> We recognize that SSI rates increase directly with the duration of surgery. We recognize that some surgeries present a marked and inescapable level of complexity that will require more time. We recognize that minimizing the duration of surgery is an important goal and a cooperative effort on the base of the entire surgical team as well as the institution. We recommend that a coordinated effort be made to minimize the duration of surgery without technical compromise of the procedure.

Delegate Vote

Agree: 96%, Disagree: 3%, Abstain: 1% (Strong Consensus)

Question 13

- **Should the scheduling of elective TJA be ordered so that clean cases are not preceded by known infected, dirty, or contaminated cases?**

<u>Consensus:</u> We recognize the concern regarding risk of infection to a clean surgery following a contaminated surgery. We recognize that studies have not demonstrated increased infection rates in clean surgery performed subsequent to contaminated cases. We recommend thorough cleaning after contaminated surgery and before further sur-

gery, as defined by local institutional standards.

Delegate Vote

Agree: 89%, Disagree: 8%, Abstain: 3% (Strong Consensus)

Question 14

- **Does patient normothermia have an essential role in preventing infectious complications?**

Consensus: We recognize the significance of patient normothermia and the data from nonorthopaedic rocedures. We support general recommendations from the general surgery literature and identify this as a field that requires further research.

Delegate Vote

Agree: 92%, Disagree: 1%, Abstain: 7% (Strong Consensus)

Question 15

- **Do FAW blankets increase the risk of SSI?**

Consensus: We recognize the theoretical risk posed by FAW blankets and that no studies have shown an increase in SSI related to the use of these devices. We recommend further study but no change to current practice.

Delegate Vote

Agree: 89%, Disagree: 5%, Abstain: 6% (Strong Consensus)

Question 16

- **Should OR personnel be required to decontaminate their hands with at least an alcohol-based foam every time their hands have been in contact with inanimate objects (including medical equipment) located in the immediate vicinity of the patient?**

Consensus: We support current recommendations for hand hygiene in patient care.

Delegate Vote

Agree: 86%, Disagree: 8%, Abstain: 6% (Strong Consensus)

Question 17

- **What are the guidelines for hand hygiene and glove use for per-**

sonnel in contact with the patient for examination, manipulation, and placement on the OR table?

Consensus: We support current recommendations in patient care in accordance with the principles of Standard Precautions.

Delegate Vote
Agree: 92%, Disagree: 1%, Abstain: 7% (Strong Consensus)

Question 18

- **Should triple gloving be used to prevent contamination during TJA?**

Consensus: We recommend double gloving and recognize the theoretical advantage of triple gloving.

Delegate Vote
Agree: 89%, Disagree: 7%, Abstain: 4% (Strong Consensus)

Question 19

- **How frequently should gloves be changed during surgery?**

Consensus: We recognize the advantage of glove changes at least every 90 minutes or more frequently and the necessity of changing perforated gloves. Permeability appears to be compromised by the exposure to methacrylate cement and gloves should be changed after cementation.

Delegate Vote
Agree: 89%, Disagree: 6%, Abstain: 5% (Strong Consensus)

Question 20

- **When should instrument trays be opened?**

Consensus: We recommend that the timing of opening trays should occur as close to the start of the surgical procedure as possible with the avoidance of any delays between tray opening and the start of surgery.

Delegate Vote
Agree: 98%, Disagree: 1%, Abstain: 1% (Strong Consensus)

Question 21

- **Should trays be covered with sterile drapes/towels when not in use?**

Consensus: We recognize a theoretical advantage to covering trays when not in use for extended periods, and that larger covers may be disadvantageous, if they are moved from contaminated areas across the sterile field. We recommend further study of this question regarding timing and techniques.

Delegate Vote

Agree: 90%, Disagree: 4%, Abstain: 6% (Strong Consensus)

Question 22

- **After skin incision, should the knife blade be changed for deeper dissections?**

Consensus: We recognize high contamination rates in studies of scalpel blades that have been used for the skin incision and recommend changes after skin incision.

Delegate Vote

Agree: 88%, Disagree: 8%, Abstain: 4% (Strong Consensus)

Question 23

- **Should electrocautery tips be changed during TJA? If so, how often?**

Consensus: In the absence of evidence we recommend further study and no specific behavior.

Delegate Vote

Agree: 95%, Disagree: 0%, Abstain: 5% (Strong Consensus)

Question 24

- **Should suction tips be regularly changed during surgery? If so, how frequently? Should suction tips enter the femoral canal?**

Consensus: We recommend changing suction tips every 60 minutes based on studies showing higher rates of contamination. Suction tips can be introduced into the femoral canal for the time necessary to evacuate fluid but should not be left in the canal, where they circulate large amounts of ambient air and particles that may contaminate the surgery.

Delegate Vote
Agree: 85%, Disagree: 8%, Abstain: 7% (Strong Consensus)

Question 25

- **Should splash basins be used, as they are known to be a source of contamination?**

<u>Consensus:</u> We recommend against the use of fluid filled basins that sit open during the surgery.

Delegate Vote
Agree: 88%, Disagree: 3%, Abstain: 9% (Strong Consensus)

Question 26

- **Do disposable instruments and cutting guides reduce contamination and subsequent PJI?**

<u>Consensus:</u> We recognize the possible theoretical advantages of disposable instrumentation but in the absence of data we can make no recommendations.

Delegate Vote
Agree: 95%, Disagree: 2%, Abstain: 3% (Strong Consensus)

Question 27

- **Is there a role for incise draping? What type of incise draping should be used (impregnated or clear)?**

<u>Consensus:</u> We recognize the presence of studies that show iodine-impregnated skin incise drapes decreased skin bacterial counts but that no correlation has been established with SSI. We do not make any recommendations regarding the use of skin barriers but do recommend further study.

Delegate Vote
Agree: 89%, Disagree: 7%, Abstain: 4% (Strong Consensus)

Question 28

- **Does the application of towels or other sterile materials to** wound edges and subcutaneous fat during an operation, clipped securely to the edges of the wound, diminish the chances of wound contamination and wound infection?

Consensus: We recognize the traditional practice of covering skin edges with sterile draping but there is wide variation in clinical practice and we make no recommendations.

Delegate Vote

Agree: 94%, Disagree: 2%, Abstain: 4% (Strong Consensus)

Question 29

- **What type of draping should be used (reusable or disposable)?**

Consensus: We recognize that penetration of drapes by liquids is believed to be equivalent to contamination and recommend impervious drapes. In the absence of data on disposable versus cloth drapes, we make no recommendation except for further study.

Delegate Vote

Agree: 90%, Disagree: 6%, Abstain: 4% (Strong Consensus)

Question 30

- **Is there evidence that the use of sticky U drapes, applied before and after prepping, effectively seals the non-prepped area from the operative field?**

Consensus: We recognize that adhesive U-drapes to isolate the perineum has been traditional practice but in the absence of data we make no recommendations.

Delegate Vote

Agree: 83%, Disagree: 11%, Abstain: 6% (Strong Consensus)

Question 31

- **Is irrigation useful? How should the delivery method for irrigation fluid be (high pulse, low pulse or bulb)?**

Consensus: We recognize the theoretical basis for irrigation to dilute contamination and nonviable tissue and that a greater volume of irrigation would be expected to achieve greater dilution. We recognize advantages and disadvantages of different methods of delivering fluid but make no recommendations of one method over another.

Delegate Vote

Agree: 91%, Disagree: 4%, Abstain: 5% (Strong Consensus)

Question 32

- **What type of irrigation solution should be used? Should antibiotics be added to the irrigation solution?**

Consensus: We recognize the mechanical advantage of irrigation as per question 31 but that conflicting evidence exists supporting the use of one agent over the other and make no recommendation regarding type of solution.

Delegate Vote

Agree: 90%, Disagree: 7%, Abstain: 3% (Strong Consensus)

Question 33

- **Is there a role for intraoperative application of autologous blood-derived products to the wound in preventing infection?**

Consensus: In the absence of data we make no recommendation regarding autologous blood derived products to the wound to prevent infection.

Delegate Vote

Agree: 94%, Disagree: 2%, Abstain: 4% (Strong Consensus)

Question 34

- **Do staples or the type of suture have an effect on infectious events? If so, what is the best closure method to prevent infectious events?**

Consensus: In the absence of conclusive data and the wide variability in surgical practice, we make no recommendation regarding specific sutures or staples to prevent infection.

Delegate Vote

Agree: 92%, Disagree: 3%, Abstain: 5% (Strong Consensus)

Question 35

- **Does the use of a surgical safety checklist and time-out affect**

the rate of SSI in arthroplasty patients?

<u>Consensus:</u> We support the surgical checklist protocol as beneficial to patient safety, and specifically as it applies to correct administration of prophylactic antibiotics.

Delegate Vote

Agree: 97%, Disagree: 1%, Abstain: 2% (Strong Consensus)

5 血液保全

Workgroup 5：Blood Conservation

Question 1

- 輸血は手術部位感染（SSI）や人工関節周囲感染（PJI）のリスクの増大と関連するか？

コンセンサス

関連する．同種血輸血は SSI や PJI のリスクの増大と関連するが，自己血輸血については結論がでていない．（参考文献 1-3）

投票結果

同意：91％，反対：5％，棄権：4％（強いコンセンサス）

Question 2

- 人工関節全置換術（TJA）における同種血輸血の必要性をあらわす指標は何か？

コンセンサス

術前ヘモグロビンレベルの低値は TJA 術後の輸血の必要性を示唆する最も強い指標である．全身麻酔，高いチャールソン併存疾患指数，女性，長い手術時間も TJA 後の同種血輸血の必要性を表らわす指標である．

（参考文献 4-23）

投票結果

同意：90％，反対：4％，棄権：6％（強いコンセンサス）

Question 3A

- PJI に対する人工関節置換術において，出血と同種血輸血を少なくする麻酔法は？

コンセンサス

全身麻酔と比べて脊髄麻酔では人工膝関節全置換術（TKA）あるいは人工股関節全置換術（THA）での出血量が少ない．

（参考文献 24-31）

投票結果
同意:77%,反対:11%,棄権:12%(強いコンセンサス)

Question 3B

- PJI の症例に対して脊髄麻酔は行うべきでないとするエビデンスはあるか(感染拡大のリスクがありうるため)?

コンセンサス

脊髄麻酔を行うべきでないというエビデンスはない.PJI 患者に脊髄麻酔を用いるか全身麻酔を用いるかの決定は麻酔チームが行い,脊髄麻酔の多くの利点と感染性中枢神経合併症(くも膜炎,髄膜炎および膿瘍)のリスクを考慮する必要がある.
(参考文献 32-34)

投票結果
同意:83%,反対:6%,棄権:11%(強いコンセンサス)

Question 4A

- 術中洗浄式自己血回収装置,術後非洗浄式自己血回収装置,バイポーラシーラーおよび希釈式自己血輸血法などの補助技術により PJI の術中出血量は減少するか?

コンセンサス

PJI 手術中の術中洗浄式自己血回収装置,術後非洗浄式自己血回収装置,バイポーラシーラーおよび希釈式自己血輸血法などの利点は立証されていない.(参考文献 35,38)

投票結果
同意:85%,反対:8%,棄権:7%(強いコンセンサス)

Question 4B

- 術中洗浄式自己血回収装置,術後非洗浄式自己血回収装置,バイポーラシーラーおよび希釈式自己血輸血法などの補助により TJA 中の出血は減少するか?

コンセンサス

初回の片側性 TJA における術中洗浄式自己血回収装置,術後非洗浄式自己血回収装置,バイポーラシーラーおよび希釈式自己血輸血法などの利点は立証されていない.(参考文献 36,37,39,40)

投票結果
同意：80％，反対：11％，棄権：9％（強いコンセンサス）

Question 5A

- ドレーン留置は SSI や PJI に影響するか？

コンセンサス

影響しない．閉鎖式ドレーンの使用により TJA 後の SSI や PJI のリスクが増大するというエビデンスはない．（参考文献 41-42）

投票結果
同意：88％，反対：8％，棄権：4％（強いコンセンサス）

Question 5B

- ドレーン抜去のタイミングは？

コンセンサス

ドレーン抜去の最適なタイミングについて結論は出ていない．（参考文献 43）

投票結果
同意：68％，反対：22％，棄権：10％（強いコンセンサス）

Question 6A

- トラネキサム酸（TA）使用で PJI 治療を目的とした手術中の出血は減少するか？

コンセンサス

TA の静脈内および局所投与により，TJA における出血量と同種血輸血量は減少する．（参考文献 44-65）

投票結果
同意：82％，反対：5％，棄権：13％（強いコンセンサス）

Question 6B

- TA の局所投与は静脈内投与に比べて有用か？

コンセンサス

TA 局所投与の静脈内投与に対する有用性は明らかでなく，両者はともに安全である．局所投与は静脈内投与が適さない症例に用いられる．（参考文献 49, 66-79）

投票結果
同意:76%,反対:4%,棄権:20%(強いコンセンサス)

Question 7
- 多血小板血漿(PRP)やフィブリン糊のような薬剤で出血は減少するか?

コンセンサス

PRP のルーチンの使用は推奨されない.フィブリン産物が出血を減少させうるというエビデンスがある.

(参考文献 80-87)

投票結果
同意:91%,反対:1%,棄権:8%(強いコンセンサス)

Question 8
- PJI 治療での二期的再置換術の第二期における自己血回収(術中および術後)は有用か?

コンセンサス

自己血回収(術中および術後)の有用性について結論は出ておらず,自己血回収は注意深く行わなければならない.

(参考文献 35, 88, 89)

投票結果
同意:80%,反対:11%,棄権:9%(強いコンセンサス)

Question 9
- PJI 治療のための二期的再置換術の第一期と第二期の手術の間でのエリスロポエチン,造血薬などの薬剤の投与は有用か?

コンセンサス

鉄やエリスロポエチン(有りあるいは無し)による術前の貧血治療により TJA での輸血のリスクが低下する.

(参考文献 90-93)

投票結果
同意:78%,反対:9%,棄権:13%(強いコンセンサス)

Question 10

- 自己完結型の吸引装置は汚染の原因になるか？

コンセンサス

外科用吸引ドレーンの先端が汚染の原因になるとのエビデンスがある．(参考文献 94, 95)

投票結果

同意：70%，反対：9%，棄権：21%（強いコンセンサス）

Question 11

- PJI 治療のための二期的再置換術において第二期の術前自己血貯血は有用か？

コンセンサス

PJI 治療において二期的再置換術の第二期の術前自己血貯血が有用であるかは立証されていない．

投票結果

同意：83%，反対：7%，棄権：10%（強いコンセンサス）

【掲載されている論文】

Blood conservation.

Rasouli MR, Gomes LS, Parsley B, Barsoum W, Bezwada H, Cashman J, Garcia J, Hamilton W, Hume E, Kim TK, Malhotra R, Memtsoudis SG, Ong A, Orozco F, Padgett DE, Reina RJ, Teloken M, Thienpont E, Waters JH.

J Arthroplasty. 2014 Feb；29（2 Suppl）：65-70. doi：10.1016/j.arth.2013.09.032. Epub 2013 Dec 17. No abstract available.

PMID：24360495

References:

1. Healthcare Infection Control Practice Advisory Committee. CDC and HICPAC Draft Guideline for Prevention of Surgical Site Infection, Arthroplasty Section; Pending.
2. Innerhofer P, Klingler A, Klimmer C, Fries D, Nussbaumer W. Risk for postoperative infection after transfusion of white blood cell-filtered allogeneic or autologous blood components in orthopedic patients undergoing primary arthroplasty. Transfusion. 2005;45(1):103-110.
3. Frietsch T, Karger R, Scholer M, et al. Leukodepletion of autologous whole blood has no impact on perioperative infection rate and length of hospital stay. Transfusion. 2008;48(10):2133-2142.
4. Carson JL, Terrin ML, Noveck H, et al. Liberal or restrictive transfusion in high-risk patients after hip surgery. N Engl J Med. 2011;365(26):2453-2462.
5. Hebert PC, Wells G, Blajchman MA, et al. A multicenter, randomized, controlled clinical trial of transfusion requirements in critical care. Transfusion Requirements in Critical Care Investigators, Canadian Critical Care Trials Group. N Engl J Med. 1999;340(6):409-417.
6. Basora M, Pereira A, Soriano A, et al. Allogeneic blood transfusion does not increase the risk of wound infection in total knee arthroplasty. Vox Sang. 2010;98(2):124-129.

7. Brandt C, Hansen S, Sohr D, Daschner F, Ruden H, Gastmeier P. Finding a method for optimizing risk adjustment when comparing surgical-site infection rates. Infect Control Hosp Epidemiol. 2004;25(4):313-318.

8. Byrne AM, Morris S, McCarthy T, Quinlan W, O'Byrne J M. Outcome following deep wound contamination in cemented arthroplasty. Int Orthop. 2007;31(1):27-31.

9. Dale H, Hallan G, Espehaug B, Havelin LI, Engesaeter LB. Increasing risk of revision due to deep infection after hip arthroplasty. Acta Orthop. 2009;80(6):639-645.

10. Gastmeier P, Sohr D, Brandt C, Eckmanns T, Behnke M, Ruden H. Reduction of orthopaedic wound infections in 21 hospitals. Arch Orthop Trauma Surg. 2005;125(8):526-530.

11. Jamsen E, Varonen M, Huhtala H, et al. Incidence of prosthetic joint infections after primary knee arthroplasty. J Arthroplasty. 2010;25(1):87-92.

12. Mraovic B, Suh D, Jacovides C, Parvizi J. Perioperative hyperglycemia and postoperative infection after lower limb arthroplasty. J Diabetes Sci Technol. 2011;5(2):412-418.

13. Ong KL, Kurtz SM, Lau E, Bozic KJ, Berry DJ, Parvizi J. Prosthetic joint infection risk after total hip arthroplasty in the Medicare population. J Arthroplasty. 2009;24(6 Suppl):105-109.

14. Peersman G, Laskin R, Davis J, Peterson M. Infection in total knee replacement: a retrospective review of 6489 total knee replacements. Clin Orthop Relat Res. 2001(392):15-23.

15. Procter LD, Davenport DL, Bernard AC, Zwischenberger JB. General surgical operative duration is associated with increased risk-adjusted infectious complication rates and length of hospital stay. J Am Coll Surg. 2010;210(1):60-65 e61-62.

16. Pulido L, Ghanem E, Joshi A, Purtill JJ, Parvizi J. Periprosthetic joint infection: the incidence, timing, and predisposing factors. Clin Orthop Relat Res. 2008;466(7):1710-1715.

17. Willis-Owen CA, Konyves A, Martin DK. Factors affecting the incidence of infection in hip and knee replacement: an analysis of 5277 cases. J Bone Joint Surg Br. 2010;92(8):1128-1133.

18. Park JH, Rasouli MR, Mortazavi SMJ, Tokarski AT, Maltenfort MG, ., Parvizi J. Predictors of perioperative blood loss in total joint arthroplasty. J Bone Joint Surg Am. 2013;in Press.

19. Faris PM, Spence RK, Larholt KM, Sampson AR, Frei D. The predictive power of baseline hemoglobin for transfusion risk in surgery patients. Orthopedics. 1999;22(1 Suppl):s135-140.

20. Perazzo P, Vigano M, De Girolamo L, et al. Blood management and transfusion strategies in 600 patients undergoing total joint arthroplasty: an analysis of pre-operative autologous blood donation. Blood Transfus. 2013;11(7):370-376.

21. Hamaji A, Hajjar L, Caiero M, et al. Volume replacement therapy during hip arthroplasty using hydroxyethyl starch (130/0.4) compared to lactated Ringer decreases allogeneic blood transfusion and postoperative infection. Rev Bras Anestesiol. 2013;63(1):27-35.

22. Xie R, Wang L, Bao H. Crystalloid and colloid preload for maintaining cardiac output in elderly patients undergoing total hip replacement under spinal anesthesia. J Biomed Res. 2013;25(3):185-190.

23. Casutt M, Kristoffy A, Schuepfer G, Spahn DR, Konrad C. Effects on coagulation of balanced (130/0.42) and non-balanced (130/0.4) hydroxyethyl starch or gelatin compared with balanced Ringer's solution: an in vitro study using two different viscoelastic coagulation tests ROTEMTM and SONOCLOTTM. Br J Anaesth. 2010;105(3):273-281.

24. Guay J. The effect of neuraxial blocks on surgical blood loss and blood transfusion requirements: a meta-analysis. J Clin Anesth. 2006;18(2):124-128.

25. Hu S, Zhang ZY, Hua YQ, Li J, Cai ZD. A comparison of regional and general anaesthesia for total replacement of the hip or knee: a meta-analysis. J Bone Joint Surg Br. 2009;91(7):935-942.

26. Macfarlane AJ, Prasad GA, Chan VW, Brull R. Does regional anaesthesia improve outcome after total hip arthroplasty? A systematic review. Br J Anaesth. 2009;103(3):335-345.

27. Macfarlane AJ, Prasad GA, Chan VW, Brull R. Does regional anesthesia improve outcome after total knee arthroplasty? Clin Orthop Relat Res. 2009;467(9):2379-2402.

28. Mauermann WJ, Shilling AM, Zuo Z. A comparison of neuraxial block versus general anesthesia for elective total hip replacement: a meta-analysis. Anesth Analg. 2006;103(4):1018-1025.

29. Stundner O, Chiu YL, Sun X, et al. Comparative perioperative outcomes associated with neuraxial versus general anesthesia for simultaneous bilateral total knee arthroplasty. Reg Anesth Pain Med. 2012;37(6):638-644.

30. Memtsoudis SG, Sun X, Chiu YL, et al. Perioperative comparative effectiveness of anesthetic technique in orthopedic patients. Anesthesiology. 2013;118(5):1046-1058.

31. Paul JE, Ling E, Lalonde C, Thabane L. Deliberate hypotension in orthopedic surgery reduces blood loss and transfusion requirements: a meta-analysis of randomized controlled trials. Can J Anaesth. 2007;54(10):799-810.

32. Wedel DJ, Horlocker TT. Regional anesthesia in the febrile or infected patient. Reg Anesth Pain Med. 2006;31(4):324-333.

33. Gritsenko K, Marcello D, Liguori GA, Jules-Elysee K, Memtsoudis SG. Meningitis or epidural abscesses after neuraxial block for removal of infected hip or knee prostheses. Br J Anaesth. 2012;108(3):485-490.

34. Chang CC, Lin HC, Lin HW. Anesthetic management and surgical site infections in total hip or knee replacement: a population-based study. Anesthesiology. 2010;113(2):279-284.
35. Waters JH, Tuohy MJ, Hobson DF, Procop G. Bacterial reduction by cell salvage washing and leukocyte depletion filtration. Anesthesiology. 2003;99(3):652-655.
36. Barsoum WK, Klika AK, Murray TG, Higuera C, Lee HH, Krebs VE. Prospective randomized evaluation of the need for blood transfusion during primary total hip arthroplasty with use of a bipolar sealer. J Bone Joint Surg Am. 2011;93(6):513-518.
37. Zeh A, Messer J, Davis J, Vasarhelyi A, Wohlrab D. The Aquamantys system--an alternative to reduce blood loss in primary total hip arthroplasty? J Arthroplasty. 2010;25(7):1072-1077.
38. Clement RC, Kamath AF, Derman PB, Garino JP, Lee GC. Bipolar sealing in revision total hip arthroplasty for infection: efficacy and cost analysis. J Arthroplasty. 2012;27(7):1376-1381.
39. Marulanda GA, Ulrich SD, Seyler TM, Delanois RE, Mont MA. Reductions in blood loss with a bipolar sealer in total hip arthroplasty. Expert Rev Med Devices. 2008;5(2):125-131.
40. Marulanda GA, Krebs VE, Bierbaum BE, et al. Hemostasis using a bipolar sealer in primary unilateral total knee arthroplasty. Am J Orthop (Belle Mead NJ). 2009;38(12):E179-183.
41. Parker MJ, Livingstone V, Clifton R, McKee A. Closed suction surgical wound drainage after orthopaedic surgery. Cochrane Database Syst Rev. 2007(3):CD001825.
42. Parker MJ, Roberts CP, Hay D. Closed suction drainage for hip and knee arthroplasty. A meta-analysis. J Bone Joint Surg Am. 2004;86-A(6):1146-1152.
43. Zamora-Navas P, Collado-Torres F, de la Torre-Solis F. Closed suction drainage after knee arthroplasty. A prospective study of the effectiveness of the operation and of bacterial contamination. Acta Orthop Belg. 1999;65(1):44-47.
44. Alshryda S, Sarda P, Sukeik M, Nargol A, Blenkinsopp J, Mason JM. Tranexamic acid in total knee replacement: a systematic review and meta-analysis. J Bone Joint Surg Br. 2011;93(12):1577-1585.
45. Kagoma YK, Crowther MA, Douketis J, Bhandari M, Eikelboom J, Lim W. Use of antifibrinolytic therapy to reduce transfusion in patients undergoing orthopedic surgery: a systematic review of randomized trials. Thromb Res. 2009;123(5):687-696.
46. Roberts I, Perel P, Prieto-Merino D, et al. Effect of tranexamic acid on mortality in patients with traumatic bleeding: prespecified analysis of data from randomised controlled trial. BMJ. 2012;345:e5839.
47. Roberts I, Shakur H, Afolabi A, et al. The importance of early treatment with tranexamic acid in bleeding trauma patients: an exploratory analysis of the CRASH-2 randomised controlled trial. Lancet. 2011;377(9771):1096-1101, 1101 e1091-1092.
48. Shakur H, Roberts I, Bautista R, et al. Effects of tranexamic acid on death, vascular occlusive events, and blood transfusion in trauma patients with significant haemorrhage (CRASH-2): a randomised, placebo-controlled trial. Lancet. 2010;376(9734):23-32.
49. Sukeik M, Alshryda S, Haddad FS, Mason JM. Systematic review and meta-analysis of the use of tranexamic acid in total hip replacement. J Bone Joint Surg Br. 2011;93(1):39-46.
50. Zhang H, Chen J, Chen F, Que W. The effect of tranexamic acid on blood loss and use of blood products in total knee arthroplasty: a meta-analysis. Knee Surg Sports Traumatol Arthrosc. 2012;20(9):1742-1752.
51. Tan J, Chen H, Liu Q, Chen C, Huang W. A meta-analysis of the effectiveness and safety of using tranexamic acid in primary unilateral total knee arthroplasty. J Surg Res. Apr 25 2013.
52. Zhou XD, Tao LJ, Li J, Wu LD. Do we really need tranexamic acid in total hip arthroplasty? A meta-analysis of nineteen randomized controlled trials. Arch Orthop Trauma Surg. 2013;133(7):1017-1027.
53. Zufferey P, Merquiol F, Laporte S, et al. Do antifibrinolytics reduce allogeneic blood transfusion in orthopedic surgery? Anesthesiology. 2006;105(5):1034-1046.
54. Zohar E, Ellis M, Ifrach N, Stern A, Sapir O, Fredman B. The postoperative blood-sparing efficacy of oral versus intravenous tranexamic acid after total knee replacement. Anesth Analg. 2004;99(6):1679-1683, table of contents.
55. Wong J, Abrishami A, El Beheiry H, et al. Topical application of tranexamic acid reduces postoperative blood loss in total knee arthroplasty: a randomized, controlled trial. J Bone Joint Surg Am. 2010;92(15):2503-2513.
56. Zohar E, Fredman B, Ellis M, Luban I, Stern A, Jedeikin R. A comparative study of the postoperative allogeneic blood-sparing effect of tranexamic acid versus acute normovolemic hemodilution after total knee replacement. Anesth Analg. 1999;89(6):1382-1387.
57. Ellis MH, Fredman B, Zohar E, Ifrach N, Jedeikin R. The effect of tourniquet application, tranexamic acid, and desmopressin on the procoagulant and fibrinolytic systems during total knee replacement. J Clin Anesth. 2001;13(7):509-513.
58. Jansen AJ, Andreica S, Claeys M, D'Haese J, Camu F, Jochmans K. Use of tranexamic acid for an effective blood conservation strategy after total knee arthroplasty. Br J Anaesth. 1999;83(4):596-601.
59. Alvarez JC, Santiveri FX, Ramos I, Vela E, Puig L, Escolano F. Tranexamic acid

60. Benoni G, Fredin H. Fibrinolytic inhibition with tranexamic acid reduces blood loss and blood transfusion after knee arthroplasty: a prospective, randomised, double-blind study of 86 patients. J Bone Joint Surg Br. 1996;78(3):434-440.
61. Camarasa MA, Olle G, Serra-Prat M, et al. Efficacy of aminocaproic, tranexamic acids in the control of bleeding during total knee replacement: a randomized clinical trial. Br J Anaesth. 2006;96(5):576-582.
62. Engel JM, Hohaus T, Ruwoldt R, Menges T, Jurgensen I, Hempelmann G. Regional hemostatic status and blood requirements after total knee arthroplasty with and without tranexamic acid or aprotinin. Anesth Analg. 2001;92(3):775-780.
63. Hiippala S, Strid L, Wennerstrand M, et al. Tranexamic acid (Cyklokapron) reduces perioperative blood loss associated with total knee arthroplasty. Br J Anaesth. 1995;74(5):534-537.
64. Hiippala ST, Strid LJ, Wennerstrand MI, et al. Tranexamic acid radically decreases blood loss and transfusions associated with total knee arthroplasty. Anesth Analg. 1997;84(4):839-844.
65. Molloy DO, Archbold HA, Ogonda L, McConway J, Wilson RK, Beverland DE. Comparison of topical fibrin spray and tranexamic acid on blood loss after total knee replacement: a prospective, randomised controlled trial. J Bone Joint Surg Br. 2007;89(3):306-309.
66. Benoni G, Fredin H, Knebel R, Nilsson P. Blood conservation with tranexamic acid in total hip arthroplasty: a randomized, double-blind study in 40 primary operations. Acta Orthop Scand. 2001;72(5):442-448.
67. Benoni G, Lethagen S, Nilsson P, Fredin H. Tranexamic acid, given at the end of the operation, does not reduce postoperative blood loss in hip arthroplasty. Acta Orthop Scand. 2000;71(3):250-254.
68. Claeys MA, Vermeersch N, Haentjens P. Reduction of blood loss with tranexamic acid in primary total hip replacement surgery. Acta Chir Belg. 2007;107(4):397-401.
69. Ekback G, Axelsson K, Ryttberg L, et al. Tranexamic acid reduces blood loss in total hip replacement surgery. Anesth Analg. 2000;91(5):1124-1130.
70. Garneti N, Field J. Bone bleeding during total hip arthroplasty after administration of tranexamic acid. J Arthroplasty. 2004;19(4):488-492.
71. Husted H, Blond L, Sonne-Holm S, Holm G, Jacobsen TW, Gebuhr P. Tranexamic acid reduces blood loss and blood transfusions in primary total hip arthroplasty: a prospective randomized double-blind study in 40 patients. Acta Orthop Scand. 2003;74(6):665-669.
72. Ido K, Neo M, Asada Y, et al. Reduction of blood loss using tranexamic acid in total knee and hip arthroplasties. Arch Orthop Trauma Surg. 2000;120(9):518-520.
73. Johansson T, Pettersson LG, Lisander B. Tranexamic acid in total hip arthroplasty saves blood and money: a randomized, double-blind study in 100 patients. Acta Orthop. 2005;76(3):314-319.
74. Lemay E, Guay J, Cote C, Roy A. Tranexamic acid reduces the need for allogenic red blood cell transfusions in patients undergoing total hip replacement. Can J Anaesth. 2004;51(1):31-37.
75. Niskanen RO, Korkala OL. Tranexamic acid reduces blood loss in cemented hip arthroplasty: a randomized, double-blind study of 39 patients with osteoarthritis. Acta Orthop. 2005;76(6):829-832.
76. Yamasaki S, Masuhara K, Fuji T. Tranexamic acid reduces blood loss after cementless total hip arthroplasty-prospective randomized study in 40 cases. Int Orthop. 2004;28(2):69-73.
77. Lin PC, Hsu CH, Huang CC, Chen WS, Wang JW. The blood-saving effect of tranexamic acid in minimally invasive total knee replacement: is an additional pre-operative injection effective? J Bone Joint Surg Br. 2012;94(7):932-936.
78. Aguilera X, Videla S, Almenara M, Fernandez JA, Gich I, Celaya F. Effectiveness of tranexamic acid in revision total knee arthroplasty. Acta Orthop Belg. 2012;78(1):68-74.
79. Oremus K, Sostaric S, Trkulja V, Haspl M. Influence of tranexamic acid on postoperative autologous blood retransfusion in primary total hip and knee arthroplasty: a randomized controlled trial. Transfusion. Apr 25 2013.
80. Diiorio TM, Burkholder JD, Good RP, Parvizi J, Sharkey PF. Platelet-rich plasma does not reduce blood loss or pain or improve range of motion after TKA. Clin Orthop Relat Res. 2012;470(1):138-143.
81. Gardner MJ, Demetrakopoulos D, Klepchick PR, Mooar PA. The efficacy of autologous platelet gel in pain control and blood loss in total knee arthroplasty. An analysis of the haemoglobin, narcotic requirement and range of motion. Int Orthop. 2007;31(3):309-313.
82. Berghoff WJ, Pietrzak WS, Rhodes RD. Platelet-rich plasma application during closure following total knee arthroplasty. Orthopedics. 2006;29(7):590-598.
83. McConnell JS, Shewale S, Munro NA, Shah K, Deakin AH, Kinninmonth AW. Reduction of blood loss in primary hip arthroplasty with tranexamic acid or fibrin spray. Acta Orthop. 2011;82(6):660-663.

84. Mawatari M, Higo T, Tsutsumi Y, Shigematsu M, Hotokebuchi T. Effectiveness of autologous fibrin tissue adhesive in reducing postoperative blood loss during total hip arthroplasty: a prospective randomised study of 100 cases. J Orthop Surg (Hong Kong). 2006;14(2):117-121.

85. Levy O, Martinowitz U, Oran A, Tauber C, Horoszowski H. The use of fibrin tissue adhesive to reduce blood loss and the need for blood transfusion after total knee arthroplasty. A prospective, randomized, multicenter study. J Bone Joint Surg Am. 1999;81(11):1580-1588.

86. Wang GJ, Goldthwaite CA, Jr., Burks S, Crawford R, Spotnitz WD. Fibrin sealant reduces perioperative blood loss in total hip replacement. J Long Term Eff Med Implants. 2003;13(5):399-411.

87. Wang GJ, Hungerford DS, Savory CG, et al. Use of fibrin sealant to reduce bloody drainage and hemoglobin loss after total knee arthroplasty: a brief note on a randomized prospective trial. J Bone Joint Surg Am. 2001;83-A(10):1503-1505.

88. Carless PA, Henry DA, Moxey AJ, O'Connell D, Brown T, Fergusson DA. Cell salvage for minimising perioperative allogeneic blood transfusion. Cochrane Database Syst Rev. 2010(4):CD001888.

89. Waters JH. Indications and contraindications of cell salvage. Transfusion. 2004;44(12 Suppl):40S-44S.

90. Spahn DR. Anemia and patient blood management in hip and knee surgery: a systematic review of the literature. Anesthesiology. 2010;113(2):482-495.

91. Feagan BG, Wong CJ, Kirkley A, et al. Erythropoietin with iron supplementation to prevent allogeneic blood transfusion in total hip joint arthroplasty. A randomized, controlled trial. Ann Intern Med. 2000;133(11):845-854.

92. Delasotta LA, Rangavajjula A, Frank ML, Blair J, Orozco F, Ong A. The Use of Preoperative Epoetin-alpha in Revision Hip Arthroplasty. Open Orthop J. 2012;6:179-183.

93. Delasotta LA, Rangavajjula AV, Frank ML, Blair JL, Orozco FR, Ong AC. The Use of Epoetin-alpha in Revision Knee Arthroplasty. Adv Orthop. 2012;2012:595027.

94. Robinson AH, Drew S, Anderson J, Bentley G, Ridgway GL. Suction tip contamination in the ultraclean-air operating theatre. Ann R Coll Surg Engl. 1993;75(4):254-256.

95. Strange-Vognsen HH, Klareskov B. Bacteriologic contamination of suction tips during hip arthroplasty. Acta Orthop Scand. 1988;59(4):410-411.

Question 1

- **Is blood transfusion associated with an increased risk of surgical site infection (SSI)/periprosthetic joint infection (PJI)?**

<u>Consensus:</u> Yes. Allogeneic blood transfusions is associated with an increased risk of SSI/PJI. The role of autologous transfusion in the risk of SSI/PJI remains inconclusive.

Delegate Vote

Agree: 91%, Disagree: 5%, Abstain: 4% (Strong Consensus)

Question 2

- **What are the predictors of the need for allogeneic blood transfusion in patients undergoing surgery for TJA?**

<u>Consensus:</u> A lower preoperative hemoglobin level is the strongest predictor for the potential need for allogeneic transfusion after TJA. The use of general anesthesia, higher Charlson comorbidity index, female gender, and longer duration of surgery are predictors of the potential need for allogeneic blood transfusion in patients undergoing total joint arthroplasty (TJA).

Delegate Vote

Agree: 90%, Disagree: 4%, Abstain: 6% (Strong Consensus)

Question 3A

- **What is the role of the type of anesthesia in minimizing blood loss and allogeneic blood transfusion during arthroplasty surgery for PJI?**

<u>Consensus:</u> Compared to general anesthesia, neuraxial anesthesia reduces the amount of blood loss during TKA or THA.

Delegate Vote

Agree: 77%, Disagree: 11%, Abstain: 12% (Strong Consensus)

Question 3B

- **Is there evidence against neuraxial blockade in PJI cases (due to probable risk of spreading infection)?**

<u>Consensus:</u> No. The decision to use neuraxial versus general anesthesia in patients with PJI lies with the anesthesia team and needs to take

into account the numerous benefits of neuraxial anesthesia versus the potential for development of infectious central nervous system complications (arachnoiditis, meningitis, and abscess) with the use of anesthesia.

Delegate Vote

Agree: 83%, Disagree: 6%, Abstain: 11% (Strong Consensus)

Question 4A

- **What is the role for adjuvant technologies including cell salvage systems, reinfusion drains, bipolar sealers, and hemodilution for minimizing blood loss during surgery for PJI?**

Consensus: There is no defined benefit for the use of cell salvage systems, reinfusion drains, biopolar sealers, and hemodilution for management of PJI.

Delegate Vote

Agree: 85%, Disagree: 8%, Abstain: 7% (Strong Consensus)

Question 4B

- **What is the role for adjuvant technologies including cell salvage systems, reinfusion drains, bipolar sealers, and hemodilution for minimizing blood loss during TJA?**

Consensus: There is no defined benefit for the use of cell salvage systems, reinfusion drains, biopolar sealers, and hemodilution during primary, unilateral TJA.

Delegate Vote

Agree: 80%, Disagree: 11%, Abstain: 9% (Strong Consensus)

Question 5A

- **Does the use of a drain (s) influence the incidence of SSI/PJI?**

Consensus: No. There is no evidence to demonstrate that the use of closed drains increases the risk of SSI/PJI following TJA.

Delegate Vote

Agree: 88%, Disagree: 8%, Abstain: 4% (Strong Consensus)

Question 5B

- **When should drain (s) be removed?**

Consensus: There is no conclusive evidence for the optimal timing of drain removal.

Delegate Vote
Agree: 68%, Disagree: 22%, Abstain: 10% (Strong Consensus)

Question 6A

- **What is the role for tranexamic acid (TA) for minimizing blood loss during surgery for treatment of PJI?**

Consensus: : Administration of both intravenous and topical TA reduces the amount of blood loss and allogeneic blood transfusion in TJA.

Delegate Vote
Agree: 82%, Disagree: 5%, Abstain: 13% (Strong Consensus)

Question 6B

- **Does administration of topical TA have an advantage over intravenous administration?**

Consensus: Topical TA does not have any obvious advantage over intravenous administration of the drug and both are safe. However, topical TA may be used in certain group of patients in whom IV TA is considered to be inappropriate.

Delegate Vote
Agree: 76%, Disagree: 4%, Abstain: 20% (Strong Consensus)

Question 7

- **What is the role for other agents such as platelet-rich plasma (PRP), fibrin glue for minimizing blood loss?**

Consensus: The routine use of PRP is not recommended. There is some evidence that fibrin products may reduce blood loss.

Delegate Vote
Agree: 91%, Disagree: 1%, Abstain: 8% (Strong Consensus)

Question 8

- **What is the role for blood salvage (intraoperative and postoperative) during the second stage of two-stage exchange arthroplasty for treatment of PJI?**

<u>Consensus:</u> The role of blood salvage (intraoperative and postoperative) during the second stage exchange arthroplasty is inconclusive. Blood salvage should be utilized with caution.

Delegate Vote

Agree: 80%, Disagree: 11%, Abstain: 9% (Strong Consensus)

Question 9

- **What is the role of administration of erythropoietin, hematinics, or other agents between the two stages of exchange arthroplasty for the treatment of PJI?**

<u>Consensus:</u> Treatment of preoperative anemia with iron, with or without erythropoietin, will reduce the risk of transfusion in patients undergoing TJA.

Delegate Vote

Agree: 78%, Disagree: 9%, Abstain: 13% (Strong Consensus)

Question 10

- **Are self-contained suction suction devices a source of contamination?**

<u>Consensus:</u> There is evidence indicating that the tip of surgical suction drains can be a source of contamination.

Delegate Vote

Agree: 70%, Disagree: 9%, Abstain: 21% (Strong Consensus)

Question 11

- **What is the role of preoperative autologous blood donation between the two stages of exchange arthroplasty for PJI?**

<u>Consensus:</u> There is no role for autologous blood donation between the two stages of exchange arthroplasty for PJI.

Delegate Vote

Agree: 83%, Disagree: 7%, Abstain: 10% (Strong Consensus)

6 人工挿入物の選択

Workgroup 6：Prosthesis Selection

Question 1

- 人工挿入物の種類は，手術部位感染（SSI）あるいは人工関節周囲感染（PJI）の発生に影響を与えるか？

コンセンサス

人工挿入物のタイプ（セメント vs 非セメント）あるいはハイドロキシアパタイトによるコーティングは SSI あるいは PJI の発生に影響を与えない．（参考文献 1-17）

投票結果

同意：92％，反対：4％，棄権：4％（強いコンセンサス）

Question 2A

- 抗菌薬含有セメントは待機的初回人工関節全置換術（TJA）後の PJI 発生を減少させるか？

コンセンサス

減少させる．抗菌薬含有ポリメタクリル酸メチル（ABX-PMMA）セメントは TJA 後の PJI 発生を減少させるので，待機的人工関節置換術を行う PJI ハイリスク患者において用いられるべきである．

投票結果

同意：90％，反対：9％，棄権：1％（強いコンセンサス）

Question 2B

- 抗菌薬含有セメントは待機的人工関節再置換術後の PJI 発生を減少させるか？

コンセンサス

減少させる．人工関節再置換術の際に，セメント固定あるいはハイブリッド固定が行われる全ての患者においてセメントに抗菌薬を加えるべきである．（Queation 2 A，2B 参考文献 18-38）

投票結果

同意：88％，反対：9％，棄権：3％（強いコンセンサス）

Question 3

- 人工股関節全置換術（THA）における摺動面のタイプは SSI や PJI の発生に影響を与えるか？

コンセンサス

観察データでは，メタル・オン・メタルの摺動面は PJI のリスクが高くなる可能性がある．（参考文献 39-42）

投票結果

同意：78％，反対：15％，棄権：7％（強いコンセンサス）

Question 4

- 人工挿入物のサイズ（異物素材の大きさ）は TJA 後の SSI 発生に影響するか？

コンセンサス

影響する．メガプロステーシスを使用すると感染発生率はより高くなる．（参考文献 43, 44）

投票結果

同意：85％，反対：11％，棄権：4％（強いコンセンサス）

Question 5

- TJA 後の SSI や PJI の発生に関して，様々な種類のセメント間で差はあるか？

コンセンサス

異なった PMMA セメント製剤が用いられた場合でも，TJA の SSI や PJI の発生に明らかな差はない．

（参考文献 24, 28, 45）

投票結果

同意：92％，反対：3％，棄権：5％（強いコンセンサス）

Question 6

- 抗菌薬の溶出に関して各セメント間で差はあるか？

コンセンサス

PMMA セメントからの抗菌薬の溶出特性は，セメントの種類

および抗菌薬の種類と投与量により明らかな差がある.
(参考文献 23-25, 45, 46)

投票結果
同意：96％，反対：0％，棄権：4％（強いコンセンサス）

Question 7

- セメントレス人工関節の種類で SSI や PJI の発生に差はあるか？

コンセンサス

人工関節再置換術ではチタンに比較して多孔性金属（タンタル）インプラントの使用で，SSI や PJI の発生は減少する可能性がある．(参考文献 47-51)

投票結果
同意：44％，反対：33％，棄権：23％（コンセンサス得られず）

Question 8

- TJA の際，創部への抗菌薬パウダー（例えば，バンコマイシン）の使用は有用か？

コンセンサス

有用ではない．バンコマイシンパウダーを創部へ注入すること，あるいはインプラントの近傍に入れることが PJI の発生を減少させることを示唆する文献はない．人工関節置換術以外の手術で，バンコマイシンパウダーの使用が術後の SSI 発生を減少させることを示す研究がわずかながらある．今後の研究が必要である．(参考文献 50, 52, 53)

投票結果
同意：91％，反対：5％，棄権：4％（強いコンセンサス）

Question 9

- 感染後の骨欠損の再建に同種骨を用いた場合と金属補填材を用いた場合で SSI や PJI の発生に差があるか？

コンセンサス

骨欠損の再建に金属補填材を用いても，同種骨を用いても SSI や PJI の発生に差はない．

投票結果
同意:80%,反対:7%,棄権:13%(強いコンセンサス)

Question 10
- PJIの発生を最小限にするのに,人工挿入物表面の改良は有用か?

コンセンサス
細菌の定着,およびそれに続発するSSIやPJIを減少させることに役だつインプラント表面の改良が真に求められる.
(参考文献 54-64)

投票結果
同意:76%,反対:15%,棄権:9%(強いコンセンサス)

Question 11
- SSIやPJI予防のための新しい展開はあるか?

コンセンサス
整形外科学界は,SSIやPJIの発生数を減らすための試みの中で,人工挿入物の表面を改良することの可能性を探求する必要がある.(参考文献 65-70)

投票結果
同意:84%,反対:10%,棄権:6%(強いコンセンサス)

【掲載されている論文】

Prosthesis selection.

Diaz-Ledezma C, Parvizi J, Zhou Y, Antoci V, Ducheyne P, Freiberg A, Garcia Rangel G, Han SB, Hickok N, Higuera C, Ketonis C, Korkusuz F, Kruczynski J, Macule F, Markuszewski J, Marín-Peña O, Nathwani D, Noble P, Ong K, Ono N, Parvizi MS, Post Z, Rivero-Boschert S, Schaer T, Shapiro I.

J Arthroplasty. 2014 Feb:29(2 Suppl):71-6. doi:10.1016/j.arth.2013.09.039. Epub 2013 Dec 17. No abstract available.

PMID:24360496

References:

1. Corten K, Bourne RB, Charron KD, Au K, Rorabeck CH. What works best, a cemented or cementless primary total hip arthroplasty?: minimum 17-year followup of a randomized controlled trial. Clin Orthop Relat Res. 2011;469(1):209-217.
2. Morshed S, Bozic KJ, Ries MD, Malchau H, Colford JM, Jr. Comparison of cemented and uncemented fixation in total hip replacement: a meta-analysis. Acta Orthop. 2007;78(3):315-326.
3. Hailer NP, Garellick G, Karrholm J. Uncemented and cemented primary total hip arthroplasty in the Swedish Hip Arthroplasty Register. Acta Orthop. 2010;81(1):34-41.
4. Dale H, Hallan G, Espehaug B, Havelin LI, Engesaeter LB. Increasing risk of revision due to deep infection after hip arthroplasty. Acta Orthop. 2009;80(6):639-645.
5. Engesaeter LB, Espehaug B, Lie SA, Furnes O, Havelin LI. Does cement increase the risk of infection in primary total hip arthroplasty? Revision rates in 56,275 cemented and uncemented primary THAs followed for 0-16 years in the Norwegian Arthroplasty Register. Acta Orthop. 2006;77(3):351-358.
6. Dale H, Skramm I, Lower HL, et al. Infection after primary hip arthroplasty: a comparison of 3 Norwegian health registers. Acta Orthop. 2011;82(6):646-654.
7. Dale H, Fenstad AM, Hallan G, et al. Increasing risk of prosthetic joint infection after total hip arthroplasty. Acta Orthop. 2011;83(5):449-458.
8. Parker MJ, Gurusamy KS, Azegami S. Arthroplasties (with and without bone cement) for proximal femoral fractures in adults. Cochrane Database Syst Rev. 2010(6):CD001706.
9. Taylor F, Wright M, Zhu M. Hemiarthroplasty of the hip with and without cement: a randomized clinical trial. J Bone Joint Surg Am. 2012;94(7):577-583.
10. Kim YH, Kim JS, Park JW, Joo JH. Contemporary total hip arthroplasty with and without cement in patients with osteonecrosis of the femoral head: a concise follow-up, at an average of seventeen years, of a previous report. J Bone Joint Surg Am. 2011;93(19):1806-1810.
11. Weiss RJ, Stark A, Karrholm J. A modular cementless stem vs. cemented long-stem prostheses in revision surgery of the hip: a population-based study from the Swedish Hip Arthroplasty Register. Acta Orthop. 2011;82(2):136-142.
12. Nakama GY, Peccin MS, Almeida GJ, Lira Neto Ode A, Queiroz AA, Navarro RD. Cemented, cementless or hybrid fixation options in total knee arthroplasty for osteoarthritis and other non-traumatic diseases. Cochrane Database Syst Rev. 2012;10:CD006193.
13. Park JW, Kim YH. Simultaneous cemented and cementless total knee replacement in the same patients: a prospective comparison of long-term outcomes using an identical design of NexGen prosthesis. J Bone Joint Surg Br. 2011;93(11):1479-1486.
14. Khaw FM, Kirk LM, Morris RW, Gregg PJ. A randomised, controlled trial of cemented versus cementless press-fit condylar total knee replacement. Ten-year survival analysis. J Bone Joint Surg Br. 2002;84(5):658-666.
15. Baker PN, Khaw FM, Kirk LM, Esler CN, Gregg PJ. A randomised controlled trial of cemented versus cementless press-fit condylar total knee replacement: 15-year survival analysis. J Bone Joint Surg Br. 2007;89(12):1608-1614.
16. Beaupre LA, al-Yamani M, Huckell JR, Johnston DW. Hydroxyapatite-coated tibial implants compared with cemented tibial fixation in primary total knee arthroplasty. A randomized trial of outcomes at five years. J Bone Joint Surg Am. 2007;89(10):2204-2211.
17. Nilsson KG, Karrholm J, Carlsson L, Dalen T. Hydroxyapatite coating versus cemented fixation of the tibial component in total knee arthroplasty: prospective randomized comparison of hydroxyapatite-coated and cemented tibial components with 5-year follow-up using radiostereometry. J Arthroplasty. 1999;14(1):9-20.
18. Chiu FY, Chen CM, Lin CF, Lo WH. Cefuroxime-impregnated cement in primary total knee arthroplasty: a prospective, randomized study of three hundred and forty knees. J Bone Joint Surg Am. 2002;84-A(5):759-762.
19. Chiu FY, Lin CF, Chen CM, Lo WH, Chaung TY. Cefuroxime-impregnated cement at primary total knee arthroplasty in diabetes mellitus. A prospective, randomised study. J Bone Joint Surg Br. 2001;83(5):691-695.
20. Espehaug B, Engesaeter LB, Vollset SE, Havelin LI, Langeland N. Antibiotic prophylaxis in total hip arthroplasty. Review of 10,905 primary cemented total hip replacements reported to the Norwegian arthroplasty register, 1987 to 1995. J Bone Joint Surg Br. 1997;79(4):590-595.
21. Parvizi J, Saleh KJ, Ragland PS, Pour AE, Mont MA. Efficacy of antibiotic-impregnated cement in total hip arthroplasty. Acta Orthop. 2008;79(3):335-341.
22. Chiu FY, Lin CF. Antibiotic-impregnated cement in revision total knee arthroplasty. A prospective cohort study of one hundred and eighty-three knees. J Bone Joint Surg Am. 2009;91(3):628-633.
23. Dall GF, Simpson PM, Breusch SJ. In vitro comparison of Refobacin-Palacos R with Refobacin Bone Cement and Palacos R + G. Acta Orthop. 2007;78(3):404-411.
24. Greene N, Holtom PD, Warren CA, et al. In vitro elution of tobramycin and vancomycin polymethylmethacrylate beads and spacers from Simplex and Palacos. Am J Orthop (Belle Meac NJ). 1998;27(3):201-205.
25. Meyer J, Piller G, Spiegel CA, Hetzel S, Squire M. Vacuum-mixing significantly changes

antibiotic elution characteristics of commercially available antibiotic-impregnated bone cements. J Bone Joint Surg Am. 2011;93(22):2049-2056.

26. Neut D, Kluin OS, Thompson J, van der Mei HC, Busscher HJ. Gentamicin release from commercially-available gentamicin-loaded PMMA bone cements in a prosthesis-related interfacial gap model and their antibacterial efficacy. BMC Musculoskelet Disord. 2011;11:258.

27. Squire MW, Ludwig BJ, Thompson JR, Jagodzinski J, Hall D, Andes D. Premixed antibiotic bone cement: an in vitro comparison of antimicrobial efficacy. J Arthroplasty. 2008;23(6 Suppl 1):110-114.

28. Stevens CM, Tetsworth KD, Calhoun JH, Mader JT. An articulated antibiotic spacer used for infected total knee arthroplasty: a comparative in vitro elution study of Simplex and Palacos bone cements. J Orthop Res. 2005;23(1):27-33.

29. Cummins JS, Tomek IM, Kantor SR, Furnes O, Engesaeter LB, Finlayson SR. Cost-effectiveness of antibiotic-impregnated bone cement used in primary total hip arthroplasty. J Bone Joint Surg Am. 2009;91(3):634-641.

30. Parvizi J, Pawasarat IM, Azzam KA, Joshi A, Hansen EN, Bozic KJ. Periprosthetic joint infection: the economic impact of methicillin-resistant infections. J Arthroplasty. 2010;25(6 Suppl):103-107.

31. McLaren AC, Nugent M, Economopoulos K, Kaul H, Vernon BL, McLemore R. Hand-mixed and premixed antibiotic-loaded bone cement have similar homogeneity. Clin Orthop Relat Res. 2009;467(7):1693-1698.

32. Miller R, McLaren A, Leon C, McLemore R. Mixing method affects elution and strength of high-dose ALBC: a pilot study. Clin Orthop Relat Res. 2012;470(10):2677-2683.

33. Song EK, Seon JK, Jeong MS. Delayed-type hypersensitivity reaction to piperacillin/tazobactam in a patient with an infected total knee replacement. J Bone Joint Surg Br. 2010;92(11):1596-1599.

34. Fink B, Vogt S, Reinsch M, Buchner H. Sufficient release of antibiotic by a spacer 6 weeks after implantation in two-stage revision of infected hip prostheses. Clin Orthop Relat Res. 2011;469(11):3141-3147.

35. Anguita-Alonso P, Rouse MS, Piper KE, Jacofsky DJ, Osmon DR, Patel R. Comparative study of antimicrobial release kinetics from polymethylmethacrylate. Clin Orthop Relat Res. 2006;445:239-244.

36. Han CD, Oh T, Cho SN, Yang JH, Park KK. Isoniazid could be used for antibiotic-loaded bone cement for musculoskeletal tuberculosis: an in vitro study. Clin Orthop Relat Res. 2013;471(7):2400-2406.

37. Adams K, Couch L, Cierny G, Calhoun J, Mader JT. In vitro and in vivo evaluation of antibiotic diffusion from antibiotic-impregnated polymethylmethacrylate beads. Clin Orthop Relat Res. 1992;(278):244-252.

38. Australian Orthopedic Association National Joint Replacement Registry. https://aoanjrr.dmac.adelaide.edu.au/en/annual-reports-2012. Accessed July 14, 2013.

39. Milosev I, Kovac S, Trebse R, Levasic V, Pisot V. Comparison of ten-year survivorship of hip prostheses with use of conventional polyethylene, metal-on-metal, or ceramic-on-ceramic bearings. J Bone Joint Surg Am. 2012;94(19):1756-1763.

40. Nikolaou VS, Edwards MR, Bogoch E, Schemitsch EH, Waddell JP. A prospective randomised controlled trial comparing three alternative bearing surfaces in primary total hip replacement. J Bone Joint Surg Br. 2012;94(4):459-465.

41. Bozic KJ, Ong K, Lau E, et al. Risk of complication and revision total hip arthroplasty among Medicare patients with different bearing surfaces. Clin Orthop Relat Res. 2010;468(9):2357-2362.

42. Bozic KJ, Lau EC, Ong KL, Vail TP, Rubash HE, Berry DJ. Comparative effectiveness of metal-on-metal and metal-on-polyethylene bearings in Medicare total hip arthroplasty patients. J Arthroplasty. 2012;27(8 Suppl):37-40.

43. Pilge H, Gradl G, von Eisenhart-Rothe R, Gollwitzer H. Incidence and outcome after infection of megaprostheses. Hip Int. 2012;22 Suppl 8:S83-90.

44. Hardes J, Gebert C, Schwappach A, et al. Characteristics and outcome of infections associated with tumor endoprostheses. Arch Orthop Trauma Surg. 2006;126(5):289-296.

45. Moojen DJ, Hentenaar B, Charles Vogely H, Verbout AJ, Castelein RM, Dhert WJ. In vitro release of antibiotics from commercial PMMA beads and articulating hip spacers. J Arthroplasty. 2008;23(8):1152-1156.

46. Spierlings PT. Properties of bone cement: testing and performance of bone cements. In: Breusch S, Malchau H, eds. The Well-Cemented Total Hip Arthroplasty: Theory and Practice. Heidelberg: Springer Medlizin Verlag Heidelberg; 2005:67-78.

47. Del Gaizo DJ, Kancherla V, Sporer SM, Paprosky WG. Tantalum augments for Paprosky IIIA defects remain stable at midterm followup. Clin Orthop Relat Res. 2012;470(2):395-401.

48. Howard JL, Kudera J, Lewallen DG, Hanssen AD. Early results of the use of tantalum femoral cones for revision total knee arthroplasty. J Bone Joint Surg Am. 2011;93(5):478-484.

49. Lachiewicz PF, Bolognesi MP, Henderson RA, Soileau ES, Vail TP. Can tantalum cones provide fixation in complex revision knee arthroplasty? Clin Orthop Relat Res. 2012;470(1):199-204.

50. Sweet FA, Roh M, Sliva C. Intrawound application of vancomycin for prophylaxis in instrumented thoracolumbar fusions: efficacy, drug levels, and patient outcomes. Spine (Phila Pa 1976). 2011;36(24):2084-2088.
51. Villanueva-Martinez M, De la Torre-Escudero B, Rojo-Manaute JM, Rios-Luna A, Chana-Rodriguez F. Tantalum cones in revision total knee arthroplasty. A promising short-term result with 29 cones in 21 patients. J Arthroplasty. 2013;28(6):988-993.
52. Molinari RW, Khera OA, Molinari WJ, 3rd. Prophylactic intraoperative powdered vancomycin and postoperative deep spinal wound infection: 1,512 consecutive surgical cases over a 6-year period. Eur Spine J. 2012;21 Suppl 4:S476-482.
53. O'Neill KR, Smith JG, Abtahi AM, et al. Reduced surgical site infections in patients undergoing posterior spinal stabilization of traumatic injuries using vancomycin powder. Spine J. 2011;11(7):641-646.
54. Antoci V, Jr., Adams CS, Hickok NJ, Shapiro IM, Parvizi J. Vancomycin bound to Ti rods reduces periprosthetic infection: preliminary study. Clin Orthop Relat Res. 2007;461:88-95.
55. Parvizi J, Wickstrom E, Zeiger AR, et al. Frank Stinchfield Award. Titanium surface with biologic activity against infection. Clin Orthop Relat Res. 2004(429):33-38.
56. Stewart S, Barr S, Engiles J, et al. Vancomycin-modified implant surface inhibits biofilm formation and supports bone-healing in an infected osteotomy model in sheep: a proof-of-concept study. J Bone Joint Surg Am. 2012;94(15):1406-1415.
57. Adams CS, Antoci V, Jr., Harrison G, et al. Controlled release of vancomycin from thin sol-gel films on implant surfaces successfully controls osteomyelitis. J Orthop Res. 2009;27(6):701-709.
58. Fiedler P, Kolitsch A, Kleffner B, Henke D, Stenger S, Brenner RE. Copper and silver ion implantation of aluminium oxide-blasted titanium surfaces: proliferative response of osteoblasts and antibacterial effects. Int J Artif Organs. 2011;34(9):882-888.
59. Kose N, Otuzbir A, Peksen C, Kiremitci A, Dogan A. A Silver Ion-doped Calcium Phosphate-based Ceramic Nanopowder-coated Prosthesis Increased Infection Resistance. Clin Orthop Relat Res. 2013;471(8):2532-2539.
60. Chai H, Guo L, Wang X, et al. Antibacterial effect of 317L stainless steel contained copper in prevention of implant-related infection in vitro and in vivo. J Mater Sci Mater Med. 2011;22(11):2525-2535.
61. Heidenau F, Mittelmeier W, Detsch R, et al. A novel antibacterial titania coating: metal ion toxicity and in vitro surface colonization. J Mater Sci Mater Med. 2005;16(10):883-888.
62. Haenle M, Fritsche A, Zietz C, et al. An extended spectrum bactericidal titanium dioxide (TiO2) coating for metallic implants: in vitro effectiveness against MRSA and mechanical properties. J Mater Sci Mater Med. 2011;22(2):381-387.
63. Schaer TP, Stewart S, Hsu BB, Klibanov AM. Hydrophobic polycationic coatings that inhibit biofilms and support bone healing during infection. Biomaterials. 2012;33(5):1245-1254.
64. Ellenrieder M, Haenle M, Lenz R, Bader R, Mittelmeier W. Titanium-copper-nitride coated spacers for two-stage revision of infected total hip endoprotheses. GMS Krankenhhyg Interdiszip. 2011;6(1):Doc16.
65. Hansen EN, Zmistowski B, Parvizi J. Periprosthetic joint infection: what is on the horizon? Int J Artif Organs. 2012;35(10):935-950.
66. Ehrlich GD, Stoodley P, Kathju S, et al. Engineering approaches for the detection and control of orthopaedic biofilm infections. Clin Orthop Relat Res. 2005(437):59-66.
67. Uhari M, Hietala J, Tuokko H. Risk of acute otitis media in relation to the viral etiology of infections in children. Clin Infect Dis. 1995;20(3):521-524.
68. Radin S, Ducheyne P. Controlled release of vancomycin from thin sol-gel films on titanium alloy fracture plate material. Biomaterials. 2007;28(9):1721-1729.
69. Wong SY, Moskowitz JS, Veselinovic J, et al. Dual functional polyelectrolyte multilayer coatings for implants: permanent microbicidal base with controlled release of therapeutic agents. J Am Chem Soc. 2012;132(50):17840-17848.
70. Reddy ST, Chung KK, McDaniel CJ, Darouiche RO, Landman J, Brennan AB. Micropatterned surfaces for reducing the risk of catheter-associated urinary tract infection: an in vitro study on the effect of sharklet micropatterned surfaces to inhibit bacterial colonization and migration of uropathogenic Escherichia coli. J Endourol. 2012;25(9):1547-1552.

Question 1

- **Does the type of prosthesis influence the incidence of surgical site infection (SSI) or periprosthetic joint infection (PJI)?**

Consensus: The type of prosthesis (cemented versus uncemented) or coating with hydroxyapatite does not influence the incidence of SSI or PJI.

Delegate Vote

Agree: 92%, Disagree: 4%, Abstain: 4% (Strong Consensus)

Question 2A

- **Does antibiotic-impregnated cement reduce the incidence of PJI following elective primary total joint arthroplasty (TJA)?**

Consensus: Yes. Antibiotic-impregnated polymethylmethacrylate cement (ABX-PMMA) reduces the incidence of PJI following TJA and should be used in patients at high risk for PJI following elective arthroplasty.

Delegate Vote

Agree: 90%, Disagree: 9%, Abstain: 1% (Strong Consensus)

Question 2B

- **Does antibiotic-impregnated cement reduce the incidence of PJI following elective revision joint arthroplasty?**

Consensus: Yes. Antibiotic should be added to cement in all patients undergoing cemented or hybrid fixation as part of revision arthroplasty.

Delegate Vote

Agree: 88%, Disagree: 9%, Abstain: 3% (Strong Consensus)

Question 3

- **Does the type of bearing surface in THA influence the incidence of SSI/PJI?**

Consensus: Observational data suggest that metal-on-metal bearing may be associated with a higher risk of PJI.

Delegate Vote

Agree: 78%, Disagree: 15%, Abstain: 7% (Strong Consensus)

Question 4

- **Does the size of prosthesis (volume of foreign material) influence the incidence of SSI following TJA?**

<u>Consensus:</u> Yes. The incidence of infection is higher following the use of mega-prostheses.

Delegate Vote

Agree: 85%, Disagree: 11%, Abstain: 4% (Strong Consensus)

Question 5

- **Is there a difference between various types of cement with regard to the incidence of SSI/PJI after TJA?**

<u>Consensus:</u> There is no clear difference in the incidence of SSI/PJI following joint arthroplasty when different PMMA cement formulations are used.

Delegate Vote

Agree: 92%, Disagree: 3%, Abstain: 5% (Strong Consensus)

Question 6

- **Is there a difference between various types of cement with regard to antibiotic elution?**

<u>Consensus:</u> There is a clear difference in the elution profile of antibiotics from PMMA cement that is determined by the type of cement, type, and dose of antibiotic.

Delegate Vote

Agree: 96%, Disagree: 0%, Abstain: 4% (Strong Consensus)

Question 7

- **Is there a difference in the incidence of SSI/PJI with the use of different uncemented prostheses?**

<u>Consensus:</u> The incidence of SSI/PJI may be lower with the use of porous metal (tantalum) implants during revision arthroplasty compared to titanium.

Delegate Vote

Agree: 44%, Disagree: 33%, Abstain: 23% (No Consensus)

Question 8

- **Is there a role for the use of antibiotic powder (such as vancomycin) in the wound during TJA?**

<u>Consensus:</u> No. There is no literature to suggest that the use of vancomycin powder poured into the wound or placed in the vicinity of an implant reduces the incidence of PJI. A few studies have shown that the use of vancomycin powder reduces the incidence of SSI following non-arthroplasty procedures. Future studies are needed.

Delegate Vote

Agree: 91%, Disagree: 5%, Abstain: 4% (Strong Consensus)

Question 9

- **Is there a difference in the incidence of SSI/PJI with the use of metal augments compared to allograft to reconstruct bone deficiency in the setting of infection?**

<u>Consensus:</u> There is no difference in the incidence of SSI/PJI following the use of metal augments or allograft bone for reconstruction of bone defects.

Delegate Vote

Agree: 80%, Disagree: 7%, Abstain: 13% (Strong Consensus)

Question 10

- **Is there a role for modification of the prosthesis surface that may minimize PJI?**

<u>Consensus:</u> There is a real need for surface modifications of implants that can help reduce bacterial colonization and subsequent SSI/PJI.

Delegate Vote

Agree : 76%, Disagree : 15%, Abstain : 9% (Strong Consensus)

Question 11

- **Are there any novel developments for the prevention of SSI/PJI?**

<u>Consensus:</u> The orthopaedic community needs to explore the potential for surface modifications of the prosthesis in an effort to reduce the incidence of SSI/PJI.

Delegate Vote
Agree: 84%, Disagree: 10%, Abstain: 6% (Strong Consensus)

7 人工関節周囲感染の診断

Workgroup 7: Diagnosis of Periprosthetic Joint Infection

Question 1A

- 人工関節周囲感染（PJI）の診断基準は？

コンセンサス

PJIの診断基準は以下のとおりである．
* 人工関節周囲組織において，同一菌種が2カ所陽性，あるいは
* 関節に交通する瘻孔が存在すること，あるいは
* 以下の小基準のうち3つを満たすこと
―血清C反応性タンパク（CRP）および赤血球沈降速度（ESR）が高値であること
―関節液白血球（WBC）値あるいは白血球エステラーゼ試験紙の＋＋陽性反応
―関節液中多形核好中球の割合（PMN％）が高値であること
―人工関節周囲組織の病理組織所見が陽性であること
―1カ所からの細菌培養陽性

投票結果

同意：85％，反対：13％，棄権：2％（強いコンセンサス）

Question 1B

- PJIの診断基準における留意事項は？

コンセンサス

臨床的には，上記診断基準を満たさないPJIが存在し得る．具体的には毒性の低い菌種（*Propionibacterium acnes* など）によるPJIである．関節液白血球エステラーゼ試験は尿検査紙を使用し，外来や術中診断などの迅速診断に用いられる．検体に血液混入がある場合には，遠心分離により白血球エステラーゼの比色定量試験の精度を維持すると報告されている．

（参考文献 1-37）

投票結果
同意：76%，反対：14%，棄権：10%（強いコンセンサス）

Question 2

- PJI の診断に関して，米国整形外科学会（AAOS）のアルゴリズムに賛同するか？

コンセンサス

　下記は PJI の診断に関する AAOS のアルゴリズムを改変したものである．人工関節術後に疼痛やその他の問題が生じた場合には，このアルゴリズムに従い診断することが推奨される．

(参考文献　38-50)

投票結果
同意：91%，反対：0%，棄権：9%（強いコンセンサス）

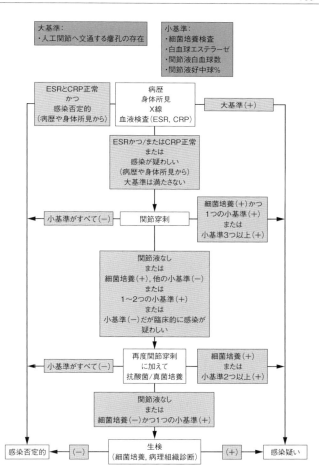

Question 3A

- 急性発症の PJI 診断における赤血球沈降速度（ESR），血清 C 反応性タンパク（CRP），多形核好中球の割合（PMN%），白血球（WBC）数のカットオフ値は？

コンセンサス

術後 6 週以内の急性期 PJI における各検査のおおよそのカッ

トオフ値は以下のとおりである.
　—ESR は急性期 PJI の診断に有用ではないため，カットオフ値は定められない.
　—CRP＞10 mg/dL（人工膝および股関節）
　—関節液 WBC 数＞10,000 cells/μL
　—関節液 PMN％＞90％

投票結果
同意：81％，反対：12％，棄権：7％（強いコンセンサス）

Question 3B

- 遅発性 PJI の診断における ESR，CRP，PMN％，WBC 数のカットオフ値は？

コンセンサス

術後 6 週以降の遅発性 PJI における各検査のおおよそのカットオフ値は以下の通りである.
　—ESR＞30 mm/hr
　—CRP＞1 mg/dL
　—関節液 WBC 数＞3,000 cells/μL
　—関節液 PMN％＞80％

投票結果
同意：81％，反対：14％，棄権：5％（強いコンセンサス）

Question 3C

- 炎症性関節症における PJI に関する ESR，CRP，PMN％，WBC 数のカットオフ値は？

コンセンサス

エビデンスが非常に限られているが，炎症性関節症の患者の PJI 診断には，上記の ESR，CRP，PMN％，WBC 数のカットオフ値は通常の PJI（急性および遅発性）と同様である．しかし，本ステートメントを裏付けるためにはさらなる研究が必要である．（参考文献　3，7-12，51-53，56）

投票結果
同意：87％，反対：9％，棄権：4％（強いコンセンサス）

Question 4

- 関節液細胞数を分析するにあたり，変動を最小限に抑えるために重要な点は？

コンセンサス

関節液細胞数を正確に分析するため，以下の点を推奨する．(1) 血液混入の影響を調整するため，関節液中の赤血球（RBC）数，血清赤血球数，血清白血球濃度を用いて関節液 WBC 数を変換する (2) metal-on-metal 人工関節では，手動での白血球分析を行う．(参考文献 3-5, 55-59)

投票結果

同意：92%，反対：1%，棄権：7%（強いコンセンサス）

Question 5

- 通常の培養はどのくらいの期間行うべきか？

コンセンサス

通常の培養期間は 5～14 日間を推奨する．低毒性の微生物による PJI が疑われる症例や，術前培養が陰性だが臨床像が PJI（培養偽陰性 PJI）と一致する場合には，14 日間以上の培養を推奨する．(参考文献 60-65)

投票結果

同意：92%，反対：1%，棄権：7%（強いコンセンサス）

Question 6A

- PJI が疑われる症例において，通常の抗酸菌（AFB）や真菌検査は必要か？

コンセンサス

PJI が確定もしくは疑われる場合において，AFB と真菌培養は，AFB や真菌感染リスクのある患者や，他の一般細菌が同定されず臨床上の疑いが残る場合に限定されるべきである．

投票結果

同意：92%，反対：6%，棄権：1%（強いコンセンサス）

Question 6B

- 無菌性ゆるみが疑われる場合,通常の AFB や真菌検査は必要か?

コンセンサス

必要ではない.AFB や真菌培養は,無菌性ゆるみが疑われる場合(術前の関節液 WBC 数や分画で PJI が疑われない症例など)は必要でない.(参考文献 66-69)

投票結果

同意:91%,反対:7%,棄権:2%(強いコンセンサス)

Question 7A

- PJI または無菌性ゆるみが疑われる症例において,細菌培養のために必要な組織検体数は?

コンセンサス

ほとんどの再置換術において,好気性菌および嫌気性菌培養として,3~6 個の術中組織検体を採取すべきである.

投票結果

同意:88%,反対:10%,棄権:2%(強いコンセンサス)

Question 7B

- 培養検体はどのように採取すべきか?

コンセンサス

感染巣,可能であればインプラント境界部分からの組織や液体を採取すべきであり,各検体は未使用の器具によって採取されるべきである.創や関節周囲の組織からのスワブ培養は推奨されない.

投票結果

同意:97%,反対:2%,棄権:1%(強いコンセンサス)

Question 7C

- すべての症例において,培養のための検体採取に先立って,抗菌薬の使用は控えるべきか?

コンセンサス

控えるべきではない.周術期の抗菌薬の予防投与を控えるのは,原因菌が同定されていなく PJI が強く疑われる症例のみで

ある．(参考文献 24, 25, 63, 70-78)

投票結果

同意：87％，反対：12％，棄権：1％（強いコンセンサス）

Question 8

- PJI 診断において通常検査として超音波処理を行う必要があるか？ あるなら，どの患者群に適用されるべきか？

コンセンサス

行う必要はない．抜去インプラントに対する通常検査としての超音波処理は推奨しない．その適応は，術前の関節液検査で培養陰性であり，2週間以内に抗菌薬を投与されていたPJI確定または疑い症例(他の検査に基づく)に限定されるべきである．(参考文献 74, 79-83)

投票結果

同意：84％，反対：9％，棄権：7％（強いコンセンサス）

Question 9

- PJI 診断に，ポリメラーゼ連鎖反応（PCR）などの分子生物学的手法が果たす役割はあるか？ もしあれば，どのような患者に対して行うべきか？

コンセンサス

PCR 法は，現時点でPJI の診断を目的とした通常検査としては推奨されていない．臨床的に感染の疑いが強いが，培養あるいは他の診断法が陰性の症例においては，PCR 法などの分子生物学的診断技術（超音波処理有りまたは無し）は，培養で同定されていない細菌の同定や抗菌薬感受性を判定するのに有用である可能性がある．(参考文献 72, 79, 81, 84-94)

投票結果

同意：96％，反対：3％，棄権：1％（強いコンセンサス）

Question 10

- PJI 診断に，画像診断法が果たす役割はあるか？

コンセンサス

単純 X 線写真はPJI が疑われる全ての症例に行われるべきである．磁気共鳴画像法(MRI)，コンピューター断層撮影(CT)，

核医学画像診断は，現時点ではPJIの診断に直接的な役割を持たないが，関節痛やインプラントゆるみの原因の特定に役だつ可能性がある．（参考文献 94-108）

投票結果

同意：93％，反対：7％，棄権：0％（強いコンセンサス）

【掲載されている論文】

Diagnosis of periprosthetic joint infection.

Zmistowski B, Della Valle C, Bauer TW, Malizos KN, Alavi A, Bedair H, Booth RE, Choong P, Deirmengian C, Ehrlich GD, Gambir A, Huang R, Kissin Y, Kobayashi H, Kobayashi N, Krenn V, Lorenzo D, Marston SB, Meermans G, Perez J, Ploegmakers JJ, Rosenberg A, Simpendorfer C, Thomas P, Tohtz S, Villafuerte JA, Wahl P, Wagenaar FC, Witzo E.

J Arthroplasty. 2014 Feb；29（2 Suppl）：77-83. doi：10.1016/j.arth.2013.09.040. Epub 2013 Dec 15. No abstract available.

PMID：24342275

References:

1. Parvizi J, Zmistowski B, Berbari EF, et al. New definition for periprosthetic joint infection: from the Workgroup of the Musculoskeletal Infection Society. Clin Orthop Relat Res. 2011;469(11):2992-2994.
2. Berbari E, Mabry T, Tsaras G, et al. Inflammatory blood laboratory levels as markers of prosthetic joint infection: a systematic review and meta-analysis. J Bone Joint Surg Am. 2010;92(11):2102-2109.
3. Cipriano CA, Brown NM, Michael AM, Moric M, Sporer SM, Della Valle CJ. Serum and synovial fluid analysis for diagnosing chronic periprosthetic infection in patients with inflammatory arthritis. J Bone Joint Surg Am. 2012;94(7):594-600.
4. Ghanem E, Antoci V, Jr., Pulido L, Joshi A, Hozack W, Parvizi J. The use of receiver operating characteristics analysis in determining erythrocyte sedimentation rate and C-reactive protein levels in diagnosing periprosthetic infection prior to revision total hip arthroplasty. Int J Infect Dis. 2009;13(6):e444-449.
5. Greidanus NV, Masri BA, Garbuz DS, et al. Use of erythrocyte sedimentation rate and C-reactive protein level to diagnose infection before revision total knee arthroplasty. A prospective evaluation. J Bone Joint Surg Am. 2007;89(7):1409-1416.
6. Olshaker JS, Jerrard DA. The erythrocyte sedimentation rate. J Emerg Med. 1997;15(6):869-874.
7. Schinsky MF, Della Valle CJ, Sporer SM, Paprosky WG. Perioperative testing for joint infection in patients undergoing revision total hip arthroplasty. J Bone Joint Surg Am. 2008;90(9):1869-1875.
8. Bedair H, Ting N, Jacovides C, et al. The Mark Coventry Award: diagnosis of early postoperative TKA infection using synovial fluid analysis. Clin Orthop Relat Res. 2011;469(1):34-40.
9. Dinneen A, Guyot A, Clements J, Bradley N. Synovial fluid white cell and differential count in the diagnosis or exclusion of prosthetic joint infection. Bone Joint J. 2013;95-B(4):554-557.
10. Mason JB, Fehring TK, Odum SM, Griffin WL, Nussman DS. The value of white blood cell counts before revision total knee arthroplasty. J Arthroplasty. 2003;18(8):1038-1043.
11. Trampuz A, Hanssen AD, Osmon DR, Mandrekar J, Steckelberg JM, Patel R. Synovial fluid leukocyte count and differential for the diagnosis of prosthetic knee infection. Am J Med. 2004;117(8):556-562.

12. Zmistowski B, Restrepo C, Huang R, Hozack WJ, Parvizi J. Periprosthetic joint infection diagnosis: a complete understanding of white blood cell count and differential. J Arthroplasty. 2012;27(9):1589-1593.
13. Tsaras G, Maduka-Ezeh A, Inwards CY, et al. Utility of intraoperative frozen section histopathology in the diagnosis of periprosthetic joint infection: a systematic review and meta-analysis. J Bone Joint Surg Am. 19 2012;94(18):1700-1711.
14. Fehring TK, McAlister JA, Jr. Frozen histologic section as a guide to sepsis in revision joint arthroplasty. Clin Orthop Relat Res. 1994(304):229-237.
15. Ko PS, Ip D, Chow KP, Cheung F, Lee OB, Lam JJ. The role of intraoperative frozen section in decision making in revision hip and knee arthroplasties in a local community hospital. J Arthroplasty. 2005;20(2):189-195.
16. Lonner JH, Desai P, Dicesare PE, Steiner G, Zuckerman JD. The reliability of analysis of intraoperative frozen sections for identifying active infection during revision hip or knee arthroplasty. J Bone Joint Surg Am. 1996;78(10):1553-1558.
17. Morawietz L, Tiddens O, Mueller M, et al. Twenty-three neutrophil granulocytes in 10 high-power fields is the best histopathological threshold to differentiate between aseptic and septic endoprosthesis loosening. Histopathology. 2009;54(7):847-853.
18. Nunez LV, Buttaro MA, Morandi A, Pusso R, Piccaluga F. Frozen sections of samples taken intraoperatively for diagnosis of infection in revision hip surgery. Acta Orthop. 2007;78(2):226-230.
19. Stroh DA, Johnson AJ, Naziri Q, Mont MA. How do frozen and permanent histopathologic diagnoses compare for staged revision after periprosthetic hip infections? J Arthroplasty. 2012;27(9):1663-1668 e1661.
20. Krenn V, Morawietz L, Kienapfel H, et al. [Revised consensus classification. Histopathological classification of diseases associated with joint endoprostheses]. Z Rheumatol. 2013;72(4):383-392.
21. Parvizi J, Jacovides C, Antoci V, Ghanem E. Diagnosis of periprosthetic joint infection: the utility of a simple yet unappreciated enzyme. J Bone Joint Surg Am. 2012;93(24):2242-2248.
22. Wetters NG, Berend KR, Lombardi AV, Morris MJ, Tucker TL, Della Valle CJ. Leukocyte esterase reagent strips for the rapid diagnosis of periprosthetic joint infection. J Arthroplasty. 2012;27(8 Suppl):8-11.
23. Aggarwal VK, Tischler E, Ghanem E, Parvizi J. Leukocyte esterase from synovial fluid aspirate: a technical note. J Arthroplasty. 2013;28(1):193-195.
24. Atkins BL, Athanasou N, Deeks JJ, et al. Prospective evaluation of criteria for microbiological diagnosis of prosthetic-joint infection at revision arthroplasty. The OSIRIS Collaborative Study Group. J Clin Microbiol. 1998;36(10):2932-2939.
25. Mikkelsen DB, Pedersen C, Hojbjerg T, Schonheyder HC. Culture of multiple peroperative biopsies and diagnosis of infected knee arthroplasties. APMIS. 2006;114(6):449-452.
26. Muller M, Morawietz L, Hasart O, Strube P, Perka C, Tohtz S. Diagnosis of periprosthetic infection following total hip arthroplasty--evaluation of the diagnostic values of pre- and intraoperative parameters and the associated strategy to preoperatively select patients with a high probability of joint infection. J Orthop Surg Res. 2008;3:31.
27. Ghanem E, Ketonis C, Restrepo C, Joshi A, Barrack R, Parvizi J. Periprosthetic infection: where do we stand with regard to Gram stain? Acta Orthop. 2009;80(1):37-40.
28. Johnson AJ, Zywiel MG, Stroh DA, Marker DR, Mont MA. Should gram stains have a role in diagnosing hip arthroplasty infections? Clin Orthop Relat Res. 2010;468(9):2387-2391.
29. Morgan PM, Sharkey P, Ghanem E, et al. The value of intraoperative Gram stain in revision total knee arthroplasty. J Bone Joint Surg Am. 2009;91(9):2124-2129.
30. Oethinger M, Warner DK, Schindler SA, Kobayashi H, Bauer TW. Diagnosing periprosthetic infection: false-positive intraoperative Gram stains. Clin Orthop Relat Res. 2011;469(4):954-960.
31. Spangehl MJ, Masterson E, Masri BA, O'Connell JX, Duncan CP. The role of intraoperative gram stain in the diagnosis of infection during revision total hip arthroplasty. J Arthroplasty. 1999;14(8):952-956.
32. Zywiel MG, Stroh DA, Johnson AJ, Marker DR, Mont MA. Gram stains have limited application in the diagnosis of infected total knee arthroplasty. Int J Infect Dis. 2011;15(10):e702-705.
33. Deirmengian GK, Zmistowski B, Jacovides C, O'Neil J, Parvizi J. Leukocytosis is common after total hip and knee arthroplasty. Clin Orthop Relat Res. 2011;469(11):3031-3036.
34. Toossi N, Adeli B, Rasouli MR, Huang R, Parvizi J. Serum white blood cell count and differential do not have a role in the diagnosis of periprosthetic joint infection. J Arthroplasty. 2012;27(8 Suppl):51-54 e51.
35. Engh CA, Jr., Ho H, Engh CA. Metal-on-metal hip arthroplasty: does early clinical outcome justify the chance of an adverse local tissue reaction? Clin Orthop Relat Res. 2009;468(2):406-412.
36. Mikhael MM, Hanssen AD, Sierra RJ. Failure of metal-on-metal total hip arthroplasty

mimicking hip infection. A report of two cases. J Bone Joint Surg Am. 2009;91(2):443-446.
37. Molvik H, Hanna SA, de Roeck NJ. Failed metal-on-metal total hip arthroplasty presenting as painful groin mass with associated weight loss and night sweats. Am J Orthop (Belle Mead NJ). 2010;39(5):E46-49.
38. Diaz-Ledezma C, Lichstein PM, Dolan JH, Parvizi J. What is the best strategy to diagnose hip/ knee periprosthetic joint infections in Medicare patients seen in the ambulatory setting? . CORR.Publication Pending.
39. Della Valle C, Parvizi J, Bauer TW, et al. Diagnosis of periprosthetic joint infections of the hip and knee. J Am Acad Orthop Surg. 2010;18(12):760-770.
40. Fink B, Gebhard A, Fuerst M, Berger I, Schafer P. High diagnostic value of synovial biopsy in periprosthetic joint infection of the hip. Clin Orthop Relat Res. 2013;471(3):956-964.
41. Fink B, Makowiak C, Fuerst M, Berger I, Schafer P, Frommelt L. The value of synovial biopsy, joint aspiration and C-reactive protein in the diagnosis of late peri-prosthetic infection of total knee replacements. J Bone Joint Surg Br. 2008;90(7):874-878.
42. Fuerst M, Fink B, Ruther W. [The value of preoperative knee aspiration and arthroscopic biopsy in revision total knee arthroplasty]. Z Orthop Ihre Grenzgeb. 2005;143(1):36-41.
43. Malhotra R, Morgan DA. Role of core biopsy in diagnosing infection before revision hip arthroplasty. J Arthroplasty. 2004;19(1):78-87.
44. Meermans G, Haddad FS. Is there a role for tissue biopsy in the diagnosis of periprosthetic infection? Clin Orthop Relat Res. 2010;468(5):1410-1417.
45. Sadiq S, Wootton JR, Morris CA, Northmore-Ball MD. Application of core biopsy in revision arthroplasty for deep infection. J Arthroplasty. 2005;20(2):196-201.
46. Williams JL, Norman P, Stockley I. The value of hip aspiration versus tissue biopsy in diagnosing infection before exchange hip arthroplasty surgery. J Arthroplasty. 2004;19(5):582-586.
47. Berbari EF, Hanssen AD, Duffy MC, et al. Risk factors for prosthetic joint infection: case-control study. Clin Infect Dis. 1998;27(5):1247-1254.
48. Bozic KJ, Lau E, Kurtz S, Ong K, Berry DJ. Patient-related risk factors for postoperative mortality and periprosthetic joint infection in medicare patients undergoing TKA. Clin Orthop Relat Res. 2012;470(1):130-137.
49. Bozic KJ, Lau E, Kurtz S, et al. Patient-related risk factors for periprosthetic joint infection and postoperative mortality following total hip arthroplasty in Medicare patients. J Bone Joint Surg Am. 2012;94(9):794-800.
50. Pulido L, Ghanem E, Joshi A, Purtill JJ, Parvizi J. Periprosthetic joint infection: the incidence, timing, and predisposing factors. Clin Orthop Relat Res. 2008;466(7):1710-1715.
51. Della Valle CJ, Sporer SM, Jacobs JJ, Berger RA, Rosenberg AG, Paprosky WG. Preoperative testing for sepsis before revision total knee arthroplasty. J Arthroplasty. 2007;22(6 Suppl 2):90-93.
52. Ghanem E, Parvizi J, Burnett RS, et al. Cell count and differential of aspirated fluid in the diagnosis of infection at the site of total knee arthroplasty. J Bone Joint Surg Am. 2008;90(8):1637-1643.
53. Parvizi J, Ghanem E, Sharkey P, Aggarwal A, Burnett RS, Barrack RL. Diagnosis of infected total knee: findings of a multicenter database. Clin Orthop Relat Res. 2008;466(11):2628-2633.
54. Parvizi J, Jacovides C, Zmistowski B, Jung KA. Definition of periprosthetic joint infection: is there a consensus? Clin Orthop Relat Res. 2011;469(11):3022-3030.
55. Schumacher HR, Jr., Sieck MS, Rothfuss S, et al. Reproducibility of synovial fluid analyses. A study among four laboratories. Arthritis Rheum. 1986;29(6):770-774.
56. Wyles CC, Larson DR, Houdek MT, Sierra RJ, Trousdale RT. Utility of synovial fluid aspirations in failed metal-on-metal total hip arthroplasty. J Arthroplasty. 2013;28(5):818-823.
57. Diagnosis of periprosthetic joint infection after unicompartmental knee arthroplasty. J Arthroplasty. 2012;27(8 Suppl):46-50.
58. Bottner F, Wegner A, Winkelmann W, Becker K, Erren M, Gotze C. Interleukin-6, procalcitonin and TNF-alpha: markers of peri-prosthetic infection following total joint replacement. J Bone Joint Surg Br. 2007;89(1):94-99.
59. Ghanem E, Houssock C, Pulido L, Han S, Jaberi FM, Parvizi J. Determining "true" leukocytosis in bloody joint aspiration. J Arthroplasty. 2008;23(2):182-187.
60. Butler-Wu SM, Burns EM, Pottinger PS, et al. Optimization of periprosthetic culture for diagnosis of Propionibacterium acnes prosthetic joint infection. J Clin Microbiol. 2011;49(7):2490-2495.
61. Larsen LH, Lange J, Xu Y, Schonheyder HC. Optimizing culture methods for diagnosis of prosthetic joint infections: a summary of modifications and improvements reported since 1995. J Med Microbiol. 2012;61(Pt 3):309-316.
62. Neut D, van Horn JR, van Kooten TG, van der Mei HC, Busscher HJ. Detection of biomaterial-associated infections in orthopaedic joint implants. Clin Orthop Relat Res. 2003(413):261-268.
63. Schafer P, Fink B, Sandow D, Margull A, Berger I, Frommelt L. Prolonged bacterial culture to identify late periprosthetic joint infection: a promising strategy. Clin Infect Dis.

2008;47(11):1403-1409.
64. Barrack RL, Aggarwal A, Burnett RS, et al. The fate of the unexpected positive intraoperative cultures after revision total knee arthroplasty. J Arthroplasty. 2007;22(6 Suppl 2):94-99.
65. Marculescu CE, Berbari EF, Hanssen AD, Steckelberg JM, Osmon DR. Prosthetic joint infection diagnosed postoperatively by intraoperative culture. Clin Orthop Relat Res. 2005;439:38-42.
66. Azzam K, Parvizi J, Jungkind D, et al. Microbiological, clinical, and surgical features of fungal prosthetic joint infections: a multi-institutional experience. J Bone Joint Surg Am. 2009;91 Suppl 6:142-149.
67. Hwang BH, Yoon JY, Nam CH, et al. Fungal peri-prosthetic joint infection after primary total knee replacement. J Bone Joint Surg Br. 2012;94(5):656-659.
68. Marculescu CE, Berbari EF, Cockerill FR, 3rd, Osmon DR. Fungi, mycobacteria, zoonotic and other organisms in prosthetic joint infection. Clin Orthop Relat Res. 2006;451:64-72.
69. Tokarski AT, O'Neil J, Deirmengian CA, Ferguson J, Deirmengian GK. The Routine use of atypical cultures in presumed aseptic revisions Is unnecessary. Clin Orthop Relat Res. 2013.
70. Kamme C, Lindberg L. Aerobic and anaerobic bacteria in deep infections after total hip arthroplasty: differential diagnosis between infectious and non-infectious loosening. Clin Orthop Relat Res. 1981(154):201-207.
71. Zappe B, Graf S, Ochsner PE, Zimmerli W, Sendi P. Propionibacterium spp. in prosthetic joint infections: a diagnostic challenge. Arch Orthop Trauma Surg. 2008;128(10):1039-1046.
72. Jacovides CL, Kreft R, Adeli B, Hozack B, Ehrlich GD, Parvizi J. Successful identification of pathogens by polymerase chain reaction (PCR)-based electron spray ionization time-of-flight mass spectrometry (ESI-TOF-MS) in culture-negative periprosthetic joint infection. J Bone Joint Surg Am. 19 2012;94(24):2247-2254.
73. Trampuz A, Piper KE, Hanssen AD, et al. Sonication of explanted prosthetic components in bags for diagnosis of prosthetic joint infection is associated with risk of contamination. J Clin Microbiol. 2006;44(2):628-631.
74. Trampuz A, Piper KE, Jacobson MJ, et al. Sonication of removed hip and knee prostheses for diagnosis of infection. N Engl J Med. 2007;357(7):654-663.
75. Aggarwal VK, Higuera C, Deirmengian G, Parvizi J, Austin MS. Swab Cultures Are Not As Effective As Tissue Cultures for Diagnosis of Periprosthetic Joint Infection. Clin Orthop Relat Res. Apr 9 2013. Epub before print.
76. Font-Vizcarra L, Garcia S, Martinez-Pastor JC, Sierra JM, Soriano A. Blood culture flasks for culturing synovial fluid in prosthetic joint infections. Clin Orthop Relat Res. 2010;468(8):2238-2243.
77. Burnett RS, Aggarwal A, Givens SA, McClure JT, Morgan PM, Barrack RL. Prophylactic antibiotics do not affect cultures in the treatment of an infected TKA: a prospective trial. Clin Orthop Relat Res. 2010;468(1):127-134.
78. Tetreault MW, Wetters NG, Aggarwal V, Mont M, Parvizi J, Della Valle CJ. The Chitranjan Ranawat Award: Should Prophylactic Antibiotics Be Withheld Before Revision Surgery to Obtain Appropriate Cultures? Clin Orthop Relat Res. Apr 30 2013. Epub before print.
79. Achermann Y, Vogt M, Leunig M, Wust J, Trampuz A. Improved diagnosis of periprosthetic joint infection by multiplex PCR of sonication fluid from removed implants. J Clin Microbiol. 2010;48(4):1208-1214.
80. Bjerkan G, Witso E, Bergh K. Sonication is superior to scraping for retrieval of bacteria in biofilm on titanium and steel surfaces in vitro. Acta Orthop. 2009;80(2):245-250.
81. Kobayashi H, Oethinger M, Tuohy MJ, Hall GS, Bauer TW. Improving clinical significance of PCR: use of propidium monoazide to distinguish viable from dead Staphylococcus aureus and Staphylococcus epidermidis. J Orthop Res. 2009;27(9):1243-1247.
82. Monsen T, Lovgren E, Widerstrom M, Wallinder L. In vitro effect of ultrasound on bacteria and suggested protocol for sonication and diagnosis of prosthetic infections. J Clin Microbiol. 2009;47(8):2496-2501.
83. Piper KE, Jacobson MJ, Cofield RH, et al. Microbiologic diagnosis of prosthetic shoulder infection by use of implant sonication. J Clin Microbiol. 2009;47(6):1878-1884.
84. Clarke MT, Roberts CP, Lee PT, Gray J, Keene GS, Rushton N. Polymerase chain reaction can detect bacterial DNA in aseptically loose total hip arthroplasties. Clin Orthop Relat Res. 2004(427):132-137.
85. Esteban J, Alonso-Rodriguez N, del-Prado G, et al. PCR-hybridization after sonication improves diagnosis of implant-related infection. Acta Orthop. 2012;83(3):299-304.
86. Gallo J, Kolar M, Dendis M, et al. Culture and PCR analysis of joint fluid in the diagnosis of prosthetic joint infection. New Microbiol. 2008;31(1):97-104.
87. Gomez E, Cazanave C, Cunningham SA, et al. Prosthetic joint infection diagnosis using broad-range PCR of biofilms dislodged from knee and hip arthroplasty surfaces using sonication. J Clin Microbiol. 2012;50(11):3501-3508.
88. Mariani BD, Martin DS, Levine MJ, Booth RE, Jr., Tuan RS. The Coventry Award.

Polymerase chain reaction detection of bacterial infection in total knee arthroplasty. Clin Orthop Relat Res. 1996(331):11-22.
89. Panousis K, Grigoris P, Butcher I, Rana B, Reilly JH, Hamblen DL. Poor predictive value of broad-range PCR for the detection of arthroplasty infection in 92 cases. Acta Orthop. 2005;76(3):341-346.
90. Rak M, Barlic-Maganja D, Kavcic M, Trebse R, Cor A. Comparison of molecular and culture method in diagnosis of prosthetic joint infection. FEMS Microbiol Lett. 2013;343(1):42-48.
91. Rasouli MR, Harandi AA, Adeli B, Purtill JJ, Parvizi J. Revision total knee arthroplasty: infection should be ruled out in all cases. J Arthroplasty. 2012;27(6):1239-1243 e1231-1232.
92. Tunney MM, Patrick S, Curran MD, et al. Detection of prosthetic hip infection at revision arthroplasty by immunofluorescence microscopy and PCR amplification of the bacterial 16S rRNA gene. J Clin Microbiol. 1999;37(10):3281-3290.
93. Portillo ME, Salvado M, Sorli L, et al. Multiplex PCR of sonication fluid accurately differentiates between prosthetic joint infection and aseptic failure. J Infect. 2012;65(6):541-548.
94. Kobayashi N, Inaba Y, Choe H, et al. Simultaneous intraoperative detection of methicillin-resistant Staphylococcus and pan-bacterial infection during revision surgery: use of simple DNA release by ultrasonication and real-time polymerase chain reaction. J Bone Joint Surg Am. 2009;91(12):2896-2902.
95. Tigges S, Stiles RG, Roberson JR. Appearance of septic hip prostheses on plain radiographs. AJR Am J Roentgenol. 1994;163(2):377-380.
96. Love C, Tomas MB, Marwin SE, Pugliese PV, Palestro CJ. Role of nuclear medicine in diagnosis of the infected joint replacement. Radiographics. 2001;21(5):1229-1238.
97. Cyteval C, Hamm V, Sarrabere MP, Lopez FM, Maury P, Taourel P. Painful infection at the site of hip prosthesis: CT imaging. Radiology. 2002;224(2):477-483.
98. Chryssikos T, Parvizi J, Ghanem E, Newberg A, Zhuang H, Alavi A. FDG-PET imaging can diagnose periprosthetic infection of the hip. Clin Orthop Relat Res. 2008;466(6):1338-1342.
99. Delank KS, Schmidt M, Michael JW, Dietlein M, Schicha H, Eysel P. The implications of 18F-FDG PET for the diagnosis of endoprosthetic loosening and infection in hip and knee arthroplasty: results from a prospective, blinded study. BMC Musculoskelet Disord. 2006;7:20.
100. Glithero PR, Grigoris P, Harding LK, Hesslewood SR, McMinn DJ. White cell scans and infected joint replacements. Failure to detect chronic infection. J Bone Joint Surg Br. 1993;75(3):371-374.
101. Graute V, Feist M, Lehner S, et al. Detection of low-grade prosthetic joint infections using 99mTc-antigranulocyte SPECT/CT: initial clinical results. Eur J Nucl Med Mol Imaging. 2010;37(9):1751-1759.
102. Love C, Marwin SE, Tomas MB, et al. Diagnosing infection in the failed joint replacement: a comparison of coincidence detection 18F-FDG and 111In-labeled leukocyte/99mTc-sulfur colloid marrow imaging. J Nucl Med. 2004;45(11):1864-1871.
103. Magnuson JE, Brown ML, Hauser MF, Berquist TH, Fitzgerald RH, Jr., Klee GG. In-111-labeled leukocyte scintigraphy in suspected orthopedic prosthesis infection: comparison with other imaging modalities. Radiology. 1988;168(1):235-239.
104. Nagoya S, Kaya M, Sasaki M, Tateda K, Yamashita T. Diagnosis of peri-prosthetic infection at the hip using triple-phase bone scintigraphy. J Bone Joint Surg Br. 2008;90(2):140-144.
105. Savarino L, Baldini N, Tarabusi C, Pellacani A, Giunti A. Diagnosis of infection after total hip replacement. J Biomed Mater Res B Appl Biomater. 2004;70(1):139-145.
106. Scher DM, Pak K, Lonner JH, Finkel JE, Zuckerman JD, Di Cesare PE. The predictive value of indium-111 leukocyte scans in the diagnosis of infected total hip, knee, or resection arthroplasties. J Arthroplasty. 2000;15(3):295-300.
107. Segura AB, Munoz A, Brulles YR, et al. What is the role of bone scintigraphy in the diagnosis of infected joint prostheses? Nucl Med Commun. 2004;25(5):527-532.
108. Sousa R, Massada M, Pereira A, Fontes F, Amorim I, Oliveira A. Diagnostic accuracy of combined 99mTc-sulesomab and 99mTc-nanocolloid bone marrow imaging in detecting prosthetic joint infection. Nucl Med Commun. 2011;32(9):834-839.

Question 1A

- **What is the definition of periprosthetic joint infection (PJI)?**

Consensus: PJI is defined as :

* Two positive periprosthetic cultures with phenotypically identical organisms, or * A sinus tract communicating with the joint, or * Having three of the following minor criteria :

—Elevated serum C-reactive protein (CRP) AND erythrocyte sedimentation rate (ESR)

—Elevated synovial fluid white blood cell (WBC) count OR + + change on leukocyte esterase test strip

—Elevated synovial fluid polymorphonuclear neutrophil percentage (PMN%) —Positive histological analysis of periprosthetic tissue—A single positive culture

Delegate Vote

Agree: 85%, Disagree: 13%, Abstain: 2% (Strong Consensus)

Question 1B

- **What are some considerations for the definition of periprosthetic joint infection (PJI)?**

Consensus: Clinically, PJI may be present without meeting these criteria, specifically in the case of less virulent organisms (eg P. acnes). Synovial leukocyte esterase can be performed as a rapid office or intraoperative point of care test using urinalysis strips. In the case of a bloody aspiration, centrifugation has been shown to preserve the accuracy of the colorimetric test for leukocyte esterase

Delegate Vote

Agree: 76%, Disagree: 14%, Abstain: 10% (Strong Consensus)

Question 2

- **Do you agree with the American Academy of Orthopaedic Surgeons's (AAOS) algorithm for diagnosis of PJI?**

Consensus: The following is an adaptation of the AAOS's algorithm for the diagnosis of PJI. This algorithm should be applied to patients who present with a painful or failed arthroplasty.

Delegate Vote

Agree: 91%, Disagree: 0%, Abstain: 9% (Strong Consensus)

Question 3A

- **What should the threshold be for ESR, serum CRP, PMN%, and WBC count for ACUTE PJI?**

Consensus: The approximate cutoffs listed below apply to tests obtained less than 6 weeks from most recent surgery：

—No threshold for ESR could be determined as it is not useful in diagnosis of acute PJI.

—CRP＞100 mg/L (knee and hip), —Synovial WBC count＞10,000 cells/μL, and —Synovial PMN% ＞90%.

Delegate Vote

Agree: 81%, Disagree: 12%, Abstain: 7% (Strong Consensus)

Question 3B

- **What should the threshold be for ESR, serum CRP, PMN%, and WBC count for CHRONIC PJI?**

Consensus: The approximate cutoffs listed below apply to tests obtained more than 6 weeks from the most recent surgery：

—ESR＞30 mm/hr, —CRP＞10 mg/L, —Synovial WBC count＞3,000 cells per μL, and —Synovial PMN% ＞80%.

Delegate Vote

Agree: 81%, Disagree: 14%, Abstain: 5% (Strong Consensus)

Question 3C

- **What should the threshold be for ESR, serum CRP, PMN%, and WBC count for PJI in inflammatory arthropathies?**

Consensus: Based upon very limited evidence, we recommend no change from the above thresholds for ESR, serum CRP, PMN%, and WBC count for PJI diagnosis in patients who have underlying inflammatory arthropathies. However, further research is needed to confirm this statement.

Delegate Vote

Agree: 87%, Disagree: 9%, Abstain: 4% (Strong Consensus)

Question 4

- **In analyzing synovial fluid cell count, what are important techniques to minimize variation?**

<u>Consensus:</u> To accurately analyze synovial fluid cell count we recommend that (1) synovial fluid WBC count results be transformed using the synovial red blood cell (RBC), serum RBC, and serum WBC concentrations to adjust for traumatic aspirations and (2) in joints with metal-on-metal components a manual WBC analysis should be performed.

Delegate Vote

Agree: 92%, Disagree: 1%, Abstain: 7%. (Strong Consensus)

Question 5

- **How long should routine cultures be kept?**

<u>Consensus:</u> We recommend that routine cultures should be maintained between 5 and 14 days. In cases of suspected PJI with low virulence organisms or if preoperative cultures have failed to show bacterial growth and the clinical picture is consistent with PJI (suspected culture-negative PJI) the cultures should be maintained for 14 days or longer.

Delegate Vote

Agree: 92%, Disagree: 1%, Abstain: 7%. (Strong Consensus)

Question 6A

- **Is there a role for routine acid-fast bacillus (AFB) and fungal testing in suspected PJI?**

<u>Consensus:</u> In proven or suspected PJI, AFB and fungal cultures should be limited to those patients at risk for such infections or when other traditional pathogens have not been identified and clinical suspicion persists.

Delegate Vote

Agree: 92%, Disagree: 6%, Abstain: 1% (Strong Consensus)

Question 6B

- **Is there a role for routine acid-fast bacillus (AFB) and fungal**

testing in suspected aseptic failure?

Consensus: No. AFB and fungal cultures do not play a role in presumed aseptic cases (eg cases where a synovial fluid WBC count and differential performed preoperatively were not suggestive of infection).

Delegate Vote

Agree: 91%, Disagree: 7%, Abstain: 2% (Strong Consensus)

Question 7A

- **How many intraoperative tissue samples should be sent for culture in suspected PJI cases and cases of suspected aseptic failure?**

Consensus: In most revision procedures, more than three but not more than six distinct intraoperative tissue samples should be sent for aerobic and anaerobic culture.

Delegate Vote

Agree: 88%, Disagree: 10%, Abstain: 2% (Strong Consensus)

Question 7B

- **How should culture samples be obtained?**

Consensus: Tissue or fluid samples from representative area should be taken, preferably from the interface, each sample taken with an unused instrument. We strongly recommend against swab cultures from wound or periarticular tissues.

Delegate Vote

Agree: 97%, Disagree: 2%, Abstain: 1% (Strong Consensus)

Question 7C

- **Should antibiotic be withheld prior to obtaining samples for culture in all cases?**

Consensus: No. Perioperative prophylactic antibiotics should be withheld only in cases with a high suspicion for PJI in which an infecting organism has not been isolated.

Delegate Vote

Agree: 87%, Disagree: 12%, Abstain: 1% (Strong Consensus)

Question 8

- **Is there a role for routine sonication of the prosthesis? If so, in which group of patients should this be done?**

<u>Consensus:</u> NO. We do not recommend routine sonication of explants. Its use should be limited to cases of suspected or proven PJI (based upon presentation and other testing) in which preoperative aspiration does not yield positive culture and antibiotics have been administered within the previous 2 weeks.

Delegate Vote

Agree: 84%, Disagree: 9%, Abstain: 7% (Strong Consensus)

Question 9

- **Is there a role for molecular techniques such as polymerase chain reaction (PCR) for diagnosis of PJI? If so, in which group of patients should this be done?**

<u>Consensus:</u> Nucleic acid based testing is not currently a recommended routine diagnostic test for PJI. In cases with high clinical suspicion of infection but negative cultures or other diagnostic tests, molecular techniques with or without sonication may help identify the unknown pathogens or antibiotic sensitivity for targeting antimicrobial therapies.

Delegate Vote

Agree: 96%, Disagree: 3%, Abstain: 1% (Strong Consensus)

Question 10

- **Is there a role for imaging modalities in the diagnosis of PJI?**

<u>Consensus:</u> Plain radiographs should be performed in all cases of suspected PJI. Magnetic resonance imaging (MRI), computed tomography (CT), and nuclear imaging currently DO NOT have a direct role in the diagnosis of PJI but may be helpful in the identification of other causes of joint pain/failure.

Delegate Vote

Agree: 93%, Disagree: 7%, Abstain: 0% (Strong Consensus)

8

術後創管理

Workgroup 8 : Wound Management

Question 1A

- 人工関節全置換術（TJA）後の創に対する最適なドレッシング材は何か？

コンセンサス

入手できれば，アルギン酸塩（ソーブサン®など）やハイドロファイバー（アクアセル®など）を含有した閉鎖性ドレッシング材の使用を推奨する．(参考文献 1-8)

投票結果

同意：63％，反対：25％，棄権：12％（弱いコンセンサス）

Question 1B

- 銀含浸ドレッシング材の使用は手術部位感染（SSI）や人工関節周囲感染（PJI）を減少させるか？

コンセンサス

銀含浸ドレッシング材の使用がSSIやPJIを減少させるという確証的な結果は示されていない．(参考文献 9-16)

投票結果

同意：87％，反対：5％，棄権：7％（強いコンセンサス）

Question 2

- TJA後どのような状態を創から浸出が持続していると考えるべきか？

コンセンサス

TJA後の創からの浸出の持続は，手術切開部位から72時間以上浸出が続くことと定義される．(参考文献 17-25)

投票結果

同意：80％，反対：15％，棄権：5％（強いコンセンサス）

Question 3A

- TJA 後の浸出が続く創に対処するための非外科的治療法は？

コンセンサス

TJA 後の 72 時間以上持続する創浸出は創処置によって対処されるべきである．(参考文献 17, 18, 20, 21, 24, 26-29)

投票結果

同意：65％，反対：26％，棄権：9％（弱いコンセンサス）

Question 3B

- TJA 後の浸出が続く創に対処するための外科的治療法は？

コンセンサス

もし創浸出が初回手術後 5〜7 日間持続するようであれば，筋膜の開放や，モジュラーコンポーネントの交換を伴う徹底的な洗浄デブリドマン（I & D）といった外科的治療が考慮されるべきである．(参考文献 17, 20, 22, 26, 30-32)

投票結果

同意：77％，反対：16％，棄権：7％（強いコンセンサス）

Question 3C

- 創から浸出が持続している患者に経口あるいは静脈内抗菌薬投与を行うべきか？

コンセンサス

われわれは，創から浸出が持続している患者に対して，経口あるいは静脈内抗菌薬投与を行うことについて反対である．

投票結果

同意：80％，反対：17％，棄権：3％（強いコンセンサス）

Question 4

- TJA 後に浸出が持続する創に対する再手術の適応は？

コンセンサス

診断時から 5〜7 日以上浸出が持続する創に対しては遅滞なく再手術を行うべきである．(参考文献 17, 21, 24, 26, 27, 33)

投票結果

同意：77％，反対：19％，棄権：4％（強いコンセンサス）

Question 5

- SSI 軽減のためどのようにして再手術前に患者状態を改善できるか？

コンセンサス

再手術前の患者状態は改善する必要がある．低栄養，抗凝固状態，貧血および糖尿病の是正は適切に行われるべきである．
(参考文献 17, 24, 33-44)

投票結果

同意：95%，反対：3%，棄権：2%（強いコンセンサス）

Question 6

- TJA 後に浸出が持続する創に対して I&D を行う際，術中培養は採取されるべきか？

コンセンサス

採取するべきである．浸出が持続する創に対して I&D の手術を行う際，術中培養（最低3つ）は採取するべきである．
(参考文献 17, 26, 45)

投票結果

同意：98%，反対：1%，棄権：1%（強いコンセンサス）

Question 7

- TJA の I&D の際に，皮膚切開前の周術期抗菌薬投与は控えるべきか？

コンセンサス

控えるべきでない．I&D の再手術前1時間以内に投与される周術期抗菌薬は皮膚切開前の使用を控えてはならない（皮膚切開前に使用すべきである）．(参考文献 46, 47)

投票結果

同意：82%，反対：14%，棄権：4%（強いコンセンサス）

Question 8

- TJA後，SSIとPJIのリスクを軽減するための最適な創閉鎖法は？

コンセンサス

特定の創閉鎖法が他の方法（ステープル，縫合，接着，あるいはテープ）より優れていることを支持するエビデンスはない．しかし，初回人工関節置換術の術後早期に，創トラブルに対し再手術を行う患者の創閉鎖は，モノフィラメント縫合糸の使用を推奨する．(参考文献 48-52)

投票結果

同意：75％，反対：15％，棄権：10％（強いコンセンサス）

【掲載されている論文】

Wound management.

Ghanem E, Heppert V, Spangehl M, Abraham J, Azzam K, Barnes L, Burgo FJ, Ebeid W, Goyal N, Guerra E, Hitt K, Kallel S, Klein G, Kosashvili Y, Levine B, Matsen L, Morris MJ, Purtill JJ, Ranawat C, Sharkey PF, Sierra R, Stefansdottir A.

J Arthroplasty. 2014 Feb；29（2 Suppl）：84-92. doi：10.1016/j.arth.2013.09.041. Epub 2013 Dec 15. No abstract available.

PMID：24342276

References:

1. Clarke JV, Deakin AH, Dillon JM, Emmerson S, Kinninmonth AW. A prospective clinical audit of a new dressing design for lower limb arthroplasty wounds. J Wound Care. 2009;18(1):5-8, 10-11.
2. Burke NG, Green C, McHugh G, McGolderick N, Kilcoyne C, Kenny P. A prospective randomised study comparing the jubilee dressing method to a standard adhesive dressing for total hip and knee replacements. J Tissue Viability. 2012;21(3):84-87.
3. Hopper GP, Deakin AH, Crane EO, Clarke JV. Enhancing patient recovery following lower limb arthroplasty with a modern wound dressing: a prospective, comparative audit. J Wound Care. 2012;21(4):200-203.
4. Abuzakuk TM, Coward P, Shenava Y, Kumar VS, Skinner JA. The management of wounds following primary lower limb arthroplasty: a prospective, randomised study comparing hydrofibre and central pad dressings. Int Wound J. 2006;3(2):133-137.
5. Ravenscroft MJ, Harker J, Buch KA. A prospective, randomised, controlled trial comparing wound dressings used in hip and knee surgery: Aquacel and Tegaderm versus Cutiplast. Ann R Coll Surg Engl. 2006;88(1):18-22.
6. Ubbink DT, Vermeulen H, Goossens A, Kelner RB, Schreuder SM, Lubbers MJ. Occlusive vs gauze dressings for local wound care in surgical patients: a randomized clinical trial. Arch Surg. 2008;143(10):950-955.
7. Foster L, Moore P, Clark S. A comparison of hydrofibre and alginate dressings on open acute surgical wounds. J Wound Care. 2000;9(9):442-445.
8. Ravnskog FA, Espehaug B, Indrekvam K. Randomised clinical trial comparing Hydrofiber and alginate dressings post-hip replacement. J Wound Care. 2011;20(3):136-142.
9. Trial C, Darbas H, Lavigne JP, et al. Assessment of the antimicrobial effectiveness of a new silver alginate wound dressing: a RCT. J Wound Care. 2010;19(1):20-26.
10. Jude EB, Apelqvist J, Spraul M, Martini J. Prospective randomized controlled study of Hydrofiber dressing containing ionic silver or calcium alginate dressings in non-ischaemic

diabetic foot ulcers. Diabet Med. 2007;24(3):280-288.
11. Jurczak F, Dugre T, Johnstone A, Offori T, Vujovic Z, Hollander D. Randomised clinical trial of Hydrofiber dressing with silver versus povidone-iodine gauze in the management of open surgical and traumatic wounds. Int Wound J. 2007;4(1):66-76.
12. Beele H, Meuleneire F, Nahuys M, Percival SL. A prospective randomised open label study to evaluate the potential of a new silver alginate/carboxymethylcellulose antimicrobial wound dressing to promote wound healing. Int Wound J. 2010;7(4):262-270.
13. Vermeulen H, van Hattem JM, Storm-Versloot MN, Ubbink DT. Topical silver for treating infected wounds. Cochrane Database Syst Rev. 2007(1):CD005486.
14. Storm-Versloot MN, Vos CG, Ubbink DT, Vermeulen H. Topical silver for preventing wound infection. Cochrane Database Syst Rev. (3):CD006478.
15. Saba SC, Tsai R, Glat P. Clinical evaluation comparing the efficacy of aquacel ag hydrofiber dressing versus petrolatum gauze with antibiotic ointment in partial-thickness burns in a pediatric burn center. J Burn Care Res. 2009;30(3):380-385.
16. Springer BD, Odum S, Griffin WL, Beaver WB, Mason JB. The role of surgical dressing in total joint arthroplasty: Level 1 randomized clinical trial. Clin Orthop Relat Res.in Press.
17. Jaberi FM, Parvizi J, Haytmanek CT, Joshi A, Purtill J. Procrastination of wound drainage and malnutrition affect the outcome of joint arthroplasty. Clin Orthop Relat Res. 2008;466(6):1368-1371.
18. Hansen E, Durinka JB, Costanzo JA, Austin MS, Deirmengian GK. Negative Pressure Wound Therapy Is Associated With Resolution of Incisional Drainage in Most Wounds After Hip Arthroplasty. Clin Orthop Relat Res. Mar 29 2013. Epub before print.
19. Butt U, Ahmad R, Aspros D, Bannister GC. Factors affecting wound ooze in total knee replacement. Ann R Coll Surg Engl. 2011;93(1):54-56.
20. Lonner JH, Lotke PA. Aseptic complications after total knee arthroplasty. J Am Acad Orthop Surg. 1999;7(5):311-324.
21. Saleh K, Olson M, Resig S, et al. Predictors of wound infection in hip and knee joint replacement: results from a 20 year surveillance program. J Orthop Res. 2002;20(3):506-515.
22. Vince K, Chivas D, Droll KP. Wound complications after total knee arthroplasty. J Arthroplasty. 2007;22(4 Suppl 1):39-44.
23. Dennis DA. Wound complications in total knee arthroplasty. Instr Course Lect. 1997;46:165-169.
24. Patel VP, Walsh M, Sehgal B, Preston C, DeWal H, Di Cesare PE. Factors associated with prolonged wound drainage after primary total hip and knee arthroplasty. J Bone Joint Surg Am. 2007;89(1):33-38.
25. Surin VV, Sundholm K, Backman L. Infection after total hip replacement. With special reference to a discharge from the wound. J Bone Joint Surg Br. 1983;65(4):412-418.
26. Weiss AP, Krackow KA. Persistent wound drainage after primary total knee arthroplasty. J Arthroplasty. 1993;8(3):285-289.
27. Pachowsky M, Gusinde J, Klein A, et al. Negative pressure wound therapy to prevent seromas and treat surgical incisions after total hip arthroplasty. Int Orthop. 2012;36(4):719-722.
28. Masden D, Goldstein J, Endara M, Xu K, Steinberg J, Attinger C. Negative pressure wound therapy for at-risk surgical closures in patients with multiple comorbidities: a prospective randomized controlled study. Ann Surg. 2012;255(6):1043-1047.
29. Webster J, Scuffham P, Sherriff KL, Stankiewicz M, Chaboyer WP. Negative pressure wound therapy for skin grafts and surgical wounds healing by primary intention. Cochrane Database Syst Rev.4:CD009261.
30. Kelm J, Schmitt E, Anagnostakos K. Vacuum-assisted closure in the treatment of early hip joint infections. Int J Med Sci. 2009;6(5):241-246.
31. Wilson MG, Kelley K, Thornhill TS. Infection as a complication of total knee-replacement arthroplasty. Risk factors and treatment in sixty-seven cases. J Bone Joint Surg Am. 1990;72(6):878-883.
32. Gardner J, Gioe TJ, Tatman P. Can this prosthesis be saved?: implant salvage attempts in infected primary TKA. Clin Orthop Relat Res. 2011;469(4):970-976.
33. Galat DD, McGovern SC, Larson DR, Harrington JR, Hanssen AD, Clarke HD. Surgical treatment of early wound complications following primary total knee arthroplasty. J Bone Joint Surg Am. 2009;91(1):48-54.
34. Gherini S, Vaughn BK, Lombardi AV, Jr., Mallory TH. Delayed wound healing and nutritional deficiencies after total hip arthroplasty. Clin Orthop Relat Res. 1993(293):188-195.
35. Lavernia CJ, Sierra RJ, Baerga L. Nutritional parameters and short term outcome in arthroplasty. J Am Coll Nutr. 1999;18(3):274-278.
36. Pedersen AB, Mehnert F, Johnsen SP, Sorensen HT. Risk of revision of a total hip replacement in patients with diabetes mellitus: a population-based follow up study. J Bone Joint Surg Br. 2010;92(7):929-934.
37. Jamsen E, Nevalainen P, Eskelinen A, Huotari K, Kalliovalkama J, Moilanen T. Obesity, diabetes, and preoperative hyperglycemia as predictors of periprosthetic joint infection: a single-center analysis of 7181 primary hip and knee replacements for osteoarthritis. J Bone Joint Surg Am. 2012;94(14):e101.

38. Golden SH, Peart-Vigilance C, Kao WH, Brancati FL. Perioperative glycemic control and the risk of infectious complications in a cohort of adults with diabetes. Diabetes Care. 1999;22(9):1408-1414.
39. Iorio R, Williams KM, Marcantonio AJ, Specht LM, Tilzey JF, Healy WL. Diabetes mellitus, hemoglobin A1C, and the incidence of total joint arthroplasty infection. J Arthroplasty. 2012;27(5):726-729 e721.
40. Adams AL, Paxton EW, Wang JQ, et al. Surgical outcomes of total knee replacement according to diabetes status and glycemic control, 2001 to 2009. J Bone Joint Surg Am. 2013;95(6):481-487.
41. Parvizi J, Ghanem E, Joshi A, Sharkey PF, Hozack WJ, Rothman RH. Does "excessive" anticoagulation predispose to periprosthetic infection? J Arthroplasty. 2007;22(6 Suppl 2):24-28.
42. Mortazavi SM, Hansen P, Zmistowski B, Kane PW, Restrepo C, Parvizi J. Hematoma following primary total hip arthroplasty: a grave complication. J Arthroplasty. 2013;28(3):498-503.
43. Kotze A, Carter LA, Scally AJ. Effect of a patient blood management programme on preoperative anaemia, transfusion rate, and outcome after primary hip or knee arthroplasty: a quality improvement cycle. Br J Anaesth. 2012;108(6):943-952.
44. Greenky M, Gandhi K, Pulido L, Restrepo C, Parvizi J. Preoperative anemia in total joint arthroplasty: is it associated with periprosthetic joint infection? Clin Orthop Relat Res. 2012;470(10):2695-2701.
45. Atkins BL, Athanasou N, Deeks JJ, et al. Prospective evaluation of criteria for microbiological diagnosis of prosthetic-joint infection at revision arthroplasty. The OSIRIS Collaborative Study Group. J Clin Microbiol. 1998;36(10):2932-2939.
46. Burnett RS, Aggarwal A, Givens SA, McClure JT, Morgan PM, Barrack RL. Prophylactic antibiotics do not affect cultures in the treatment of an infected TKA: a prospective trial. Clin Orthop Relat Res. 2010;468(1):127-134.
47. Tetreault MW, Wetters NG, Aggarwal V, Mont M, Parvizi J, Della Valle CJ. The Chitranjan Ranawat Award: Should Prophylactic Antibiotics Be Withheld Before Revision Surgery to Obtain Appropriate Cultures? Clin Orthop Relat Res. Apr 30, 2013. Epub before print.
48. Khan RJ, Fick D, Yao F, et al. A comparison of three methods of wound closure following arthroplasty: a prospective, randomised, controlled trial. J Bone Joint Surg Br. 2006;88(2):238-242.
49. Eggers MD, Fang L, Lionberger DR. A comparison of wound closure techniques for total knee arthroplasty. J Arthroplasty. 2011;26(8):1251-1258 e1251-1254.
50. Livesey C, Wylde V, Descamps S, et al. Skin closure after total hip replacement: a randomised controlled trial of skin adhesive versus surgical staples. J Bone Joint Surg Br. 2009;91(6):725-729.
51. Smith TO, Sexton D, Mann C, Donell S. Sutures versus staples for skin closure in orthopaedic surgery: meta-analysis. BMJ. 2010;340:c1199.
52. Coulthard P, Worthington H, Esposito M, Elst M, Waes OJ. Tissue adhesives for closure of surgical incisions. Cochrane Database Syst Rev. 2004(2):CD004287.

Question 1A

- **What is the optimal dressing for a wound after total joint arthroplasty (TJA) ?**

Consensus: We recommend the use of occlusive dressings with alginated hydrofiber, when available.

Delegate Vote

Agree: 63%, Disagree: 25%, Abstain: 12% (Weak Consensus)

Question 1B

- **Does the use of silver-impregnated dressings reduce SSI/PJI?**

Consensus: Silver-impregnated dressings have not been conclusively shown to reduce SSI/PJI.

Delegate Vote

Agree: 87%, Disagree: 5%, Abstain: 7% (Strong Consensus)

Question 2

- **What is considered to be persistent drainage from a wound after TJA?**

Consensus: Persistent wound drainage after TJA is defined as continued drainage from the operative incision site for greater than 72 hours.

Delegate Vote

Agree: 80%, Disagree: 15%, Abstain: 5% (Strong Consensus)

Question 3A

- **What are non-surgical strategies to address a draining wound after TJA?**

Consensus: Persistent wound drainage for greater than 72 hours after TJA should be managed by wound care.

Delegate Vote

Agree: 65%, Disagree: 26%, Abstain: 9% (Weak Consensus)

Question 3B

- **What are surgical strategies to address a draining wound after TJA?**

Consensus: Surgical management consisting of opening the fascia, performing a thorough irrigation and debridement (I & D) with exchange of modular components should be considered if wound drainage has persisted for 5 to 7 days after the index procedure.

Delegate Vote

Agree: 77%, Disagree: 16%, Abstain: 7% (Strong Consensus)

Question 3C

- **Should oral or intravenous antibiotics be administered to patients with persistent wound drainage?**

Consensus: We recommend against administration of oral or intravenous antibiotics to patients with persistent wound drainage.

Delegate Vote

Agree: 80%, Disagree: 17%, Abstain: 3% (Strong Consensus)

Question 4

- **What are the indications for reoperation for a persistently draining wound after TJA?**

Consensus: A wound that has been persistently draining for greater than 5 to 7 days from the time of diagnosis should be reoperated on without delay.

Delegate Vote

Agree: 77%, Disagree: 19%, Abstain: 4% (Strong Consensus)

Question 5

- **How can we optimize patient status prior to reoperation to minimize SSI?**

Consensus: We recommend that patients should be optimized prior to undergoing reoperation. Correction of malnutrition, anticoagulation, anemia, and diabetes should be reasonably pursued.

Delegate Vote

Agree: 95%, Disagree: 3%, Abstain: 2% (Strong Consensus)

Question 6

- **Should intraoperative cultures be taken when performing I & D**

for a persistently draining wound after TJA?

Consensus: Yes. Intraoperative cultures (minimum of 3) should be taken when performing I & D reoperation for a persistently draining wound.

Delegate Vote

Agree: 98%, Disagree: 1%, Abstain: 1% (Strong Consensus)

Question 7

- **Should perioperative antibiotics be withheld prior to skin incision for I & D of TJA?**

Consensus: No. Perioperative antibiotics given within one hour prior to I & D reoperation should not be withheld prior to skin incision.

Delegate Vote

Agree: 82%, Disagree: 14%, Abstain: 4% (Strong Consensus)

Question 8

- **What is the optimal method for wound closure after TJA to minimize the risk of SSI and PJI?**

Consensus: Despite the lack of evidence supporting the superiority of one technique of skin closure over others (staples, suture, adhesive, or tapes), we recommend the use of monofilament suture for wound closure in patients who undergo reoperation for wound-related problems during the early postoperative period after index arthroplasty.

Delegate Vote

Agree: 75%, Disagree: 15%, Abstain: 10% (Strong Consensus)

9

スペーサー

Workgroup 9：Spacers

Question 1

- 人工膝関節周囲感染に対する治療で，インプラントを抜去してから再置換を行うまでの待機期間において，非人工関節型スペーサーと人工関節型スペーサーに機能的な差はあるか？

コンセンサス

人工膝関節全置換術（TKA）の二期的再置換術の待機期間中において，非人工関節型スペーサーよりも人工関節型スペーサーの方が機能的予後は良い．特にスペーサーの留置期間が3カ月を超えることが見込まれる患者に人工関節型スペーサーは有用である．（参考文献 1-46）

投票結果

同意：89％，反対：6％，棄権：5％（強いコンセンサス）

Question 2

- TKAの治療において非人工関節型スペーサーもしくは人工関節型スペーサーを使用することで，再置換術後少なくとも2年以降の機能的予後に差はあるか？

コンセンサス

人工関節型スペーサーを非人工関節型スペーサーと比較して，可動域の改善に有意な差はないが，委員会はなお人工関節型スペーサーが患者にとって有用であると考えている．

（参考文献 1-46）

投票結果

同意：82％，反対：12％，棄権：6％（強いコンセンサス）

Question 3

- 人工股関節周囲感染に対する治療でインプラントを抜去してから再置換を行うまでの待機期間中，非人工関節型スペーサーと人工関節型スペーサーに機能的な差はあるか？

コンセンサス

人工股関節全置換術（THA）の二期的再置換術の待機期間中では，人工関節型スペーサーの方が機能的予後が良い．特にスペーサーの留置期間が3カ月を超えることが見込まれる患者には人工関節型スペーサーは有用である．（参考文献 42, 47-71）

投票結果

同意：89％，反対：7％，棄権：4％（強いコンセンサス）

Question 4

- THA の治療において，非人工関節型スペーサーもしくは人工関節型スペーサーを使用することで，再置換術後少なくとも2年以降における機能的予後に差はあるか？

コンセンサス

人工関節型スペーサーを非人工関節型スペーサーと比較して，機能改善に有意な差はないが，委員会はなお人工関節型スペーサーが患者にとって有用であると考えている．

（参考文献 42, 47-71）

投票結果

同意：81％，反対：12％，棄権：7％（強いコンセンサス）

Question 5

- 膝および股関節の人工関節周囲感染（PJI）の治療に対し，非人工関節型スペーサーと人工関節型スペーサーでは，再置換術の手技上の難易度に差はあるか？

コンセンサス

差はある．非人工関節型スペーサーと比較して，人工関節型スペーサーを使用する方が，概して再置換術は容易である．

投票結果

同意：81％，反対：8％，棄権：11％（強いコンセンサス）

Question 6

- 膝関節の人工関節型スペーサーと非人工関節型スペーサーでは,感染制御に関して差はあるか?

コンセンサス

差はない.膝関節の二期的再置換術において,スペーサーの種類は感染の治癒率に影響しない.(参考文献 1-59, 72-85)

投票結果

同意:89%,反対:6%,棄権:5%(強いコンセンサス)

Question 7

- 股関節の人工関節型スペーサーと非人工関節型スペーサーの使用では,感染制御に関して差はあるか?

コンセンサス

差はない.股関節の二期的再置換術において,スペーサーの種類は感染治癒率に影響しない.

(参考文献 9, 42, 47-72, 74, 78, 86-120)

投票結果

同意:95%,反対:3%,棄権:2%(強いコンセンサス)

Question 8

- 膝関節に使用される人工関節型スペーサーの種類の違いにより,感染制御に関して差はあるか?

コンセンサス

人工膝関節周囲感染の治療において,人工関節型スペーサーの種類の違いによって,感染制御に差はない.

(参考文献 1, 3-6, 8-10, 12-14, 16-18, 21-25, 27, 29, 30, 32, 33, 35-38, 40-45, 51, 72-73, 77, 79-82, 85)

投票結果

同意:90%,反対:5%,棄権:5%(強いコンセンサス)

Question 9

- 非人工関節型スペーサーや人工関節型スペーサーの使用において禁忌はあるか?

コンセンサス

手技上技術的に問題がなければ,非人工関節型スペーサーと

人工関節型スペーサーの使用に関する明らかな禁忌はない．しかし，巨大な骨欠損や軟部組織の欠損や靱帯機能不全のある患者では，非人工関節型スペーサーの使用は非常に慎重に考慮すべきである．(参考文献 9, 47-72, 74, 78, 86-120)

投票結果
同意：92％，反対：3％，棄権：5％（強いコンセンサス）

Question 10

- 膝の手術において，製品として市販されているスペーサーと術者が手作りした可動性のあるスペーサーでは，機能的予後に差はあるか？

コンセンサス

膝関節の手術で，製品として市販されているスペーサーと術者が手作りした可動性のあるスペーサーでは，機能的予後に差はない．(参考文献 1-50, 72, 73, 75, 77, 79-82, 84, 85, 108)

しかし，費用の問題，使いやすさ，抗菌薬の溶出について考慮する必要がある．

投票結果
同意：89％，反対：5％，棄権：6％（強いコンセンサス）

Question 11

- 膝関節の手術で，製品として市販されているスペーサーと術者が手作りした可動性のあるスペーサーでは，感染制御率に差はあるか？

コンセンサス

膝関節の手術で，製品として市販されているスペーサーと術者が手作りした可動性のあるスペーサーでは，感染制御率に差はない．(参考文献 1-50, 72, 73, 75, 77, 79-82, 84, 85, 108)

しかし，費用の問題，使いやすさ，抗菌薬の溶出について考慮する必要がある．

投票結果
同意：93％，反対：2％，棄権：5％（強いコンセンサス）

Question 12

- 股関節の手術で,製品として市販されているスペーサーと術者が手作りした可動性のあるスペーサーでは,機能的予後に差はあるか?

コンセンサス

股関節に使用される製品として市販されているスペーサーと術者が手作りした可動性のあるスペーサーでは,機能的予後に差はない.

(参考文献 9,47-54,56-59,61-67,70-72,74,78,86-88,90-98,100-108,110-113,115,117,119,120,123)

しかし,費用の問題,使いやすさ,抗菌薬の溶出について考慮する必要がある.

投票結果

同意:89%,反対:7%,棄権:4%(強いコンセンサス)

Question 13

- 股関節の手術で,製品として市販されているスペーサーと術者が手作りした可動性のあるスペーサーでは,感染制御率に差はあるか.

コンセンサス

股関節の手術で,製品として市販されているスペーサーと術者が手作りした可動性のあるスペーサーでは,感染制御率に差はない.

(参考文献 9,47-54,56-59,61-67,70-72,74,78,86-88,90-98,100-108,110-113,115,117,119,120,123)

しかし,費用の問題,使いやすさ,抗菌薬の溶出について考慮する必要がある.

投票結果

同意:94%,反対:3%,棄権:3%(強いコンセンサス)

Question 14

- どの抗菌薬を使用し,どのくらいの量をセメントスペーサーに加えるべきか?

コンセンサス

抗菌薬の種類と量は,(入手可能であれば)細菌培養結果やア

ンチバイオグラム（1菌種の各種抗菌薬に対する感受性をまとめたもの）の結果ならびに患者の腎機能，アレルギー歴に基づいて個別化される必要がある．しかし，ほとんどの感染症は，バンコマイシン（40 g 包のセメントにつき 1～4 g）とゲンタマイシン，もしくはトブラマイシン（40 g 包のセメントにつき 2.4～4.8 g）を加えたスペーサーで治療できる．われわれは，通常の原因菌に対する入手可能な抗菌薬とその推奨量の一覧表を提供する．(参考文献 1-134)

投票結果
同意：89％，反対：7％，棄権：4％（強いコンセンサス）

スペーサーに使用可能な抗菌薬と抗真菌薬

抗菌薬の分類	薬物名	対象菌群	骨セメント40 gあたりの投与量
アミノグリコシド	トブラマイシン	緑膿菌などのグラム陰性菌	1～4.8 g
	ゲンタマイシン	グラム陰性大腸菌 大腸菌、クレブシエラ、特に緑膿菌 嫌気性菌（偏性/通性嫌気性菌でないての）	0.25～4.8 g
セファロスポリン第1世代	セファゾリン	グラム陽性菌感染症（グラム陰性のカバーは限られる）	1～2 g
セファロスポリン第2世代	セフロキシム	グラム陽性菌のカバーは減るが、グラム陰性菌のカバーは拡大する	1.5～2 g
セファロスポリン第3世代	セフタジジム	グラム陰性菌、特に緑膿菌	2 g
セファロスポリン第4世代	セフォタキシム	グラム陰性菌、緑膿菌への抗菌活性はない	2 g
セファロスポリン第5世代	セフタロロン	グラム陰性菌、緑膿菌への抗菌活性はない	2～4 g
フルオロキノロン	シプロフロキサシン	グラム陰性菌（エンテロバクターを含む）	0.2～3 g
グリコペプチド	バンコマイシン	メチシリン耐性菌を含むグラム陽性菌	0.5～4 g
リンコマイシン	クリンダマイシン	グラム陽性菌、嫌気性菌	1～2 g
マクロライド	エリスロマイシン	好気性のグラム陽性球菌および桿菌	0.5～1 g
ポリミキシン	コリスチン	グラム陰性菌	0.24 g
β-ラクタム系	ピペラシリン（ピペトノバクタム は使用不能）	グラム陰性菌（特に緑膿菌、エンテロバクター、嫌気性菌	4～8 g
	アズトレオナム	グラム陰性菌のみ	4 g
β-ラクタマーゼ阻害薬	タゾバクタム	グラム陰性菌（特に緑膿菌）、エンテロバクター、ピペラシリンとの併用により嫌気性菌に有効	0.5 g
オキサゾリジノン系	リネゾリド	MRSAのような多剤耐性グラム陽性球菌	1.2 g
カルバペネム系	メロペナム	グラム陽性菌およびグラム陰性菌 嫌気性菌 緑膿菌	0.5～4 g
リポペプチド	ダプトマイシン	グラム陽性菌のみ	2 g
抗真菌薬	アムホテリシン	真菌のほとんど	200 mg
	ボリカナゾール	真菌のほとんど	300～600 mg

投与量は分析結果に記載されたので推奨投与量ではない。（参考文献：1-134）
抗菌薬の種類と濃度は、患者ごとに検出された微生物のプロファイルとアンチバイオグラム、さらには患者の腎機能やアレルギーによって個々に決定される必要がある。

Question 15

- 高用量の抗菌薬含有セメントスペーサーを準備するのに，最適な方法は（混合の仕方，抗菌薬を加えるタイミングと方法，多孔性）？

コンセンサス

高用量の抗菌薬含有セメントスペーサーの最適な準備方法に関するコンセンサスはない．（参考文献 108, 122, 124-127, 130-134）

投票結果

同意：93％，反対：3％，棄権：4％（強いコンセンサス）

【掲載されている論文】

Spacers.

Citak M, Argenson JN, Masri B, Kendoff D, Springer B, Alt V, Baldini A, Cui Q, Deirmengian GK, Del Sel H, Harrer MF, Israelite CL, Jahoda D, Jutte PC, Levicoff E, Meani E, Motta F, Pena OR, Ranawat AS, Safir O, Squire MW, Taunton MJ, Vogely CH, Wellman SS.

J Arthroplasty. 2014 Feb；29（2 Suppl）：93-9. doi：10.1016/j.arth.2013.09.042. Epub 2013 Dec 15. No abstract available.

PMID：24342279

References:

1. Anderson JA, Sculco PK, Heitkemper S, Mayman DJ, Bostrom MP, Sculco TP. An articulating spacer to treat and mobilize patients with infected total knee arthroplasty. J Arthroplasty. 2009;24(4):631-635.
2. Booth RE Jr, Lotke PA. The results of spacer block technique in revision of infected total knee arthroplasty. Clin Orthop Relat Res. 1989;(248):57-60.
3. Brunnekreef J, Hannink G, Malefijt Mde W. Recovery of knee mobility after a non-articulating or mobile spacer in total knee infection. Acta Orthop Belg. 2013;79(1):83-89.
4. Chiang ER, Su YP, Chen TH, Chiu FY, Chen WM. Comparison of articulating and non-articulating spacers regarding infection with resistant organisms in total knee arthroplasty. Acta Orthop. 2011;82(4):460-464.
5. Choi HR, Malchau H, Bedair H. Are prosthetic spacers safe to use in 2-stage treatment for infected total knee arthroplasty? J Arthroplasty. 2012;27(8):1474-1479 e1471.
6. Cuckler JM. The infected total knee: management options. J Arthroplasty. 2005;20(4 Suppl 2):33-36.
7. Durbhakula SM, Czajka J, Fuchs MD, Uhl RL. Antibiotic-loaded articulating cement spacer in the 2-stage exchange of infected total knee arthroplasty. J Arthroplasty. 2004;19(6):768-774.
8. Emerson RH Jr, Muncie M, Tarbox TR, Higgins LL. Comparison of a non-articulating with a mobile spacer in total knee infection. Clin Orthop Relat Res. 2002;(404):132-138.
9. Evans RP. Successful treatment of total hip and knee infection with articulating antibiotic components: a modified treatment method. Clin Orthop Relat Res. 2004;(427):37-46.
10. Fehring TK, Odum S, Calton TF, Mason JB. Articulating versus non-articulating spacers in revision total knee arthroplasty for sepsis. The Ranawat Award. Clin Orthop Relat Res. 2000;(380):9-16.
11. Gacon G, Laurencon M, Van de Velde D, Giudicelli DP. Two stages reimplantation for infection after knee arthroplasty. Apropos of a series of 29 cases. Rev Chir Orthop Reparatrice Appar Mot. 1997;83(4):313-323.

12. Garg P, Ranjan R, Bandyopadhyay U, Chouksey S, Mitra S, Gupta SK. Antibiotic-impregnated articulating cement spacer for infected total knee arthroplasty. Indian J Orthop. 2011;45(6):535-540.
13. Gooding CR, Masri BA, Duncan CP, Greidanus NV, Garbuz DS. Durable infection control and function with the PROSTALAC spacer in two-stage revision for infected knee arthroplasty. Clin Orthop Relat Res. 2011;469(4):985-993.
14. Haddad FS, Masri BA, Campbell D, McGraw RW, Beauchamp CP, Duncan CP. The PROSTALAC functional spacer in two-stage revision for infected knee replacements. Prosthesis of antibiotic-loaded acrylic cement. J Bone Joint Surg Br. 2000;82(6):807-812.
15. Haleem AA, Berry DJ, Hanssen AD. Mid-term to long-term followup of two-stage reimplantation for infected total knee arthroplasty. Clin Orthop Relat Res. 2004;(428):35-39.
16. Hart WJ, Jones RS. Two-stage revision of infected total knee replacements using articulating cement spacers and short-term antibiotic therapy. J Bone Joint Surg Br. 2006;88(8):1011-1015.
17. Hofmann AA, Goldberg T, Tanner AM, Kurtin SM. Treatment of infected total knee arthroplasty using an articulating spacer: 2- to 12-year experience. Clin Orthop Relat Res. 2005;(430):125-131.
18. Hofmann AA, Kane KR, Tkach TK, Plaster RL, Camargo MP. Treatment of infected knee arthroplasty using an articulating spacer. Clin Orthop Relat Res. 1995;(321):45-54.
19. Huang HT, Su JY, Chen SK. The results of articulating spacer technique for infected total knee arthroplasty. J Arthroplasty. 2006;21(8):1163-1168.
20. Hsu CS, Hsu CC, Wang JW, Lin PC. Two-stage revision of infected total knee arthroplasty using an antibiotic-impregnated non-articulating cement-spacer. Chang Gung Med J. 2008;31(6):583-591.
21. Hsu YC, Cheng HC, Ng TP, Chiu KY. Antibiotic-loaded cement articulating spacer for 2-stage reimplantation in infected total knee arthroplasty: a simple and economic method. J Arthroplasty. 2007;22(7):1060-1066.
22. Hwang BH, Yoon JY, Nam CH, et al. Fungal peri-prosthetic joint infection after primary total knee replacement. J Bone Joint Surg Br. 2012;94(5):656-659.
23. Jamsen E, Sheng P, Halonen P, et al. Spacer prostheses in two-stage revision of infected knee replacement. Int Orthop. 2006;30(4):257-261.
24. Jia YT, Zhang Y, Ding C, et al. Antibiotic-loaded articulating cement spacers in two-stage revision for infected total knee arthroplasty: individual antibiotic treatment and early results of 21 cases. Chin J Traumatol. 2012;15(4):212-221.
25. Johnson AJ, Sayeed SA, Naziri Q, Khanuja HS, Mont MA. Minimizing articulating knee spacer complications in infected revision arthroplasty. Clin Orthop Relat Res. 2012;470(1):220-227.
26. Kotwal SY, Farid YR, Patil SS, Alden KJ, Finn HA. Intramedullary rod and cement non-articulating spacer construct in chronically infected total knee arthroplasty. J Arthroplasty. 2012;27(2):253-259 e254.
27. Lee JK, Choi CH. Two-stage reimplantation in infected total knee arthroplasty using a re-sterilized tibial polyethylene insert and femoral component. J Arthroplasty. 2012;27(9):1701-1706 e1701.
28. Logoluso N, Champlon C, Melegati G, Dell'Oro F, Romano CL. Gait analysis in patients with a preformed articulated knee spacer. Knee. 2012;19(4):370-372.
29. MacAvoy MC, Ries MD. The ball and socket articulating spacer for infected total knee arthroplasty. J Arthroplasty. 2005;20(6):757-762.
30. Macheras GA, Kateros K, Galanakos SP, Koutsostathis SD, Kontou E, Papadakis SA. The long-term results of a two-stage protocol for revision of an infected total knee replacement. J Bone Joint Surg Br. 2011;93(11):1487-1492.
31. Macmull S, Bartlett W, Miles J, et al. Custom-made hinged spacers in revision knee surgery for patients with infection, bone loss and instability. Knee. 2010;17(6):403-406.
32. Meek RM, Dunlop D, Garbuz DS, McGraw R, Greidanus NV, Masri BA. Patient satisfaction and functional status after aseptic versus septic revision knee arthroplasty using the PROSTALAC articulating spacer. J Arthroplasty. 2004;19(7):874-879.
33. Meek RM, Masri BA, Dunlop D, et al. Patient satisfaction and functional status after treatment of infection at the site of a total knee arthroplasty with use of the PROSTALAC articulating spacer. J Bone Joint Surg Am. 2003;85-A(10):1888-1892.
34. Ocguder A, Firat A, Tecimel O, Solak S, Bozkurt M. Two-stage total infected knee arthroplasty treatment with articulating cement spacer. Arch Orthop Trauma Surg. 2010;130(6):719-725.
35. Park SJ, Song EK, Seon JK, Yoon TR, Park GH. Comparison of non-articulating and mobile antibiotic-impregnated cement spacers for the treatment of infected total knee arthroplasty. Int Orthop. 2010;34(8):1181-1186.
36. Pietsch M, Hofmann S, Wenisch C. Treatment of deep infection of total knee arthroplasty using a two-stage procedure. Oper Orthop Traumatol. 2006;18(1):66-87.
37. Pitto RP, Castelli CC, Ferrari R, Munro J. Pre-formed articulating knee spacer in two-stage revision for the infected total knee arthroplasty. Int Orthop. 2005;29(5):305-308.

38. Qiu XS, Sun X, Chen DY, Xu ZH, Jiang Q. Application of an articulating spacer in two-stage revision for severe infection after total knee arthroplasty. Orthop Surg. 2010;2(4):299-304.
39. Shen H, Zhang X, Jiang Y, Wang Q, Chen Y, Shao J. Intraoperatively-made cement-on-cement antibiotic-loaded articulating spacer for infected total knee arthroplasty. Knee. 2010;17(6):407-411.
40. Siebel T, Kelm J, Porsch M, Regitz T, Neumann WH. Two-stage exchange of infected knee arthroplasty with an prosthesis-like interim cement spacer. Acta Orthop Belg. 2002;68(2):150-156.
41. Su YP, Lee OK, Chen WM, Chen TH. A facile technique to make articulating spacers for infected total knee arthroplasty. J Chin Med Assoc. 2009;72(3):138-145.
42. Thabe H, Schill S. Two-stage reimplantation with an application spacer and combined with delivery of antibiotics in the management of prosthetic joint infection. Oper Orthop Traumatol. 2007;19(1):78-100.
43. Tigani D, Trisolino G, Fosco M, Ben Ayad R, Costigliola P. Two-stage reimplantation for periprosthetic knee infection: Influence of host health status and infecting microorganism. Knee. 2013;20(1):9-18.
44. Van Thiel GS, Berend KR, Klein GR, Gordon AC, Lombardi AV, Della Valle CJ. Intraoperative molds to create an articulating spacer for the infected knee arthroplasty. Clin Orthop Relat Res. 2011;469(4):994-1001.
45. Villanueva M, Rios A, Pereiro J, Chana F, Fahandez-Saddi H. Hand-made articulating spacers for infected total knee arthroplasty: a technical note. Acta Orthop. 2006;77(2):329-332.
46. Wilde AH, Ruth JT. Two-stage reimplantation in infected total knee arthroplasty. Clin Orthop Relat Res. 1988;(236):23-35.
47. Cabrita HB, Croci AT, Camargo OP, Lima AL. Prospective study of the treatment of infected hip arthroplasties with or without the use of an antibiotic-loaded cement spacer. Clinics (Sao Paulo). 2007;62(2):99-108.
48. D'Angelo F, Negri L, Binda T, Zatti G, Cherubino P. The use of a preformed spacer in two-stage revision of infected hip arthroplasties. Musculoskelet Surg. 2011;95(2):115-120.
49. D'Angelo F, Negri L, Zatti G, Grassi FA. Two-stage revision surgery to treat an infected hip implant. A comparison between a custom-made spacer and a pre-formed one. Chir Organi Mov. 2005;90(3):271-279.
50. Diwanji SR, Kong IK, Park YH, Cho SG, Song EK, Yoon TR. Two-stage reconstruction of infected hip joints. J Arthroplasty. 2008;23(5):656-661.
51. Durbhakula SM, Czajka J, Fuchs MD, Uhl RL. Spacer endoprosthesis for the treatment of infected total hip arthroplasty. J Arthroplasty. 2004;19(6):760-767.
52. Fei J, Liu GD, Yu HJ, Zhou YG, Wang Y. Antibiotic-impregnated cement spacer versus antibiotic irrigating metal spacer for infection management after THA. Orthopedics. 2011;34(3):172.
53. Fink B, Grossmann A, Fuerst M, Schafer P, Frommelt L. Two-stage cementless revision of infected hip endoprostheses. Clin Orthop Relat Res. 2009;467(7):1848-1858.
54. Fleck EE, Spangehl MJ, Rapuri VR, Beauchamp CP. An articulating antibiotic spacer controls infection and improves pain and function in a degenerative septic hip. Clin Orthop Relat Res. 2011;469(11):3055-3064.
55. Haddad FS, Muirhead-Allwood SK, Manktelow AR, Bacarese-Hamilton I. Two-stage uncemented revision hip arthroplasty for infection. J Bone Joint Surg Br. 2000;82(5):689-694.
56. Hofmann AA, Goldberg TD, Tanner AM, Cook TM. Ten-year experience using an articulating antibiotic cement hip spacer for the treatment of chronically infected total hip. J Arthroplasty. 2005;20(7):874-879.
57. Hsieh PH, Shih CH, Chang YH, Lee MS, Shih HN, Yang WE. Two-stage revision hip arthroplasty for infection: comparison between the interim use of antibiotic-loaded cement beads and a spacer prosthesis. J Bone Joint Surg Am. 2004;86-A(9):1989-1997.
58. Jahoda D, Sosna A, Landor I, Vavrik P, Pokorny D. A cannulated articulating spacer--a functional implant for treatment of infected hip joint prostheses. Acta Chir Orthop Traumatol Cech. 2004;71(2):73-79.
59. Kamath AF, Anakwenze O, Lee GC, Nelson CL. Staged custom, intramedullary antibiotic spacers for severe segmental bone loss in infected total hip arthroplasty. Adv Orthop. 2011:398954.
60. Masri BA, Panagiotopoulos KP, Greidanus NV, Garbuz DS, Duncan CP. Cementless two-stage exchange arthroplasty for infection after total hip arthroplasty. J Arthroplasty. 2007;22(1):72-78.
61. McKenna PB, O'Shea K, Masterson EL. Two-stage revision of infected hip arthroplasty using a shortened post-operative course of antibiotics. Arch Orthop Trauma Surg. 2009;129(4):489-494.
62. Morshed S, Huffman GR, Ries MD. Extended trochanteric osteotomy for 2-stage revision of infected total hip arthroplasty. J Arthroplasty. 2005;20(3):294-301.
63. Neumann DR, Hofstaedter T, List C, Dorn U. Two-stage cementless revision of late total hip arthroplasty infection using a premanufactured spacer. J Arthroplasty. 2012;27(7):1397-1401.
64. Romano CL, Romano D, Albisetti A, Meani E. Preformed antibiotic-loaded cement

spacers for two-stage revision of infected total hip arthroplasty. Long-term results. Hip Int. 2012;22(Suppl 8):S46-53.
65. Romano CL, Romano D, Logoluso N, Meani E. Long-stem versus short-stem preformed antibiotic-loaded cement spacers for two-stage revision of infected total hip arthroplasty. Hip Int. 2010;20(1):26-33.
66. Romano CL, Romano D, Meani E, Logoluso N, Drago L. Two-stage revision surgery with preformed spacers and cementless implants for septic hip arthritis: a prospective, non-randomized cohort study. BMC Infect Dis.2011;11:129.
67. Toulson C, Walcott-Sapp S, Hur J, et al. Treatment of infected total hip arthroplasty with a 2-stage reimplantation protocol: update on "our institution's" experience from 1989 to 2003. J Arthroplasty. 2009;24(7):1051-1060.
68. Wang L, Hu Y, Dai Z, Zhou J, Li M, Li K. Mid-term effectiveness of two-stage hip prosthesis revision in treatment of infection after hip arthroplasty. Zhongguo Xiu Fu Chong Jian Wai Ke Za Zhi. 2011;25(6):646-649.
69. Wei W, Kou BL, Ju RS, Lu HS. The second stage revision for infected total hip arthroplasty using antibiotic-loaded cement prosthesis. Zhonghua Wai Ke Za Zhi. 2007;45(4):246-248.
70. Younger AS, Duncan CP, Masri BA, McGraw RW. The outcome of two-stage arthroplasty using a custom-made interval spacer to treat the infected hip. J Arthroplasty. 1997;12(6):615-623.
71. Zou YG, Feng ZQ, Xing JS, Peng ZH, Luo X. Two-stage revision for treatment of periprosthetic infection following hip arthroplasty. Nan Fang Yi Ke Da Xue Xue Bao. 2011;31(4):690-693.
72. Babiak I. Application of individually performed acrylic cement spacers containing 5% of antibiotic in two-stage revision of hip and knee prosthesis due to infection. Pol Orthop Traumatol. 2012;77:29-37.
73. Babis GC, Zahos KA, Tsailas P, Karaliotas GI, Kanellakopoulou K, Soucacos PN. Treatment of stage III-A-1 and III-B-1 periprosthetic knee infection with two-stage exchange arthroplasty and articulating spacer. J Surg Orthop Adv. 2008;17(3):173-178.
74. Borowski M, Kusz D, Wojciechowski P, Cielinski L. Treatment for periprosthetic infection with two-stage revision arthroplasty with a gentamicin loaded spacer. The clinical outcomes. Ortop Traumatol Rehabil. 2012;14(1):41-54.
75. Cai P, Hu Y, Xie L, Wang L. Two-stage revision of infected total knee arthroplasty using antibiotic-impregnated articulating cement spacer. Zhongguo Xiu Fu Chong Jian Wai Ke Za Zhi. 2012;26(10):1169-1173.
76. Calton TF, Fehring TK, Griffin WL. Bone loss associated with the use of spacer blocks in infected total knee arthroplasty. Clin Orthop Relat Res. 1997;(345):148-154.
77. Freeman MG, Fehring TK, Odum SM, Fehring K, Griffin WL, Mason JB. Functional advantage of articulating versus non-articulating spacers in 2-stage revision for total knee arthroplasty infection. J Arthroplasty. 2007;22(8):1116-1121.
78. Incavo SJ, Russell RD, Mathis KB, Adams H. Initial results of managing severe bone loss in infected total joint arthroplasty using customized articulating spacers. J Arthroplasty. 2009;24(4):607-613.
79. Kalore NV, Maheshwari A, Sharma A, Cheng E, Gioe TJ. Is there a preferred articulating spacer technique for infected knee arthroplasty? A preliminary study. Clin Orthop Relat Res. 2012;470(1):228-235.
80. Nettrour JF, Polikandriotis JA, Bernasek TL, Gustke KA, Lyons ST. Articulating spacers for the treatment of infected total knee arthroplasty: effect of antibiotic combinations and concentrations. Orthopedics. 2013;36(1):e19-24.
81. Pietsch M, Wenisch C, Traussnig S, Trnoska R, Hofmann S. Temporary articulating spacer with antibiotics-impregnated cement for an infected knee endoprosthesis. Orthopade. 2003;32(6):490-497.
82. Souillac V, Costes S, Aunoble S, Langlois V, Dutronc H, Chauveaux D. Evaluation of an articulated spacer for two-stage reimplantation for infected total knee arthroplasty: 28 cases. Rev Chir Orthop Reparatrice Appar Mot. 2006;92(5):485-489.
83. Springer BD, Lee GC, Osmon D, Haidukewych GJ, Hanssen AD, Jacofsky DJ. Systemic safety of high-dose antibiotic-loaded cement spacers after resection of an infected total knee arthroplasty. Clin Orthop Relat Res. 2004;(427):47-51.
84. Trezies A, Parish E, Dixon P, Cross M. The use of an articulating spacer in the management of infected total knee arthroplasties. J Arthroplasty. 2006;21(5):702-704.
85. Wan Z, Karim A, Momaya A, Incavo SJ, Mathis KB. Preformed articulating knee spacers in 2-stage total knee revision arthroplasty: minimum 2-year follow-up. J Arthroplasty. 2012;27(8):1469-1473.
86. Anagnostakos K, Jung J, Kelm J, Schmitt E. Two-stage treatment protocol for isolated septic acetabular cup loosening. Hip Int. 2010;20(3):320-326.
87. Anagnostakos K, Kelm J, Schmitt E, Jung J. Fungal periprosthetic hip and knee joint infections clinical experience with a 2-stage treatment protocol. J Arthroplasty. 2012;27(2):293-298.
88. Ben-Lulu O, Farno A, Gross AE, Backstein DJ, Kosashvili Y, Safir OA. A modified

cement spacer technique for infected total hip arthroplasties with significant bone loss. J Arthroplasty. 2012;27(4):613-619.
89. Berend KR, Lombardi AV Jr., Morris MJ, Bergeson AG, Adams JB, Sneller MA. Two-stage treatment of hip periprosthetic joint infection is associated with a high rate of infection control but high mortality. Clin Orthop Relat Res. 2013;471(2):510-518.
90. Biring GS, Kostamo T, Garbuz DS, Masri BA, Duncan CP. Two-stage revision arthroplasty of the hip for infection using an interim articulated Prostalac hip spacer: a 10- to 15-year follow-up study. J Bone Joint Surg Br. 2009;91(11):1431-1437.
91. Dairaku K, Takagi M, Kawaji H, Sasaki K, Ishii M, Ogino T. Antibiotics-impregnated cement spacers in the first step of two-stage revision for infected totally replaced hip joints: report of ten trial cases. J Orthop Sci. 2009;14(6):704-710.
92. Degen RM, Davey JR, Howard JL, McCalden RW, Naudie DD. Does a prefabricated gentamicin-impregnated, load-bearing spacer control periprosthetic hip infection? Clin Orthop Relat Res. 2012;470(10):2724-2729.
93. Flores X, Corona PS, Cortina J, Guerra E, Amat C. Temporary cement tectoplasty: a technique to improve prefabricated hip spacer stability in two-stage surgery for infected hip arthroplasty. Arch Orthop Trauma Surg. 2012;132(5):719-724.
94. Gil Gonzalez S, Marques Lopez F, Rigol Ramon P, Mestre Cortadellas C, Caceres Palou E, Leon Garcia A. Two-stage revision of hip prosthesis infection using a hip spacer with stabilising proximal cementation. Hip Int. 2010;20 Suppl 7:128-134.
95. Hsieh PH, Chen LH, Chen CH, Lee MS, Yang WE, Shih CH. Two-stage revision hip arthroplasty for infection with a custom-made, antibiotic-loaded, cement prosthesis as an interim spacer. J Trauma. 2004;56(6):1247-1252.
96. Hsieh PH, Huang KC, Lee PC, Lee MS. Two-stage revision of infected hip arthroplasty using an antibiotic-loaded spacer: retrospective comparison between short-term and prolonged antibiotic therapy. J Antimicrob Chemother. 2009;64(2):392-397.
97. Hsieh PH, Huang KC, Tai CL. Liquid gentamicin in bone cement spacers: in vivo antibiotic release and systemic safety in two-stage revision of infected hip arthroplasty. J Trauma. 2009;66(3):804-808.
98. Hsieh PH, Shih CH, Chang YH, Lee MS, Yang WE, Shih HN. Treatment of deep infection of the hip associated with massive bone loss: two-stage revision with an antibiotic-loaded interim cement prosthesis followed by reconstruction with allograft. J Bone Joint Surg Br. 2005;87(6):770-775.
99. Jahoda D, Sosna A, Landor I, Vavrik P, Pokorny D, Hudec T. Two-stage reimplantation using spacers--the method of choice in treatment of hip joint prosthesis-related infections. Comparison with methods used from 1979 to 1998. Acta Chir Orthop Traumatol Cech. 2003;70(1):17-24.
100. Jung J, Schmid NV, Kelm J, Schmitt E, Anagnostakos K. Complications after spacer implantation in the treatment of hip joint infections. Int J Med Sci. 2009;6(5):265-273.
101. Kalra KP, Lin KK, Bozic KJ, Ries MD. Repeat 2-stage revision for recurrent infection of total hip arthroplasty. J Arthroplasty. 2010;25(6):880-884.
102. Kent M, Rachha R, Sood M. A technique for the fabrication of a reinforced moulded articulating cement spacer in two-stage revision total hip arthroplasty. Int Orthop. 2010;34(7):949-953.
103. Koo KH, Yang JW, Cho SH, et al. Impregnation of vancomycin, gentamicin, and cefotaxime in a cement spacer for two-stage cementless reconstruction in infected total hip arthroplasty. J Arthroplasty. 2001;16(7):882-892.
104. Leung F, Richards CJ, Garbuz DS, Masri BA, Duncan CP. Two-stage total hip arthroplasty: how often does it control methicillin-resistant infection? Clin Orthop Relat Res. 2011;469(4):1009-1015.
105. Leunig M, Chosa E, Speck M, Ganz R. A cement spacer for two-stage revision of infected implants of the hip joint. Int Orthop. 1998;22(4):209-214.
106. Liu XC, Zhou YG, Wang Y, et al. Antibiotic-loaded cement articulating spacer made by a self-made mold system in the treatment of the infected hip replacement. Zhonghua Wai Ke Za Zhi. 2010;48(14):1050-1054.
107. Magnan B, Regis D, Biscaglia R, Bartolozzi P. Preformed acrylic bone cement spacer loaded with antibiotics: use of two-stage procedure in 10 patients because of infected hips after total replacement. Acta Orthop Scand. 2001;72(6):591-594.
108. Masri BA, Duncan CP, Beauchamp CP. Long-term elution of antibiotics from bone-cement: an in vivo study using the prosthesis of antibiotic-loaded acrylic cement (PROSTALAC) system. J Arthroplasty. 1998;13(3):331-338.
109. Mortazavi SM, O'Neil JT, Zmistowski B, Parvizi J, Purtill JJ. Repeat 2-stage exchange for infected total hip arthroplasty: a viable option? J Arthroplasty. 2012;27(6):923-926 e921.
110. Pattyn C, De Geest T, Ackerman P, Audenaert E. Preformed gentamicin spacers in two-stage revision hip arthroplasty: functional results and complications. Int Orthop. 2011;35(10):1471-1476.
111. Peng KT, Hsu WH, Hsu RW. Improved antibiotic impregnated cement prosthesis for treating deep hip infection: a novel design using hip compression screw. J Arthroplasty.

2010;25(8):1304-1306.
112. Peng KT, Kuo LT, Hsu WH, Huang TW, Tsai YH. The effect of endoskeleton on antibiotic impregnated cement spacer for treating deep hip infection. BMC Musculoskelet Disord. 2011;12:10.
113. Pignatti G, Nitta S, Rani N, et al. Two stage hip revision in periprosthetic infection: results of 41 cases. Open Orthop J. 2010;4:193-200.
114. Regis D, Sandri A, Rizzo A, Bartolozzi P. A performed temporary antibiotic-loaded cement spacer for the treatment of destructive septic hip arthritis: a case report. Int J Infect Dis. 2010;14(3):e259-261.
115. Romano CL, Romano D, Logoluso N, Meani E. Septic versus aseptic hip revision: how different? J Orthop Traumatol. 2010;11(3):167-174.
116. Stockley I, Mockford BJ, Hoad-Reddick A, Norman P. The use of two-stage exchange arthroplasty with depot antibiotics in the absence of long-term antibiotic therapy in infected total hip replacement. J Bone Joint Surg Br. 2008;90(2):145-148.
117. Takahira N, Itoman M, Higashi K, Uchiyama K, Miyabe M, Naruse K. Treatment outcome of two-stage revision total hip arthroplasty for infected hip arthroplasty using antibiotic-impregnated cement spacer. J Orthop Sci. 2003;8(1):26-31.
118. Takigami I, Ito Y, Ishimaru D, et al. Two-stage revision surgery for hip prosthesis infection using antibiotic-loaded porous hydroxyapatite blocks. Arch Orthop Trauma Surg. 2010;130(10):1221-1226.
119. Whittaker JP, Warren RE, Jones RS, Gregson PA. Is prolonged systemic antibiotic treatment essential in two-stage revision hip replacement for chronic Gram-positive infection? J Bone Joint Surg Br. 2009;91(1):44-51.
120. Yamamoto K, Miyagawa N, Masaoka T, Katori Y, Shishido T, Imakiire A. Clinical effectiveness of antibiotic-impregnated cement spacers for the treatment of infected implants of the hip joint. J Orthop Sci. 2003;8(6):823-828.
121. Fink B, Vogt S, Reinsch M, Buchner H. Sufficient release of antibiotic by a spacer 6 weeks after implantation in two-stage revision of infected hip prostheses. Clin Orthop Relat Res. 2011;469(11):3141-3147.
122. McLaren AC, McLaren SG, Hickmon MK. Sucrose, xylitol, and erythritol increase PMMA permeability for depot antibiotics. Clin Orthop Relat Res. 2007;461:60-63.
123. Garcia-Oltra E, Bori G, Tomas X, Gallart X, Garcia S, Soriano A. Radiological evaluation of acetabular erosion after antibiotic-impregnated polymethylmethacrylate spacer (spacer-g). J Arthroplasty. 2013;28(6):1021-1024.
124. Kühn KD. Antibiotic loaded bone cements- antibiotic release and influence on mechanical properties. In: Walenkamp G, ed. Local Antibiotics in Arthroplasty: Thieme; 2007.
125. Masri BA, Duncan CP, Beauchamp CP. The modified two staged exchange arthroplasty in the treatment of infected total knee replacement: The Prostalac system and other articulated spacers. In: Engh GA, Rorabeck CH, eds. Revision Total Knee Arthroplasty. Vol 13. 1998/05/20 ed. Baltimore: Willams & Wilkins; 1997:394-424.
126. Bertazzoni Minelli E, Benini A, Magnan B, Bartolozzi P. Release of gentamicin and vancomycin from temporary human hip spacers in two-stage revision of infected arthroplasty. J Antimicrob Chemother. 2004;53(2):329-334.
127. Frommelt L. Properties of bone cement: antibiotic loaded cement. The Well-Cemented Total Hip Arthroplasty, Part II. Berlin: Springer; 2006:86-92.
128. Frommelt L. Antibiotic choices in bone surgery- local therapy using antibiotic loaded bone cement. In: Walenkamp G, ed. Local Antibiotics in Arthroplasty: Thieme; 2007.
129. Frommelt L. Local antibiotic therapy. Septic Bone and Joint Surgery: Thieme; 2010:78-83.
130. Meyer J, Piller G, Spiegel CA, Hetzel S, Squire M. Vacuum-mixing significantly changes antibiotic elution characteristics of commercially available antibiotic-impregnated bone cements. J Bone Joint Surg Am. 2011;93(22):2049-2056.
131. McLaren AC, McLaren SG, Smeltzer M. Xylitol and glycine fillers increase permeability of PMMA to enhance elution of daptomycin. Clin Orthop Relat Res. 2006;(451):25-28.
132. McLaren AC, Nelson CL, McLaren SG, De CGR. The effect of glycine filler on the elution rate of gentamicin from acrylic bone cement: a pilot study. Clin Orthop Relat Res. 2004;(427):25-27.
133. McLaren AC, Nelson CL, McLaren SG, Wassell DL. Phenolphthalein used to assess permeability of antibiotic-laden polymethylmethacrylate: a pilot study. Clin Orthop Relat Res. 2005;(439):48-51.
134. Amin TJ, Lamping JW,Hendricks KJ, McIff TE. Increasing the elution of vancomycin from high-dose antibiotic-loaded bone cement: a novel preparation technique. J Bone Joint Surg Am. 2012;94(21):1946-1951.

Question 1

- **Is there a functional difference in the use of non-articulating or articulating spacers for the treatment of periprosthetic joint infection (PJI) in the knee, in between of two-stage exchange arthroplasty?**

<u>Consensus:</u> Articulating spacers provide better function than non-articulating spacers for the patient in between the stages of total knee arthroplasty (TKA). An articulating spacer is especially preferred for patients who are likely to have a spacer in place for longer than 3 months.

Delegate Vote

Agree: 89%, Disagree: 6%, Abstain: 5% (Strong Consensus)

Question 2

- **Is there a functional difference in the use of non-articulating or articulating spacers for treatment of periprosthetic joint infection (PJI) in the knee at minimum two years after reimplantation?**

<u>Consensus:</u> There is a non-significant trend in range of motion improvement with articulating compared to non-articulating spacers, but the panels believes that this is still of value to the patient

Delegate Vote

Agree: 82%, Disagree: 12%, Abstain: 6% (Strong Consensus)

Question 3

- **Is there a functional difference in the use of non-articulating or articulating spacers for the treatment of PJI in the hip, in between stages of two-stage exchange arthroplasty?**

<u>Consensus:</u> A well performing articulating spacer provides better function for the patient in between the stages of total hip arthroplasty (THA). These are especially preferred for patients who are likely to have a spacer in place for longer than 3 months.

Delegate Vote

Agree: 89%, Disagree: 7%, Abstain: 4% (Strong Consensus)

Question 4

- **Is there a functional difference in the use of non-articulating or articulating spacers for the treatment of PJI in the hip, at minimum two years after reimplantation?**

<u>Consensus:</u> There is a non-significant trend in functional improvement with articulating compared to non-articulating spacers, but the panels believes that this is still of value to the patient.

Delegate Vote

Agree: 81%, Disagree: 12%, Abstain: 7% (Strong Consensus)

Question 5

- **Is there a difference in reimplantation (surgical ease) with the use of non-articulating or articulating spacers for the treatment of PJI in the knee and hip?**

<u>Consensus:</u> Yes. Reimplantation surgery is easier overall in patients receiving articulating spacers compared to non-articulating spacers.

Delegate Vote

Agree: 81%, Disagree: 8%, Abstain: 11% (Strong Consensus)

Question 6

- **Is there a difference with regards to control of infection with the use of articulating or non-articulating spacers in the knee?**

<u>Consensus:</u> No. The type of spacer does not influence the rate of infection eradication in two-stage exchange arthroplasty of the knee.

Delegate Vote

Agree: 89%, Disagree: 6%, Abstain: 5% (Strong Consensus)

Question 7

- **Is there a difference with regards to control of infection with the use of articulating or non-articulating spacers in the hip?**

<u>Consensus:</u> No. The type of spacer does not influence the rate of infection eradication in two-stage exchange arthroplasty of the hip.

Delegate Vote

Agree: 95%, Disagree: 3%, Abstain: 2% (Strong Consensus)

Question 8

- **Is there a difference with regards to control of infection between different types of articulating spacers used in the knee?**

Consensus: Control of the infection is no different between different types of articulating spacers in the treatment of infected TKA.

Delegate Vote

Agree: 90%, Disagree: 5%, Abstain: 5% (Strong Consensus)

Question 9

- **Are there contraindications for the use of non-articulating and/or articulating spacers?**

Consensus: There are no clear contraindications for the use of non-articulating or articulating spacers, other than the technical feasibility of the procedure. In patients with massive bone loss and/or lack of integrity of soft-tissues or ligamentous restraint, strong consideration should be given to the use of non-articulating spacers.

Delegate Vote

Agree: 92%, Disagree: 3%, Abstain: 5% (Strong Consensus)

Question 10

- **Are there any differences in functional outcome between manufactured spacers versus surgeon-made dynamic spacers used in the knee?**

Consensus: There is no difference in functional outcome between manufactured spacers versus surgeon-made articulating spacers used in the knee. However, issues of cost, ease of use, and antibiotic delivery should be considered.

Delegate Vote

Agree: 89%, Disagree: 5%, Abstain: 6% (Strong Consensus)

Question 11

- **Are there any differences in the rate of infection control between manufactured spacers versus surgeon-made articulating spacers used in the knee?**

Consensus: There are no differences in the rate of infection control between manufactured spacers and surgeon-made articulating spacers used in the knee. However, issues of cost, ease of use, and antibiotic delivery should be considered.

Delegate Vote
Agree: 93%, Disagree: 2%, Abstain: 5% (Strong Consensus)

Question 12

- **Are there any differences in functional outcome between manufactured spacers versus surgeon-made dynamic spacers used in the hip?**

Consensus: There is no difference in functional outcome between manufactured spacers versus surgeon-made articulating spacers used in the hip. However, issues of cost, ease of use, and antibiotic delivery should be considered.

Delegate Vote
Agree: 89%, Disagree: 7%, Abstain: 4% (Strong Consensus)

Question 13

- **Are there any differences in the rate of infection control between manufactured spacers versus surgeon-made dynamic spacers used in the hip?**

Consensus: There is no difference in the rate of infection control between manufactured spacers versus surgeon-made articulating spacers used in the hip. However, issues of cost, ease of use, and antibiotic delivery should be considered.

Delegate Vote
Agree: 94%, Disagree: 3%, Abstain: 3% (Strong Consensus)

Question 14

- **Which antibiotic should be used and how much of it should be added to cement spacers?**

Consensus: The type of antibiotic and the dose needs to be individualized for each patient based on the organism profile and antibiogram (if available) as well as the patient's renal function and allergy profile.

However, most infections can be treated with a spacer with vancomycin (1 to 4 g per 40 g package of cement) and gentamicin or tobramycin (2.4 to 4.8 g per 40 g package of cement). We provide a list of all available antibiotics and the range of doses to be used against common infecting organisms.

Delegate Vote
Agree: 89%, Disagree: 7%, Abstain: 4% (Strong Consensus)

Question 15

- **What is the optimal technique for preparing a high-dose antibiotic cement spacer (mixing, when and how to add antibiotics, and porosity)?**

Consensus: There is no consensus on the best method of preparation of high-dose antibiotic cement spacers.

Delegate Vote
Agree: 93%, Disagree: 3%, Abstain: 4% (Strong Consensus)

10 洗浄デブリドマン

Workgroup 10：Irrigation and Debridement

Question 1A
- 洗浄デブリドマン（I&D）はどの段階で考慮されるべきか？

コンセンサス

最初に行われた人工関節置換術の術後3カ月以内に発症した早期感染に対して，症状発生から3週間以内であればI&Dを施行してもよい．

投票結果

同意：84％，反対：13％，棄権：3％（強いコンセンサス）

Question 1B
- 晩期の血行性感染に対する治療として，I&Dを行ってもよいか？

コンセンサス

感染の誘因となったイベント発生から3週間以内の，または症状が出てから3週間以内の晩期血行性感染に対して，I&Dは施行してもよい．（参考文献 1-25）

投票結果

同意：88％，反対：9％，棄権：3％（強いコンセンサス）

Question 2
- I&Dの禁忌は？

コンセンサス

創を閉鎖できない，または瘻孔を形成している患者では，I&Dや人工関節の温存は絶対禁忌である．人工関節のゆるみを認める場合も絶対禁忌である．（参考文献 13, 25-29）

投票結果

同意：95％，反対：4％，棄権：1％（強いコンセンサス）

Question 3A

- 人工膝関節全置換術（TKA）後の血腫に対してI&Dを施行する際，深筋膜を切開するべきか？

コンセンサス

TKA後で血腫を形成している患者に対しては，筋膜や関節切開は常に行うべきである．（参考文献 15, 18, 30）

投票結果

同意：87％，反対：8％，棄権：5％（強いコンセンサス）

Question 3B

- 人工股関節全置換術（THA）後の血腫に対してI&Dを施行する際，深筋膜を切開するべきか？

コンセンサス

術前またはI&Dの際に関節穿刺を行うべきである．明らかな筋膜の欠損のある場合，または穿刺によって筋膜より深部に血腫や液体貯留が確認された場合は，筋膜切開を施行するべきである．（参考文献 15, 18, 30）

投票結果

同意：87％，反対：9％，棄権：4％（強いコンセンサス）

Question 4

- I&Dは，人工関節周囲感染（PJI）でどのように行うべきか？

コンセンサス

人工関節のI&Dは，細心の注意払いながら詳細なプロトコールに従って行われる必要がある．簡単にまとめると：
　―術前に患者を最良な状態にする．
　―良い視野を確保し，十分なデブリドマンを行う．
　―細菌培養用に多くのサンプルを採取する．
　―大量の洗浄液（6～9L）を用いて関節を洗浄する．
　―必要であれば人工関節の抜去を行う．
（参考文献 30-32）

投票結果

同意：90％，反対：6％，棄権：4％（強いコンセンサス）

Question 5

- モジュラーパーツはI&Dの際に常に交換するべきか?

コンセンサス

交換するべきである．I&Dの際には，可能な限りすべてのモジュラーコンポーネントを抜去し交換するべきである．

(参考文献 1, 6, 7, 11, 13, 17, 25, 26, 30, 33-35)

投票結果

同意：92％，反対：8％，棄権：0％（強いコンセンサス）

Question 6

- I&Dの適応を決める際に有用な分類システム（例：Tsukayama分類）はあるか？

コンセンサス

現在ある分類システムの中で，外科医が早期PJIに対して適切な外科的治療法を決めるために有用な分類システムはない．急性発症のPJI患者に対しI&Dが奏効しないリスクファクターを特定するにはさらなる研究が必要である．

(参考文献 17, 23, 30, 36-43)

投票結果

同意：84％，反対：5％，棄権：11％（強いコンセンサス）

Question 7

- I&Dは緊急処置なのか？ それとも術前に患者を最良な状態にしてから望むべきか？

コンセンサス

緊急処置ではない．敗血症に罹患していない患者において，I&Dは緊急処置ではない．外科的介入よりも優先して，患者状態を良くするためのあらゆる努力がなされるべきである．

投票結果

同意：92％，反対：6％，棄権：2％（強いコンセンサス）

Question 8

- 関節鏡検査はI&Dにおいて何かしら意味があるか？

コンセンサス

関節鏡検査はPJIに対しI&Dを行う上で必要でない．

(参考文献 6, 35, 44)
投票結果
同意：91％，反対：7％，棄権：2％（強いコンセンサス）

Question 9
- インプラント抜去を行う前のI&Dは，何度まで行うのが妥当か？

コンセンサス

1度でもI&Dに失敗したら，執刀医はインプラント抜去を考慮すべきである．(参考文献 13, 19, 45-47)

投票結果
同意：94％，反対：6％，棄権：0％（強いコンセンサス）

Question 10
- I&D施行中に細菌培養用のサンプルを採取するべきか？ もしそうであればどこからどのくらい採取するべきか？

コンセンサス

I&D施行中に人工関節周囲から3～6個の代表的な組織または液体をサンプルとして採取すべきである．(参考文献 48, 49)

投票結果
同意：98％，反対：2％，棄権：0％（強いコンセンサス）

Question 11
- I&D後の患者に抗菌薬の長期投与は行うべきか？ もしそうであれば，その適応，抗菌薬のタイプ，投与量と治療期間は？

コンセンサス

行うべきでない．PJIの診断基準を満たす患者にのみ抗菌薬の長期投与を行うべきである（Workgroup 7参照）．感染した患者に対しては，感染症専門医（ID専門医）へコンサルテーションを行い抗菌薬の種類，投与量と治療期間を決定するべきである．

投票結果
同意：75％，反対：20％，棄権：5％（強いコンセンサス）

Question 12

- I & D 後の関節内局所抗菌薬投与は有用か？ 有用であるとすればその適応は？

コンセンサス

有用であるとは言えない．PJI の治療として，持続的な関節内抗菌薬投与のエビデンスは不十分である．（参考文献 4, 50-53）

投票結果

同意：89％，反対：7％，棄権：4％（強いコンセンサス）

Question 13

- 吸収性抗菌薬含有剤（硫酸カルシウムなど）は有用か？ 有用であるとすれば，その適応は？

コンセンサス

有用であるとは言えない．吸収性抗菌薬含有材が I & D のアウトカムを好転させるとした決定的なエビデンスは現在ない．

（参考文献 53-57）

投票結果

同意：88％，反対：6％，棄権：6％（強いコンセンサス）

【掲載されている論文】

Irrigation and debridement.

Haasper C, Buttaro M, Hozack W, Aboltins CA, Borens O, Callaghan JJ, de Carvalho PI, Chang Y, Corona P, Da Rin F, Esposito S, Fehring TK, Sanchez XF, Lee GC, Martinez-Pastor JC, Mortazavi SM, Noiseux NO, Peng KT, Schutte HD, Schweitzer D, Trebše R, Tsiridis E, Whiteside L.

J Arthroplasty. 2014 Feb；29（2 Suppl）：100-3. doi：10.1016/j.arth.2013.09.043. Epub 2013 Dec 17. No abstract available.

PMID:24360491

References:

1. Odum SM, Fehring TK, Lombardi AV, et al. Irrigation and debridement for periprosthetic infections: does the organism matter? J Arthroplasty. 2011;26(6 Suppl):114-118.
2. Romano CL, Manzi G, Logoluso N, Romano D. Value of debridement and irrigation for the treatment of peri-prosthetic infections. A systematic review. Hip Int. 2012;22(Suppl 8):S19-24.
3. Aboltins CA, Page MA, Buising KL, et al. Treatment of staphylococcal prosthetic joint infections with debridement, prosthesis retention and oral rifampicin and fusidic acid. Clin Microbiol Infect. 2007;13(6):586-591.

4. Berdal JE, Skramm I, Mowinckel P, Gulbrandsen P, Bjornholt JV. Use of rifampicin and ciprofloxacin combination therapy after surgical debridement in the treatment of early manifestation prosthetic joint infections. Clin Microbiol Infect. 2005;11(10):843-845.
5. Burger RR, Basch T, Hopson CN. Implant salvage in infected total knee arthroplasty. Clin Orthop Relat Res. 1991;(273):105-112.
6. Byren I, Bejon P, Atkins BL, et al. One hundred and twelve infected arthroplasties treated with 'DAIR' (debridement, antibiotics and implant retention): antibiotic duration and outcome. J Antimicrob Chemother. 2009;63(6):1264-1271.
7. Giuliери SG, Graber P, Ochsner PE, Zimmerli W. Management of infection associated with total hip arthroplasty according to a treatment algorithm. Infection. 2004;32(4):222-228.
8. Hartman MB, Fehring TK, Jordan L, Norton HJ. Periprosthetic knee sepsis. The role of irrigation and debridement. Clin Orthop Relat Res. 1991;(273):113-118.
9. Klouche S, Lhotellier L, Mamoudy P. Infected total hip arthroplasty treated by an irrigation-debridement/component retention protocol. A prospective study in a 12-case series with minimum 2 years' follow-up. Orthop Traumatol Surg Res. 2011;97(2):134-138.
10. Kotwal SY, Farid YR, Patil SS, Alden KJ, Finn HA. Intramedullary rod and cement static spacer construct in chronically infected total knee arthroplasty. J Arthroplasty. 2012;27(2):253-259 e254.
11. Koyonos L, Zmistowski B, Della Valle CJ, Parvizi J. Infection control rate of irrigation and debridement for periprosthetic joint infection. Clin Orthop Relat Res. 2011;469(11):3043-3048.
12. Legout L, Stern R, Assal M, et al. Suction drainage culture as a guide to effectively treat musculoskeletal infection. Scand J Infect Dis. 2006;38(5):341-345.
13. Lora-Tamayo J, Murillo O, Iribarren JA, et al. A large multicenter study of methicillin-susceptible and methicillin-resistant Staphylococcus aureus prosthetic joint infections managed with implant retention. Clin Infect Dis. 2013;56(2):182-194.
14. Martinez-Pastor JC, Munoz-Mahamud E, Vilchez F, et al. Outcome of acute prosthetic joint infections due to gram-negative bacilli treated with open debridement and retention of the prosthesis. Antimicrob Agents Chemother. 2009;53(11):4772-4777.
15. Segawa H, Tsukayama DT, Kyle RF, Becker DA, Gustilo RB. Infection after total knee arthroplasty. A retrospective study of the treatment of eighty-one infections. J Bone Joint Surg Am. 1999;81(10):1434-1445.
16. Trebse R, Pisot V, Trampuz A. Treatment of infected retained implants. J Bone Joint Surg Br. 2005;87(2):249-256.
17. Tsukayama DT, Estrada R, Gustilo RB. Infection after total hip arthroplasty. A study of the treatment of one hundred and six infections. J Bone Joint Surg Am. 1996;78(4):512-523.
18. Van Kleunen JP, Knox D, Garino JP, Lee GC. Irrigation and debridement and prosthesis retention for treating acute periprosthetic infections. Clin Orthop Relat Res. 2010;468(8):2024-2028.
19. Vilchez F, Martinez-Pastor JC, Garcia-Ramiro S, et al. Outcome and predictors of treatment failure in early post-surgical prosthetic joint infections due to Staphylococcus aureus treated with debridement. Clin Microbiol Infect. 2011;17(3):439-444.
20. Vilchez F, Martinez-Pastor JC, Garcia-Ramiro S, et al. Efficacy of debridement in hematogenous and early post-surgical prosthetic joint infections. Int J Artif Organs. 2011;34(9):863-869.
21. Widmer AF, Gaechter A, Ochsner PE, Zimmerli W. Antimicrobial treatment of orthopedic implant-related infections with rifampin combinations. Clin Infect Dis. 1992;14(6):1251-1253.
22. Zimmerli W, Ochsner PE. Management of infection associated with prosthetic joints. Infection. 2003;31(2):99-108.
23. Zimmerli W, Trampuz A, Ochsner PE. Prosthetic-joint infections. N Engl J Med. 2004;351(16):1645-1654.
24. Zimmerli W, Widmer AF, Blatter M, Frei R, Ochsner PE. Role of rifampin for treatment of orthopedic implant-related staphylococcal infections: a randomized controlled trial. Foreign-Body Infection (FBI) Study Group. JAMA. 1998;279(19):1537-1541.
25. Zmistowski B, Fedorka CJ, Sheehan E, Deirmengian G, Austin MS, Parvizi J. Prosthetic joint infection caused by gram-negative organisms. J Arthroplasty. 2013;26(6 Suppl):104-108.
26. Buller LT, Sabry FY, Easton RW, Klika AK, Barsoum WK. The preoperative prediction of success following irrigation and debridement with polyethylene exchange for hip and knee prosthetic joint infections. J Arthroplasty. 2012;27(6):857-864 e851-854.
27. Westberg M, Grogaard B, Snorrason F. Early prosthetic joint infections treated with debridement and implant retention: 38 primary hip arthroplasties prospectively recorded and followed for median 4 years. Acta Orthop. 2012;83(3):227-232.
28. Peel TN, Cheng AC, Choong PF, Buising KL. Early onset prosthetic hip and knee joint infection: treatment and outcomes in Victoria, Australia. J Hosp Infect. 2012;82(4):248-253.
29. Marculescu CE, Berbari EF, Hanssen AD, et al. Outcome of prosthetic joint infections treated with debridement and retention of components. Clin Infect Dis. 2006;42(4):471-478.
30. Schwechter EM, Folk D, Varshney AK, Fries BC, Kim SJ, Hirsh DM. Optimal irrigation and debridement of infected joint implants: an in vitro methicillin-resistant Staphylococcus aureus biofilm model. J Arthroplasty. 2011;26(6 Suppl):109-113.

31. Kalteis T, Lehn N, Schroder HJ, et al. Contaminant seeding in bone by different irrigation methods: an experimental study. J Orthop Trauma. 2005;19(9):591-596.
32. Munoz-Mahamud E, Garcia S, Bori G, et al. Comparison of a low-pressure and a high-pressure pulsatile lavage during debridement for orthopaedic implant infection. Arch Orthop Trauma Surg. 2011;131(9):1233-1238.
33. Engesaeter LB, Dale H, Schrama JC, Hallan G, Lie SA. Surgical procedures in the treatment of 784 infected THAs reported to the Norwegian Arthroplasty Register. Acta Orthop. 2011;82(5):530-537.
34. Suke k M, Patel S, Haddad FS. Aggressive early debridement for treatment of acutely infected cemented total hip arthroplasty. Clin Orthop Relat Res. 2012;470(11):3164-3170.
35. Laffe RR, Graber P, Ochsner PE, Zimmerli W. Outcome of prosthetic knee-associated infection: evaluation of 40 consecutive episodes at a single centre. Clin Microbiol Infect. 2006;12(5):433-439.
36. Osmon DR, Berbari EF, Berendt AR, et al. Diagnosis and management of prosthetic joint infection: clinical practice guidelines by the Infectious Diseases Society of America. Clin Infect Dis. 2013;56(1):e1-e25.
37. Senneville E, Joulie D, Legout L, et al. Outcome and predictors of treatment failure in total hip/knee prosthetic joint infections due to Staphylococcus aureus. Clin Infect Dis. 2009;53(4):334-340.
38. Garvin KL, Hanssen AD. Infection after total hip arthroplasty. Past, present, and future. J Bone Joint Surg Am. 1995;77(10):1576-1588.
39. Garvin KL, Konigsberg BS. Infection following total knee arthroplasty: prevention and management. J Bone Joint Surg Am. 2011;93(12):1167-1175.
40. McPherson EJ, Woodson C, Holtom P, Roidis N, Shufelt C, Patzakis M. Periprosthetic total hip infection: outcomes using a staging system. Clin Orthop Relat Res. 2002;(403):8-15.
41. Bradbury T, Fehring TK, Taunton M, et al. The fate of acute methicillin-resistant Staphylococcus aureus periprosthetic knee infections treated by open debridement and retention of components. J Arthroplasty. 2009;24(6 Suppl):101-104.
42. Fehring TK, Odum SM, Berend KR, et al. Failure of irrigation and debridement for early postoperative periprosthetic infection. Clin Orthop Relat Res. 2013;471(1):250-257.
43. Zimmerli W, Moser C. Pathogenesis and treatment concepts of orthopaedic biofilm infections. FEMS Immunol Med Microbiol. 2012;65(2):158-168.
44. Waldman BJ, Hostin E, Mont MA, Hungerford DS. Infected total knee arthroplasty treated by arthroscopic irrigation and debridement. J Arthroplasty. 2000;15(4):430-436.
45. Peel TN, Buising KL, Dowsey MM, et al. Outcome of debridement and retention in prosthetic joint infections by methicillin-resistant staphylococci, with special reference to rifampin and fusidic acid combination therapy. Antimicrob Agents Chemother. 2013;57(1):350-355.
46. Mont MA, Waldman B, Banerjee C, Pacheco IH, Hungerford DS. Multiple irrigation, debridement, and retention of components in infected total knee arthroplasty. J Arthroplasty. 1997;12(4):426-433.
47. Sherrell JC, Fehring TK, Odum S, et al. The Chitranjan Ranawat Award: fate of two-stage reimplantation after failed irrigation and debridement for periprosthetic knee infection. Clin Orthop Relat Res. 2012;469(1):18-25.
48. Atkins BL, Athanasou N, Deeks JJ, et al. Prospective evaluation of criteria for microbiological diagnosis of prosthetic-joint infection at revision arthroplasty. The OSIRIS Collaborative Study Group. J Clin Microbiol. 1998;36(10):2932-2939.
49. Ghanem E, Parvizi J, Clohisy J, Burnett S, Sharkey PF, Barrack R. Perioperative antibiotics should not be withheld in proven cases of periprosthetic infection. Clin Orthop Relat Res. 2007;461:44-47.
50. Whiteside LA, Nayfeh TA, LaZear R, Roy ME. Reinfected revised TKA resolves with an aggressive protocol and antibiotic infusion. Clin Orthop Relat Res. 2012;470(1):236-243.
51. Fukagawa S, Matsuda S, Miura H, Okazaki K, Tashiro Y, Iwamoto Y. High-dose antibiotic infusion for infected knee prosthesis without implant removal. J Orthop Sci. 2010;15(4):470-476.
52. Estes CS, Beauchamp CP, Clarke HD, Spangehl MJ. A two-stage retention debridement protocol for acute periprosthetic joint infections. Clin Orthop Relat Res. 2010;468(8):2029-2038.
53. Tintle SM, Forsberg JA, Potter BK, Islinger RB, Andersen RC. Prosthesis retention, serial debridement, and antibiotic bead use for the treatment of infection following total joint arthroplasty. Orthopedics. 2009;32(2):87.
54. Kuiper JW, Brohet RM, Wassink S, van den Bekerom MP, Nolte PA, Vergroesen DA. Implantation of resorbable gentamicin sponges in addition to irrigation and debridement in 34 patients with infection complicating total hip arthroplasty. Hip Int. 2013;23(2):173-180.
55. McGlothan KR, Gosmanova EO. A case report of acute interstitial nephritis associated with antibiotic-impregnated orthopedic bone-cement spacer. Tenn Med. 2012;105(9):37-40, 42.
56. Nelson CL, McLaren SG, Skinner RA, Smeltzer MS, Thomas JR, Olsen KM. The treatment of experimental osteomyelitis by surgical debridement and the implantation of calcium sulfate tobramycin pellets. J Orthop Res. 2002;20(4):643-647.
57. Rauschmann MA, Wichelhaus TA, Stirnal V, et al. Nanocrystalline hydroxyapatite and

calcium sulphate as biodegradable composite carrier material for local delivery of antibiotics in bone infections. Biomaterials. 2005;26(15):2677-2684.

Question 1A

- **When can irrigation and debridement (I & D) be considered?**

<u>Consensus:</u> I & D may be performed for early postoperative infections that occur within 3 months of index primary arthroplasty with less than 3 weeks of symptoms.

Delegate Vote

Agree: 84%, Disagree: 13%, Abstain: 3% (Strong Consensus)

Question 1B

- **Can irrigation and debridement (I & D) be considered for late hematogenous infections?**

<u>Consensus:</u> I & D may be performed for patients with late hematogenous infection that occurred within 3 weeks of an inciting event or with symptoms not longer than 3 weeks.

Delegate Vote

Agree: 88%, Disagree: 9%, Abstain: 3% (Strong Consensus)

Question 2

- **What are the contraindications for I & D?**

<u>Consensus:</u> The inability to close a wound or the presence of a sinus tract are absolute contraindications to performing an I & D and retention of the prosthesis. Another absolute contraindication is the presence of a loose prostheses.

Delegate Vote

Agree: 95%, Disagree: 4%, Abstain: 1% (Strong Consensus)

Question 3A

- **When performing an I & D for hematoma after TKA, should the deep fascia be opened?**

<u>Consensus:</u> The fascia/arthrotomy should always be opened in patients with total knee arthroplasty (TKA) and hematoma formation.

Delegate Vote

Agree: 87%, Disagree: 8%, Abstain: 5% (Strong Consensus)

Question 3B

- **When performing an I & D for hematoma after THA, should the deep fascia be opened?**

Consensus: Aspiration of the joint, either prior to surgery or at the time of I & D, should be performed. For patients with a clear fascial defect or hematoma/fluid deep to the fascia confirmed by aspiration, the fascia should be opened.

Delegate Vote

Agree: 87%, Disagree: 9%, Abstain: 4% (Strong Consensus)

Question 4

- **How should I & D be performed for PJI?**

Consensus: An I & D of a prosthetic joint needs to be performed meticulously and according to the detailed protocol provided. Briefly this includes :

　—Preoperative optimization of the patient

　—Good visualization and thorough debridement

　—Obtaining multiple culture samples

　—Copious irrigation (6 to 9 L) of the joint

　—Explantation of the prosthesis if indicated.

Delegate Vote

Agree: 90%, Disagree: 6%, Abstain: 4% (Strong Consensus)

Question 5

- **Should the modular part always be exchanged during I & D?**

Consensus: Yes. All modular components should be removed and exchanged, if possible, during I & D.

Delegate Vote

Agree: 92%, Disagree: 8%, Abstain: 0% (Strong Consensus)

Question 6

- **Do useful classification systems (such as the Tsukayama classification) exist that may guide a surgeon in deciding on the appropriateness of an I & D?**

Consensus: The available classification system is inadequate in guiding a surgeon in selecting the appropriate surgical intervention for management of early PJI. There is a need for further studies to identify risk factors for failure of I & D in patients with acute PJI.

Delegate Vote

Agree: 84%, Disagree: 5%, Abstain: 11% (Strong Consensus)

Question 7

- **Is I & D an emergency procedure or can the patient be optimized prior to the procedure?**

<u>Consensus</u>: No. I & D is not an emergency procedure in a patient without generalized sepsis. All efforts should be made to optimize the patients prior to surgical intervention.

Delegate Vote

Agree: 92%, Disagree: 6%, Abstain: 2% (Strong Consensus)

Question 8

- **Does arthroscopy have a role in I & D?**

<u>Consensus</u>: Arthroscopy has no role in I & D of an infected prosthetic joint.

Delegate Vote

Agree: 91%, Disagree: 7%, Abstain: 2% (Strong Consensus)

Question 9

- **How many I & Ds are reasonable before implant removal is considered?**

<u>Consensus</u>: Following failure of one I & D, the surgeon should give consideration to implant removal.

Delegate Vote

Agree: 94%, Disagree: 6%, Abstain: 0% (Strong Consensus)

Question 10

- **Should culture samples be taken during I & D? If so how many and from where?**

<u>Consensus</u>: Representative tissue and fluid samples, between 3 to 6, from the periprosthetic region should be taken during I & D.

Delegate Vote

Agree: 98%, Disagree: 2%, Abstain: 0% (Strong Consensus)

Question 11

- **Should extended antibiotic treatment be given to patients following I & D? If so, what are the indications, type of antibiotic, dose and duration of treatment?**

<u>Consensus:</u> No. Extended antibiotic should only be administered to patients that meet the criteria for PJI (see workgroup 7). The type, dose and duration of antibiotic treatment for infected cases should be determined in consultation with an ID specialist.

Delegate Vote

Agree: 75%, Disagree: 20%, Abstain: 5% (Strong Consensus)

Question 12

- **Is there a role for intra-articular local antibiotic treatment after I & D? If so, define indications.**

<u>Consensus:</u> No. There is inadequate evidence to support administration of continuous intra-articular antibiotics for the treatment of PJI.

Delegate Vote

Agree: 89%, Disagree: 7%, Abstain: 4% (Strong Consensus)

Question 13

- **Is there a role for the use of resorbable antibiotic-impregnated pellets (calcium sulfate, etc)? If so, define indications for use.**

<u>Consensus:</u> No. Currently there is no conclusive evidence that the use of antibiotic-impregnated resorbable material improves the outcome of surgical intervention for I & D.

Delegate Vote

Agree: 88%, Disagree: 6%, Abstain: 6% (Strong Consensus)

11 抗菌薬治療と再置換術のタイミング

Workgroup 11: Antibiotic Treatment and Timing of Reimplantation

Question 1

- 人工関節周囲感染（PJI）の人工関節抜去後の初期治療で，経口抗菌薬治療は点滴の代わりとなりうるか？

コンセンサス

PJIの治療法の1つとして，原因菌に特異的で生物学的利用性が高い経口抗菌薬治療を支持するエビデンスがある．

（参考文献　1-7）

投票結果

同意：79%，反対：11%，棄権：1%（強いコンセンサス）

Question 2

- 初期の抗菌薬点滴加療後に経口抗菌薬治療は適切か？

コンセンサス

点滴による抗菌薬治療を行った後のPJIの治療法の1つとして，原因菌に特異的で生物学的利用性が高い経口抗菌薬治療が適切であることを支持するエビデンスがある．（参考文献　8-11）

投票結果

同意：98%，反対：1%，棄権：1%（強いコンセンサス）

Question 3

- 感染インプラント抜去後の適切な抗菌薬投与期間はどれくらいか？

コンセンサス

適切な抗菌薬投与期間についての明らかなエビデンスはないが，2週間から6週間の抗菌薬投与を推奨する．

（参考文献　6, 8-17）

投票結果

同意：93%，反対：5%，棄権：2%（強いコンセンサス）

Question 4

- 抗菌薬投与期間はどのように決定するべきか？（炎症マーカー，臨床所見など）

コンセンサス

抗菌薬投与期間をどのように決定するべきかについての明らかなエビデンスはない．臨床徴候，臨床症状および生物学的マーカーを総合的に判断する必要がある．最適な再置換術のタイミングを判断するためのマーカーが必要である．

(参考文献 18-29)

投票結果
同意：96％，反対：3％，棄権：1％（強いコンセンサス）

Question 5

- 再置換術前に抗菌薬の休薬期間は必要か？

コンセンサス

感染の治癒を確かめるための手段として，再置換術前に抗菌薬中止後の休薬期間を設けることを支持する明らかなエビデンスはない．(参考文献 30-33)

投票結果
同意：74％，反対：22％，棄権：4％（強いコンセンサス）

Question 6

- 感染インプラント抜去後の点滴抗菌薬治療にリファンピンを併用することは，ブドウ球菌感染症（特にメチシリン耐性黄色ブドウ球菌〔MRSA〕）に対してより迅速で確実な治癒につながるか？

コンセンサス

点滴抗菌薬治療にリファンピンを併用することが，インプラント抜去後に他の抗菌薬で単剤治療を行うことよりも適切な治療オプションとなることを支持するエビデンスはない．

(参考文献 1, 34-38)

投票結果
同意：77％，反対：18％，棄権：5％（強いコンセンサス）

Question 7

- リファンピン投与を開始する最も適切なタイミングはいつか？

コンセンサス

リファンピン投与を開始する最適なタイミングについて明らかなエビデンスはない．リファンピン開始前に，初期の抗菌薬の良好な経口摂取と適切な投与法が確立されるべきである．治療開始前と治療終了前に，起こりうる副作用および薬物相互作用について評価しておくべきである．（参考文献 39，40）

投票結果

同意：83％，反対：11％，棄権：6％（強いコンセンサス）

Question 8

- PJI に対して施行された一期的（人工関節）再置換術後，どのくらいの期間抗菌薬投与を継続すべきか？

コンセンサス

一期的再置換術後の適切な抗菌薬投与期間についての明らかなエビデンスはない．一期的再置換術後，2〜6週間の点滴抗菌薬治療を行った上で，さらに経口抗菌薬をより長期間投与することの検討を推奨する．（参考文献 1，7，12，34，35，41-43）

投票結果

同意：87％，反対：10％，棄権：3％（強いコンセンサス）

Question 9

- 再置換術後の関節内局所抗菌薬投与は有用か？　もし有用であればその適応は？

コンセンサス

関節内局所抗菌薬投与を支持する明らかなエビデンスはない．関節内局所抗菌薬投与を支持するさらなるエビデンスが必要である．（参考文献 44-45）

投票結果

同意：95％，反対：4％，棄権：1％（強いコンセンサス）

Question 10
- 培養陰性のPJIに対する最適な抗菌薬の治療法は？

コンセンサス
培養陰性のPJIにおける最適な抗菌薬の治療法についての明らかなエビデンスはない．グラム陰性菌，グラム陽性菌（MRSAを含む），および嫌気性菌をカバーする広域スペクトラムの抗菌薬の投与を推奨する．真菌感染症疑いの患者では，一般的な真菌に対する治療も考慮するべきである．(参考文献 46-48)

投票結果
同意：91%，反対：8%，棄権：1%（強いコンセンサス）

Question 11
- 再置換術前の関節穿刺は必要か？

コンセンサス
再置換術前に関節穿刺を行うことを支持する明らかなエビデンスはない．症例によっては有益であろう．初回の関節穿刺で関節液貯留を認めなかった患者に対して，罹患関節への液体注入および追加穿刺を施行することは推奨しない．
(参考文献 19, 49-51)

投票結果
同意：89%，反対：8%，棄権：3%（強いコンセンサス）

【掲載されている論文】

Antibiotic treatment and timing of reimplantation.
Restrepo C, Schmitt S, Backstein D, Alexander BT, Babic M, Brause BD, Esterhai JL, Good RP, Jørgensen PH, Lee P, Marculescu C, Mella C, Perka C, Pour AE, Rubash HE, Saito T, Suarez R, Townsend R, Tözün IR, Van den Bekerom MP.
J Arthroplasty. 2014 Feb；29(2 Suppl)：104-7. doi：10.1016/j.arth.2013.09.047. Epub 2013 Oct 1. No abstract available.
PMID：24360490

References:

1. Farhad R, Roger PM, Albert C, et al. Six weeks antibiotic therapy for all bone infections: results of a cohort study. Eur J Clin Microbiol Infect Dis. 2010;29(2):217-222.
2. Gomez J, Canovas E, Banos V, et al. Linezolid plus rifampin as a salvage therapy in prosthetic joint infections treated without removing the implant. Antimicrob Agents Chemother. 2011;55(9):4308-4310.
3. Peel TN, Buising KL, Dowsey MM, et al. Outcome of debridement and retention in prosthetic joint infections by methicillin-resistant staphylococci, with special reference to rifampin and fusidic acid combination therapy. Antimicrob Agents Chemother. 2013;57(1):350-355.
4. Toma MB, Smith KM, Martin CA, Rapp RP. Pharmacokinetic considerations in the treatment of methicillin-resistant Staphylococcus aureus osteomyelitis. Orthopedics. 2006;29(6):497-501.
5. Trampuz A, Zimmerli W. Antimicrobial agents in orthopaedic surgery: Prophylaxis and treatment. Drugs. 2006;66(8):1089-1105.
6. Stockley I, Mockford BJ, Hoad-Reddick A, Norman P. The use of two-stage exchange arthroplasty with depot antibiotics in the absence of long-term antibiotic therapy in infected total hip replacement. J Bone Joint Surg Br. 2008;90(2):145-148.
7. Osmon DR, Berbari EF, Berendt AR, Dhar Diagnosis and management of prosthetic joint infection: clinical practice guidelines by the Infectious Diseases Society of America. Clin Infect Dis. 2013;56(1):e1-e25.
8. Bertazzoni Minelli E, Caveiari C, Benini A. Release of antibiotics from polymethylmethacrylate cement. J Chemother. 2002;14(5):492-500.
9. Dubee V, Zeller V, Lhotellier L, et al. Continuous high-dose vancomycin combination therapy for methicillin-resistant staphylococcal prosthetic hip infection: a prospective cohort study. Clin Microbiol Infect. 2013;19(2):E98-105.
10. Masri BA, Panagiotopoulos KP, Greidanus NV, Garbuz DS, Duncan CP. Cementless two-stage exchange arthroplasty for infection after total hip arthroplasty. J Arthroplasty. 2007;22(1):72-78.
11. Darley ES, Bannister GC, Blom AW, Macgowan AP, Jacobson SK, Alfouzan W. Role of early intravenous to oral antibiotic switch therapy in the management of prosthetic hip infection treated with one- or two-stage replacement. J Antimicrob Chemother. 2011;66(10):2405-2408.
12. Esposito S, Esposito I, Leone S. Considerations of antibiotic therapy duration in community- and hospital-acquired bacterial infections. J Antimicrob Chemother. 2012;67(11):2570-2575.
13. Hsieh PH, Shih CH, Chang YH, Lee MS, Shih HN, Yang WE. Two-stage revision hip arthroplasty for infection: comparison between the interim use of antibiotic-loaded cement beads and a spacer prosthesis. J Bone Joint Surg Am. 2004;86-A(9):1989-1997.
14. McKenna PB, O'Shea K, Masterson EL. Two-stage revision of infected hip arthroplasty using a shortened post-operative course of antibiotics. Arch Orthop Trauma Surg. 2009;129(4):489-494.
15. Senthi S, Munro JT, Pitto RP. Infection in total hip replacement: meta-analysis. Int Orthop. 2011;35(2):253-260.
16. Whittaker JP, Warren RE, Jones RS, Gregson PA. Is prolonged systemic antibiotic treatment essential in two-stage revision hip replacement for chronic Gram-positive infection? J Bone Joint Surg Br. 2009;91(1):44-51.
17. Bernard L, Legout L, Zurcher-Pfund L, et al. Six weeks of antibiotic treatment is sufficient following surgery for septic arthroplasty. J Infect. 2010;61(2):125-132.
18. Glassman AH, Lachiewicz PF, Tanzer M, eds. Orthopaedic Knowledge Update 4: Hip and Knee Reconstruction. 4th ed: American Academy of Orthopaedics; 2011.
19. Kusuma SK, Ward J, Jacofsky M, Sporer SM, Della Valle CJ. What is the role of serological testing between stages of two-stage reconstruction of the infected prosthetic knee? Clin Orthop Relat Res. 2011;469(4):1002-1008.
20. Larsson S, Thelander U, Friberg S. C-reactive protein (CRP) levels after elective orthopedic surgery. Clin Orthop Relat Res. 1992(275):237-242.
21. Schinsky MF, Della Valle CJ, Sporer SM, Paprosky WG. Perioperative testing for joint infection in patients undergoing revision total hip arthroplasty. J Bone Joint Surg Am. 2008;90(9):1869-1875.
22. Shukla SK, Ward JP, Jacofsky MC, Sporer SM, Paprosky WG, Della Valle CJ. Perioperative testing for persistent sepsis following resection arthroplasty of the hip for periprosthetic infection. J Arthroplasty. 2010;25(6 Suppl):87-91.
23. Spangehl MJ, Masri BA, O'Connell JX, Duncan CP. Prospective analysis of preoperative and intraoperative investigations for the diagnosis of infection at the sites of two hundred and two revision total hip arthroplasties. J Bone Joint Surg Am. 1999;81(5):672-683.
24. Ghanem E, Antoci V, Jr., Pulido L, Joshi A, Hozack W, Parvizi J. The use of receiver operating characteristics analysis in determining erythrocyte sedimentation rate and C-reactive protein levels in diagnosing periprosthetic infection prior to revision total hip arthroplasty. Int J Infect Dis. 2009;13(6):e444-449.

25. Pundiche M, Sarbu V, Unc OD, et al. [Role of procalcitonin in monitoring the antibiotic therapy in septic surgical patients]. Chirurgia (Bucur). 2012;107(1):71-78.
26. Jacovides CL, Parvizi J, Adeli B, Jung KA. Molecular markers for diagnosis of periprosthetic joint infection. J Arthroplasty. 2011;26(6 Suppl):99-103 e101.
27. Parvizi J, Jacovides C, Antoci V, Ghanem E. Diagnosis of periprosthetic joint infection: the utility of a simple yet unappreciated enzyme. J Bone Joint Surg Am. 2012;93(24):2242-2248.
28. Parvizi J, Walinchus L, Adeli B. Molecular diagnostics in periprosthetic joint infection. Int J Artif Organs. 2011;34(9):847-855.
29. Deirmengian C, Hallab N, Tarabishy A, et al. Synovial fluid biomarkers for periprosthetic infection. Clin Orthop Relat Res. 2010;468(8):2017-2023.
30. Bejon P, Berendt A, Atkins BL, et al. Two-stage revision for prosthetic joint infection: predictors of outcome and the role of reimplantation microbiology. J Antimicrob Chemother. 2010;65(3):569-575.
31. Hozack WJ, Parvizi J. New definition for periprosthetic joint infection. J Arthroplasty. 2011;26(8):1135.
32. Parvizi J. New definition for periprosthetic joint infection. Am J Orthop (Belle Mead NJ). 2011;40(12):614-615.
33. Parvizi J, Zmistowski B, Berbari EF, et al. New definition for periprosthetic joint infection: from the Workgroup of the Musculoskeletal Infection Society. Clin Orthop Relat Res. 2011;469(11):2992-2994.
34. Esposito S, Leone S, Bassetti M, et al. Italian guidelines for the diagnosis and infectious disease management of osteomyelitis and prosthetic joint infections in adults. Infection. 2009;37(6):478-496.
35. Zimmerli W, Widmer AF, Blatter M, Frei R, Ochsner PE. Role of rifampin for treatment of orthopedic implant-related staphylococcal infections: a randomized controlled trial. Foreign-Body Infection (FBI) Study Group. JAMA. 20 1998;279(19):1537-1541.
36. Zimmerli W, Trampuz A, Ochsner PE. Prosthetic-joint infections. N Engl J Med. 2004;351(16):1645-1654.
37. San Juan R, Garcia-Reyne A, Caba P, et al. Safety and efficacy of moxifloxacin monotherapy for treatment of orthopedic implant-related staphylococcal infections. Antimicrob Agents Chemother. 2010;54(12):5161-5166.
38. Forrest GN, Tamura K. Rifampin combination therapy for nonmycobacterial infections. Clin Microbiol Rev. 2010;23(1):14-34.
39. Lai CC, Tan CK, Lin SH, Liao CH, Huang YT, Hsueh PR. Emergence of rifampicin resistance during rifampicin-containing treatment in elderly patients with persistent methicillin-resistant Staphylococcus aureus bacteremia. J Am Geriatr Soc. 2010;58(5):1001-1003.
40. Achermann Y, Eigenmann K, Ledergerber B, et al. Factors associated with rifampin resistance in staphylococcal periprosthetic joint infections (PJI): a matched case-control study. Infection. 2013;41(2):431-437.
41. Rudelli S, Uip D, Honda E, Lima AL. One-stage revision of infected total hip arthroplasty with bone graft. J Arthroplasty. 2008;23(8):1165-1177.
42. Winkler H, Stoiber A, Kaudela K, Winter F, Menschik F. One stage uncemented revision of infected total hip replacement using cancellous allograft bone impregnated with antibiotics. J Bone Joint Surg Br. 2008;90(12):1580-1584.
43. Yoo JJ, Kwon YS, Koo KH, Yoon KS, Kim YM, Kim HJ. One-stage cementless revision arthroplasty for infected hip replacements. Int Orthop. 2009;33(5):1195-1201.
44. Whiteside LA, Nayfeh TA, LaZear R, Roy ME. Reinfected revised TKA resolves with an aggressive protocol and antibiotic infusion. Clin Orthop Relat Res. 2012;470(1):236-243.
45. Whiteside LA, Peppers M, Nayfeh TA, Roy ME. Methicillin-resistant Staphylococcus aureus in TKA treated with revision and direct intra-articular antibiotic infusion. Clin Orthop Relat Res. 2011;469(1):26-33.
46. Choi HR, Kwon YM, Freiberg AA, Nelson SB, Malchau H. Periprosthetic joint infection with negative culture results: clinical characteristics and treatment outcome. J Arthroplasty. 2013;28(6):899-903.
47. Huang R, Hu CC, Adeli B, Mortazavi J, Parvizi J. Culture-negative periprosthetic joint infection does not preclude infection control. Clin Orthop Relat Res. 2012;470(10):2717-2723.
48. Marschall J, Lane MA, Beekmann SE, Polgreen PM, Babcock HM. Current management of prosthetic joint infections in adults: results of an Emerging Infections Network survey. Int J Antimicrob Agents. 2013;41(3):272-277.
49. Ghanem E, Azzam K, Seeley M, Joshi A, Parvizi J. Staged revision for knee arthroplasty infection: what is the role of serologic tests before reimplantation? Clin Orthop Relat Res. 2009;467(7):1699-1705.
50. Lonner JH, Siliski JM, Della Valle C, DiCesare P, Lotke PA. Role of knee aspiration after resection of the infected total knee arthroplasty. Am J Orthop (Belle Mead NJ). 2001;30(4):305-309.
51. Mont MA, Waldman BJ, Hungerford DS. Evaluation of preoperative cultures before second-stage reimplantation of a total knee prosthesis complicated by infection. A comparison-group study. J Bone Joint Surg Am. 2000;82-A(11):1552-1557.

Question 1

- **Can oral antibiotic therapy be used instead of intravenous for the initial treatment of periprosthetic joint infection (PJI) following resection?**

Consensus: There is evidence to support pathogen-specific, highly bioavailable oral antibiotic therapy as a choice for the treatment of PJI.

Delegate Vote

Agree: 79%, Disagree: 11%, Abstain: 1% (Strong Consensus)

Question 2

- **Is oral antibiotic therapy appropriate after an initial IV antibiotic course?**

Consensus: There is evidence that pathogen-specific, highly bioavailable oral antibiotic therapy is an appropriate choice for the treatment of PJI after an initial IV antibiotic regimen.

Delegate Vote

Agree: 98%, Disagree: 1%, Abstain: 1% (Strong Consensus)

Question 3

- **What is the ideal length of antibiotic treatment following removal of the infected implant?**

Consensus: There is no conclusive evidence regarding the ideal duration of antibiotic therapy. However, we recommend a period of antibiotic therapy between 2 to 6 weeks.

Delegate Vote

Agree: 93%, Disagree: 5%, Abstain: 2% (Strong Consensus)

Question 4

- **How should the length of antibiotic treatment be determined? (Inflammatory markers, clinical signs, etc).**

Consensus: There is no conclusive evidence on how to determine the length of antibiotic therapy. A combination of clinical signs and symptoms and biochemical markers may be employed. There is the need for a marker that can determine the optimal timing for reimplantation.

Delegate Vote

Agree: 96%, Disagree: 3%, Abstain: 1% (Strong Consensus)

Question 5

- **Should there be an antibiotic holiday period prior to reimplantation?**

<u>Consensus:</u> There is no conclusive evidence supporting a holiday period following discontinuation of antibiotic treatment and prior to reimplantation surgery as a means of ensuring eradication of infection.

Delegate Vote

Agree: 74%, Disagree: 22%, Abstain: 4% (Strong Consensus)

Question 6

- **Does the use of rifampin in conjunction with IV antibiotic therapy following removal of the infected implant lead to a more rapid and definitive eradication of staphylococcal infection (particularly methicillin-resistant *Staphylococcus aureus* [MRSA])?**

<u>Consensus:</u> There is no evidence to support the use of rifampin in conjunction with IV antibiotic therapy as a more adequate treatment option than either agent used alone following implant removal.

Delegate Vote

Agree: 77%, Disagree: 18%, Abstain: 5% (Strong Consensus)

Question 7

- **What is the optimal time to start rifampin treatment?**

<u>Consensus:</u> There is no conclusive evidence regarding the best time to start rifampin treatment. Good oral intake and adequate administration of a primary antimicrobial agent should be well-established before starting rifampin. Potential side effects and drug interactions should be addressed prior to the start and at the conclusion of therapy.

Delegate Vote

Agree: 83%, Disagree: 11%, Abstain: 6% (Strong Consensus)

Question 8

- **How long should antibiotic treatment be given following a single-stage exchange arthroplasty performed for PJI?**

Consensus: There is no conclusive evidence regarding the ideal duration of antibiotic therapy for a single-stage exchange arthroplasty. We recommend that parenteral antibiotic be given for 2 to 6 weeks following single-stage exchange arthroplasty, with consideration for longer-term oral antibiotic therapy.

Delegate Vote

Agree: 87%, Disagree: 10%, Abstain: 3% (Strong Consensus)

Question 9

- **Is there a role for intra-articular local antibiotic treatment after reimplantation? If so, what are the indications?**

Consensus: There is no conclusive evidence to support the use of intra-articular local antibiotic therapy. Further evidence is needed to support the use of intra-articular local antibiotic therapy.

Delegate Vote

Agree: 95%, Disagree: 4%, Abstain: 1% (Strong Consensus)

Question 10

- **What is the optimal antibiotic treatment for culture-negative PJI?**

Consensus: There is no conclusive evidence on the optimal antibiotic treatment for patients with culture-negative PJI. We recommend a broad spectrum antibiotic regimen covering gram-negative and gram-positive organisms (including MRSA) as well as anaerobic organisms. In patients with suspected fungal infection, coverage against common fungi should be considered.

Delegate Vote

Agree: 91%, Disagree: 8%, Abstain: 1% (Strong Consensus)

Question 11

- **Is joint aspiration necessary prior to reimplantation?**

Consensus: There is no conclusive evidence to support mandatory joint aspiration prior to reimplantation. It may be useful in selected cases. We recommend against infiltration of any liquids into the affected joint and reaspiration in patients with an initial dry aspirate.

Delegate Vote

Agree: 89%, Disagree: 8%, Abstain: 3% (Strong Consensus)

12 一期的再置換術 vs 二期的再置換術

Workgroup 12：One-stage vs Two-stage Exchange

Question 1

- 一期的（人工関節）再置換術の適応と禁忌は？

コンセンサス

一期的再置換術は，薬剤感受性のある抗菌薬が存在する人工関節周囲感染（PJI）患者には適切であるが，全身の感染症状（敗血症）があり，切除関節形成術や汚染微生物数減少が必要と考えらえる患者には適さない．一期的再置換術を行う上での相対的禁忌は，術前に原因菌が同定できないこと，瘻孔の存在，組織片の被覆を必要とする重度の軟部組織病変が存在する場合である．（参考文献 1-33）

投票結果

同意：78％，反対：17％，棄権：5％（強いコンセンサス）

Question 2

- 二期的（人工関節）再置換術の適応は？

コンセンサス

二期的再置換術は，PJI の治療に適切な選択肢である．一期的再置換術よりも二期的再置換術が適する状態は，以下のとおりである．1）全身の感染症状（敗血症）のある患者，2）感染は明らかだが，原因菌が同定できない場合，3）術前培養により原因菌の治療が困難で耐性菌であると判明した場合，4）瘻孔が存在する場合，5）周囲軟部組織の状態が不良で被覆が困難な場合．（参考文献 4，7，9，17，18，32，34-36）

投票結果

同意：93％，反対：7％，棄権：0％（強いコンセンサス）

Question 3

- 二期的再置換術の最適な待機期間はどれくらいか？

コンセンサス

二期的再置換術の最適な待機期間について，文献では明確なエビデンスがない．報告により 2 週間から数カ月までばらつきがある．（参考文献 7, 18, 37-45）

投票結果

同意：87％，反対：9％，棄権：4％（強いコンセンサス）

Question 4

- 一期的再置換術と二期的再置換術ではコストに差があるか？

コンセンサス

実際にかかった費用に関する知識が不足していることと，比較研究がないことから，明確に回答することはできない．しかし，感染が再手術の必要なく順調に治療されれば，一期的再置換術は二期的再置換術よりも低コストである．さらなる研究が必要である．（参考文献 4, 7, 30, 46-56）

投票結果

同意：91％，反対：5％，棄権：4％（強いコンセンサス）

Question 5

- PJI 患者には，再置換術は何回行うべきか？

コンセンサス

感染部位の再置換の回数制限を裏付ける決定的なエビデンスはない．再切除後に感染が適切に管理され，患者が再手術に耐えることができ，手術により適切な軟部組織の被覆が得られ関節が機能するのであれば，再置換術は妥当である．

（参考文献 1, 3, 7, 17, 23, 25, 28, 31, 55, 57-63）

投票結果

同意：98％，反対：2％，棄権：0％（強いコンセンサス）

Question 6

- 膝関節固定術の適応は？

コンセンサス

この問題に対する提言を行うには文献が不足している．膝関

節固定術は，再建の試みに複数回失敗した患者，人工関節再置換術後の再感染リスクが非常に高い患者，あるいは膝伸筋機構が欠損している患者では適切な選択肢であると考えられる．関節固定術か切断術かの選択は，患者の臨床的状態と希望を考慮に入れる必要がある．

(参考文献　2, 7, 9, 17, 18, 25, 43, 55, 56, 59, 60, 64-66)

投票結果

同意：96%，反対：1%，棄権：3%（強いコンセンサス）

Question 7

- 感染が慢性化した関節に膝関節固定術を計画する場合，一期的か二期的のどちらで行うべきか？

コンセンサス

膝関節固定術を一期的か二期的のどちらで行うかは，患者の状態や宿主因子による．(参考文献　2, 4, 7, 11-18, 25, 40, 65, 67-82)

投票結果

同意：94%，反対：3%，棄権：3%（強いコンセンサス）

Question 8

- 切断術の適応は？

コンセンサス

膝あるいは股関節の PJI 治療として切断術が適切なのは，歩行不能な患者，積極的なデブリドマンの効果がない壊死性筋膜炎，関節固定術（膝）が不可能な重篤な骨欠損，軟部組織の被覆が不十分であること，段階的置換や切除関節形成術に複数回失敗していること，末梢血管疾患，神経血管損傷のいずれかの場合である．(参考文献　2, 3, 7, 17, 18, 25, 45, 56, 59, 83-86)

投票結果

同意：98%，反対：1%，棄権：1%（強いコンセンサス）

【掲載されている論文】

One-Stage vs Two-Stage Exchange.

Lichstein P, Gehrke T, Lombardi A, Romano C, Stockley I, Babis G, Bialecki J, Bucsi L, Cai X, Cao L, de Beaubien B, Erhardt J, Goodman S, Jiranek W, Keogh P, Lewallen D, Manner P, Marczynski W, Mason JB, Mulhall K, Paprosky W, Patel P,

Piccaluga F, Polkowski G, Pulido L, Stockley I, Suarez J, Thorey F, Tikhilov R, Velazquez JD, Winkler H.

J Arthroplasty. 2014 Feb;29(2 Suppl):108-11. doi:10.1016/j.arth.2013.09.048. Epub 2013 Oct 1. No abstract available.

PMID: 24360339

References:

1. Casanova D, Hulard O, Zalta R, Bardot J, Magalon G. Management of wounds of exposed or infected knee prostheses. Scand J Plast Reconstr Surg Hand Surg. 2001;35(1):71-77.
2. Conway JD, Mont MA, Bezwada HP. Arthrodesis of the knee. J Bone Joint Surg Am. 2004;86-A(4):835-848.
3. Hanssen AD, Trousdale RT, Osmon DR. Patient outcome with reinfection following reimplantation for the infected total knee arthroplasty. Clin Orthop Relat Res. 1995(321):55-67.
4. Jackson WO, Schmalzried TP. Limited role of direct exchange arthroplasty in the treatment of infected total hip replacements. Clin Orthop Relat Res. 2000(381):101-105.
5. Jamsen E, Sheng P, Halonen P, et al. Spacer prostheses in two-stage revision of infected knee arthroplasty. Int Orthop. 2006;30(4):257-261.
6. Nahabedian MY, Orlando JC, Delanois RE, Mont MA, Hungerford DS. Salvage procedures for complex soft tissue defects of the knee. Clin Orthop Relat Res. 1998(356):119-124.
7. Osmon DR, Berbari EF, Berendt AR, et al. Executive summary: diagnosis and management of prosthetic joint infection: clinical practice guidelines by the Infectious Diseases Society of America. Clin Infect Dis. 2013;56(1):1-10.
8. Parkinson RW, Kay PR, Rawal A. A case for one-stage revision in infected total knee arthroplasty? Knee. 2011;18(1):1-4.
9. Senthi S, Munro JT, Pitto RP. Infection in total hip replacement: meta-analysis. Int Orthop. 2011;35(2):253-260.
10. Winkler H, Stoiber A, Kaudela K, Winter F, Menschik F. One stage uncemented revision of infected total hip replacement using cancellous allograft bone impregnated with antibiotics. J Bone Joint Surg Br. 2008;90(12):1580-1584.
11. Buechel FF, Femino FP, D'Alessio J. Primary exchange revision arthroplasty for infected total knee replacement: a long-term study. Am J Orthop (Belle Mead NJ). 2004;33(4):190-198; discussion 198.
12. Callaghan JJ, Katz RP, Johnston RC. One-stage revision surgery of the infected hip. A minimum 10-year followup study. Clin Orthop Relat Res. 1999(369):139-143.
13. Cordero-Ampuero J, Esteban J, Garcia-Cimbrelo E, Munuera L, Escobar R. Low relapse with oral antibiotics and two-stage exchange for late arthroplasty infections in 40 patients after 2-9 years. Acta Orthop. 2007;78(4):511-519.
14. Engesaeter LB, Dale H, Schrama JC, Hallan G, Lie SA. Surgical procedures in the treatment of 784 infected THAs reported to the Norwegian Arthroplasty Register. Acta Orthop. 2011;82(5):530-537.
15. Goksan SB, Freeman MA. One-stage reimplantation for infected total knee arthroplasty. J Bone Joint Surg Br. 1992;74(1):78-82.
16. Kurd MF, Ghanem E, Steinbrecher J, Parvizi J. Two-stage exchange knee arthroplasty: does resistance of the infecting organism influence the outcome? Clin Orthop Relat Res. 2010;468(8):2060-2066.
17. Parvizi J, Adeli B, Zmistowski B, Restrepo C, Greenwald AS. Management of periprosthetic joint infection: the current knowledge: AAOS exhibit selection. J Bone Joint Surg Am. 2012;94(14):e104.
18. Zimmerli W, Trampuz A, Ochsner PE. Prosthetic-joint infections. N Engl J Med. 2004;351(16):1645-1654.
19. Buchholz HW, Elson RA, Engelbrecht E, Lodenkamper H, Rottger J, Siegel A. Management of deep infection of total hip replacement. J Bone Joint Surg Br. 1981;63-B(3):342-353.
20. Cordero-Ampuero J, Esteban J, Garcia-Cimbrelo E. Oral antibiotics are effective for highly resistant hip arthroplasty infections. Clin Orthop Relat Res. 2009;467(9):2335-2342.
21. Deirmengian C, Greenbaum J, Stern J, et al. Open debridement of acute gram-positive infections after total knee arthroplasty. Clin Orthop Relat Res. 2003(416):129-134.
22. Huang R, Hu CC, Adeli B, Mortazavi J, Parvizi J. Culture-negative periprosthetic joint infection does not preclude infection control. Clin Orthop Relat Res. 2012;470(10):2717-2723.

23. Leung F, Richards CJ, Garbuz DS, Masri BA, Duncan CP. Two-stage total hip arthroplasty: how often does it control methicillin-resistant infection? Clin Orthop Relat Res. 2011;469(4):1009-1015.
24. Mortazavi SM, Vegari D, Ho A, Zmistowski B, Parvizi J. Two-stage exchange arthroplasty for infected total knee arthroplasty: predictors of failure. Clin Orthop Relat Res. 2011;469(11):3049-3054.
25. Rasouli MR, Tripathi MS, Kenyon R, Wetters N, Della Valle CJ, Parvizi J. Low rate of infection control in enterococcal periprosthetic joint infections. Clin Orthop Relat Res. 2012;470(10):2708-2716.
26. Raut VV, Siney PD, Wroblewski BM. One-stage revision of infected total hip replacements with discharging sinuses. J Bone Joint Surg Br. 1994;76(5):721-724.
27. Rudelli S, Uip D, Honda E, Lima AL. One-stage revision of infected total hip arthroplasty with bone graft. J Arthroplasty. 2008;23(8):1165-1177.
28. Singer J, Merz A, Frommelt L, Fink B. High rate of infection control with one-stage revision of septic knee prostheses excluding MRSA and MRSE. Clin Orthop Relat Res. 2012;470(5):1461-1471.
29. Ueng SW, Lee CY, Hu CC, Hsieh PH, Chang Y. What is the success of treatment of hip and knee candidal periprosthetic joint infection? Clin Orthop Relat Res. 2013;471(9):3002-3009.
30. Ure KJ, Amstutz HC, Nasser S, Schmalzried TP. Direct-exchange arthroplasty for the treatment of infection after total hip replacement. An average ten-year follow-up. J Bone Joint Surg Am. 1998;80(7):961-968.
31. Walls RJ, Roche SJ, O'Rourke A, McCabe JP. Surgical site infection with methicillin-resistant Staphylococcus aureus after primary total hip replacement. J Bone Joint Surg Br. 2008;90(3):292-298.
32. Wongworawat MD. Clinical faceoff: One- versus two-stage exchange arthroplasty for prosthetic joint infections. Clin Orthop Relat Res. 2013;471(6):1750-1753.
33. Yoo JJ, Kwon YS, Koo KH, Yoon KS, Kim YM, Kim HJ. One-stage cementless revision arthroplasty for infected hip replacements. Int Orthop. 2009;33(5):1195-1201.
34. Berend KR, Lombardi AV, Jr., Morris MJ, Bergeson AG, Adams JB, Sneller MA. Two-stage treatment of hip periprosthetic joint infection is associated with a high rate of infection control but high mortality. Clin Orthop Relat Res. 2013;471(2):510-518.
35. Romano CL, Gala L, Logoluso N, Romano D, Drago L. Two-stage revision of septic knee prosthesis with articulating knee spacers yields better infection eradication rate than one-stage or two-stage revision with static spacers. Knee Surg Sports Traumatol Arthrosc. 2012;20(12):2445-2453.
36. Romano D, Drago L, Romano CL, Logoluso N. Does two-stage revision of septic hip prosthesis provides better infection eradication rate than one-stage? . Paper presented at: 14th EFFORT Congress, 2013; Istanbul.
37. Brandt CM, Duffy MC, Berbari EF, Hanssen AD, Steckelberg JM, Osmon DR. Staphylococcus aureus prosthetic joint infection treated with prosthesis removal and delayed reimplantation arthroplasty. Mayo Clin Proc. 1999;74(6):553-558.
38. Hanssen AD, Rand JA, Osmon DR. Treatment of the infected total knee arthroplasty with insertion of another prosthesis. The effect of antibiotic-impregnated bone cement. Clin Orthop Relat Res. 1994(309):44-55.
39. Segawa H, Tsukayama DT, Kyle RF, Becker DA, Gustilo RB. Infection after total knee arthroplasty. A retrospective study of the treatment of eighty-one infections. J Bone Joint Surg Am. 1999;81(10):1434-1445.
40. Westrich GH, Walcott-Sapp S, Bornstein LJ, Bostrom MP, Windsor RE, Brause BD. Modern treatment of infected total knee arthroplasty with a 2-stage reimplantation protocol. J Arthroplasty. 2013;25(7):1015-1021, 1021 e1011-1012.
41. Joseph J, Raman R, Macdonald DA. Time interval between first and second stage revision hip arthroplasty for infection, the effect on outcome. J Bone Joint Surg Br. 2003;85-B(Suppl):58.
42. Ghanem E, Azzam K, Seeley M, Joshi A, Parvizi J. Staged revision for knee arthroplasty infection: what is the role of serologic tests before reimplantation? Clin Orthop Relat Res. 2009;467(7):1699-1705.
43. Kusuma SK, Ward J, Jacofsky M, Sporer SM, Della Valle CJ. What is the role of serological testing between stages of two-stage reconstruction of the infected prosthetic knee? Clin Orthop Relat Res. 2011;469(4):1002-1008.
44. Shukla SK, Ward JP, Jacofsky MC, Sporer SM, Paprosky WG, Della Valle CJ. Perioperative testing for persistent sepsis following resection arthroplasty of the hip for periprosthetic infection. J Arthroplasty. 2010;25(6 Suppl):87-91.
45. Springer BD, Lee GC, Osmon D, Haidukewych GJ, Hanssen AD, Jacofsky DJ. Systemic safety of high-dose antibiotic-loaded cement spacers after resection of an infected total knee arthroplasty. Clin Orthop Relat Res. 2004(427):47-51.
46. Bozic KJ, Ries MD. The impact of infection after total hip arthroplasty on hospital and surgeon resource utilization. J Bone Joint Surg Am. 2005;87(8):1746-1751.
47. Parvizi J, Pawasarat IM, Azzam KA, Joshi A, Hansen EN, Bozic KJ. Periprosthetic joint

infection: the economic impact of methicillin-resistant infections. J Arthroplasty. 2010;25(6 Suppl):103-107.
48. Sculco TP. The economic impact of infected total joint arthroplasty. Instr Course Lect. 1993;42:349-351.
49. Gehrke T, Kendoff D. Peri-prosthetic hip infections: in favour of one-stage. Hip Int. 2012;22 Suppl 8:S40-45.
50. Kurtz SM, Lau E, Watson H, Schmier JK, Parvizi J. Economic burden of periprosthetic joint infection in the United States. J Arthroplasty. 2012;27(8 Suppl):61-65 e61.
51. Peel TN, Dowsey MM, Buising KL, Liew D, Choong PF. Cost analysis of debridement and retention for management of prosthetic joint infection. Clin Microbiol Infect. 2013;19(2):181-186.
52. Klouche S, Sariali E, Mamoudy P. Total hip arthroplasty revision due to infection: a cost analysis approach. Orthop Traumatol Surg Res. 2010;96(2):124-132.
53. De Man FH, Sendi P, Zimmerli W, Maurer TB, Ochsner PE, Ilchmann T. Infectiological, functional, and radiographic outcome after revision for prosthetic hip infection according to a strict algorithm. Acta Orthop. 2011;82(1):27-34.
54. Wolf CF, Gu NY, Doctor JN, Manner PA, Leopold SS. Comparison of one and two-stage revision of total hip arthroplasty complicated by infection: a Markov expected-utility decision analysis. J Bone Joint Surg Am. 2011;93(7):631-639.
55. Filice GA, Nyman JA, Lexau C, et al. Excess costs and utilization associated with methicillin resistance for patients with Staphylococcus aureus infection. Infect Control Hosp Epidemiol. 2010;31(4):365-373.
56. Parvizi J, Azzam K, Ghanem E, Austin MS, Rothman RH. Periprosthetic infection due to resistant staphylococci: serious problems on the horizon. Clin Orthop Relat Res. 2009;467(7):1732-1739.
57. Kalra KP, Lin KK, Bozic KJ, Ries MD. Repeat 2-stage revision for recurrent infection of total hip arthroplasty. J Arthroplasty. 2010;25(6):880-884.
58. Mortazavi SM, O'Neil JT, Zmistowski B, Parvizi J, Purtill JJ. Repeat 2-stage exchange for infected total hip arthroplasty: a viable option? J Arthroplasty. 2012;27(6):923-926 e921.
59. Azzam K, McHale K, Austin M, Purtill JJ, Parvizi J. Outcome of a second two-stage reimplantation for periprosthetic knee infection. Clin Orthop Relat Res. 2009;467(7):1706-1714.
60. Bejon P, Berendt A, Atkins BL, et al. Two-stage revision for prosthetic joint infection: predictors of outcome and the role of reimplantation microbiology. J Antimicrob Chemother. 2010;65(3):569-575.
61. Kubista B, Hartzler RU, Wood CM, Osmon DR, Hanssen AD, Lewallen DG. Reinfection after two-stage revision for periprosthetic infection of total knee arthroplasty. Int Orthop. 2012;36(1):65-71.
62. Maheshwari AV, Gioe TJ, Kalore NV, Cheng EY. Reinfection after prior staged reimplantation for septic total knee arthroplasty: is salvage still possible? J Arthroplasty. 2010;25(6 Suppl):92-97.
63. Pagnano MW, Trousdale RT, Hanssen AD. Outcome after reinfection following reimplantation hip arthroplasty. Clin Orthop Relat Res. 1997(338):192-204.
64. Husted H, Toftgaard Jensen T. Clinical outcome after treatment of infected primary total knee arthroplasty. Acta Orthop Belg. 2002;68(5):500-507.
65. Rand JA, Bryan RS, Chao EY. Failed total knee arthroplasty treated by arthrodesis of the knee using the Ace-Fischer apparatus. J Bone Joint Surg Am. 1987;69(1):39-45.
66. Knutson K, Lindstrand A, Lidgren L. Arthrodesis for failed knee arthroplasty. A report of 20 cases. J Bone Joint Surg Br. 1985;67(1):47-52.
67. Behr JT, Chmell SJ, Schwartz CM. Knee arthrodesis for failed total knee arthroplasty. Arch Surg. 1985;120(3):350-354.
68. Rothacker GW, Jr., Cabanela ME. External fixation for arthrodesis of the knee and ankle. Clin Orthop Relat Res. 1983(180):101-108.
69. Wade PJ, Denham RA. Arthrodesis of the knee after failed knee replacement. J Bone Joint Surg Br. 1984;66(3):362-366.
70. Wilde AH, Stearns KL. Intramedullary fixation for arthrodesis of the knee after infected total knee arthroplasty. Clin Orthop Relat Res. 1989(248):87-92.
71. Bengston S, Knutson K, Lidgren L. Treatment of infected knee arthroplasty. Clin Orthop Relat Res. 1989(245):173-178.
72. Damron TA, McBeath AA. Arthrodesis following failed total knee arthroplasty: comprehensive review and meta-analysis of recent literature. Orthopedics. 1995;18(4):361-368.
73. Knutson K, Hovelius L, Lindstrand A, Lidgren L. Arthrodesis after failed knee arthroplasty. A nationwide multicenter investigation of 91 cases. Clin Orthop Relat Res. 1984(191):202-211.
74. Schoifet SD, Morrey BF. Persistent infection after successful arthrodesis for infected total knee arthroplasty. A report of two cases. J Arthroplasty. 1990;5(3):277-279.
75. Ellingsen DE, Rand JA. Intramedullary arthrodesis of the knee after failed total knee arthroplasty. J Bone Joint Surg Am. 1994;76(6):870-877.
76. Harris CM, Froehlich J. Knee fusion with intramedullary rods for failed total knee

arthroplasty. Clin Orthop Relat Res. 1985(197):209-216.
77. Jorgensen PS, Torholm C. Arthrodesis after infected knee arthroplasty using long arthrodesis nail. A report of five cases. Am J Knee Surg. Summer 1995;8(3):110-113.
78. Lai KA, Shen WJ, Yang CY. Arthrodesis with a short Huckstep nail as a salvage procedure for failed total knee arthroplasty. J Bone Joint Surg Am. 1998;80(3):380-388.
79. Stiehl JB, Hanel DP. Knee arthrodesis using combined intramedullary rod and plate fixation. Clin Orthop Relat Res. 1993(294):238-241.
80. Waldman BJ, Mont MA, Payman KR, et al. Infected total knee arthroplasty treated with arthrodesis using a modular nail. Clin Orthop Relat Res. 1999(367):230-237.
81. Fern ED, Stewart HD, Newton G. Curved Kuntscher nail arthrodesis after failure of knee replacement. J Bone Joint Surg Br. 1989;71(4):588-590.
82. Puranen J, Kortelainen P, Jalovaara P. Arthrodesis of the knee with intramedullary nail fixation. J Bone Joint Surg Am. 1990;72(3):433-442.
83. Isiklar ZU, Landon GC, Tullos HS. Amputation after failed total knee arthroplasty. Clin Orthop Relat Res. 1994(299):173-178.
84. Sierra RJ, Trousdale RT, Pagnano MW. Above-the-knee amputation after a total knee replacement: prevalence, etiology, and functional outcome. J Bone Joint Surg Am. 2003;85-A(6):1000-1004.
85. Fedorka CJ, Chen AF, McGarry WM, Parvizi J, Klatt BA. Functional ability after above-the-knee amputation for infected total knee arthroplasty. Clin Orthop Relat Res. 2011;469(4):1024-1032.
86. Zalavras CG, Rigopoulos N, Ahlmann E, Patzakis MJ. Hip disarticulation for severe lower extremity infections. Clin Orthop Relat Res. 2009;467(7):1721-1726.

Question 1

- **What are the indications and contraindications for one-stage exchange arthroplasty?**

Consensus: One stage-exchange arthroplasty is a reasonable option for the treatment of periprosthetic joint infection (PJI) in circumstances where effective antibiotics are available but not in patients with systemic manifestations of infection (sepsis) in whom resection arthroplasty and reduction of bioburden may be necessary. Relative contraindications to performing a one-stage exchange may include lack of identification of an organism preoperatively, the presence of a sinus tract or severe soft tissue involvement that may lead to the need for flap coverage.

Delegate Vote

Agree: 78%, Disagree: 17%, Abstain: 5% (Strong Consensus)

Question 2

- **What are the indications for two-stage exchange arthroplasty?**

Consensus: Two stage-exchange arthroplasty is a reasonable option for the treatment of periprosthetic joint infection (PJI). Specific conditions where two-stage exchange may be indicated over one-stage exchange include: 1) patients with systemic manifestations of infection (sepsis); 2) the scenario where infection appears ovious but no organism has been identified; 3) preoperative cultures identifying difficult to treat and antibiotic-resistant organisms; 4) presence of a sinus tract, 5) inadequate and non-viable soft tissue coverage.

Delegate Vote

Agree: 93%, Disagree: 7%, Abstain: 0% (Strong Consensus)

Question 3

- **What is the optimal interval between two stages?**

Consensus: There is no definitive evidence in the literature as to the optimal time interval between the two stages. Reports vary from 2 weeks to several months.

Delegate Vote

Agree: 87%, Disagree: 9%, Abstain: 4% (Strong Consensus)

Question 4

- **Is there a difference in cost between one-stage and two-stage exchange arthroplasty?**

Consensus: Due to the lack of knowledge about the real costs and the absence of comparative studies we are not able to give a clear statement. If, however, infection is effectively treated without the need for reoperation, one-stage exchange arthroplasty is less expensive than two- stage exchange. Further studies are required.

Delegate Vote

Agree: 91%, Disagree: 5%, Abstain: 4% (Strong Consensus)

Question 5

- **How many exchange arthroplasty should be attempted in patients with PJI?**

Consensus: There is no definitive evidence that supports limiting the number of septic exchanges that should be attempted. Reimplantation is appropriate if the infection is adequately controlled following repeat resection, the patient is able to tolerate additional surgery, and such surgery will allow for a functioning joint with adequate soft tissue coverage.

Delegate Vote

Agree: 98%, Disagree: 2%, Abstain: 0% (Strong Consensus)

Question 6

- **What are the indications for knee arthrodesis?**

Consensus: The literature is deficient in providing guidance on this issue. Knee arthrodesis may be an appropriate option for patients who have had failed multiple attempts at reconstruction and stand an unacceptably high risk of recurrent infection with repeat arthroplasty procedures and/or has a deficient extensor mechanism. The choice between arthrodesis and amputation needs to take into account the clinical situation of the individual and patient preference.

Delegate Vote

Agree: 96%, Disagree: 1%, Abstain: 3% (Strong Consensus)

Question 7

- **If knee arthrodesis is planned for a chronically infected joint, should this be performed in a single stage or two stages?**

Consensus: Knee arthrodesis may be performed as one stage or two stage, but the decision depends on the individual circumstances and the host factors.

Delegate Vote

Agree: 94%, Disagree: 3%, Abstain: 3% (Strong Consensus)

Question 8

- **What are the indications for amputation?**

Consensus: Amputation for treatment of PJI affecting the knee or the hip may be appropriate in selected cases involving a non-ambulatory patient, necrotizing fasciitis resistant to aggressive debridement, severe bone loss that precludes arthrodesis (knee), inadequate soft tissue coverage, and multiple failed attempts at staged exchange and resection arthroplasty, or peripheral vascular disease and neurovascular injury.

Delegate Vote

Agree: 98%, Disagree: 1%, Abstain: 1% (Strong Consensus)

13 真菌性あるいは非定型的人工関節周囲感染の治療

Workgroup 13：Management of Fungal or Atypical Periprosthetic Joint Infections

Question 1

- 真菌性あるいは非定型的人工関節周囲感染（PJI）の定義は何か？

コンセンサス

真菌性および非定型的 PJI は真菌および非定型細菌によって引き起こされた人工関節の感染である．(参考文献 1-3)

投票結果

同意：89％，反対：7％，棄権：4％（強いコンセンサス）

Question 2

- どのような場合に真菌微生物が PJI の原因だとみなすべきか？

コンセンサス

血清や関節穿刺液の異常所見（好中球数や分画の異常）がある患者において人工関節周囲組織培養や関節穿刺から真菌が同定されたとき，真菌による PJI を考慮するべきである．真菌 PJI を疑う臨床症状があれば，関節穿刺を繰り返す必要がある．
(参考文献 4-10)

投票結果

同意：94％，反対：4％，棄権：2％（強いコンセンサス）

Question 3

- 真菌性 PJI を起こしやすい宿主側の因子（合併症や他の因子）は何か？

コンセンサス

真菌性 PJI を起こしやすい宿主側の因子は，免疫抑制（細胞性免疫減少，好中球減少，コルチコステロイドあるいは他の免疫抑制薬，臓器移植歴，後天性免疫不全症候群），悪性腫瘍，抗がん剤薬の使用，薬物乱用，抗菌薬の長期使用，体内留置カテーテル（静脈内，尿管あるいは経静脈栄養），糖尿病，栄養不

良，関節リウマチ，頻回の腹部手術歴，重度の熱傷，結核，人工挿入物の細菌感染の既往などである．

投票結果
同意：95％，反対：2％，棄権：3％（強いコンセンサス）

人工膝関節置換術後の真菌性人工関節周囲感染46件における併存疾患の頻度（36論文の集計）

併存症	症例数	％
糖尿病	10	22
自己免疫性疾患	6	13
長期間の抗菌薬投与を要した人工関節周囲感染の既往	10	22
投薬による免疫抑制	7	15
悪性疾患	4	9
HIV	1	2

Question 4

- 真菌微生物が対象として考慮される場合，どのような検体が収集されるべきか？ どのような追加診断方法を用いるべきか？ 診断の最適化のために，それらをいかに用いるべきか？

コンセンサス

真菌培養に特有な培地の使用が必須であり，長期間培養が必要であろう．臨床的に真菌感染の疑いが強い一定の症例では，組織サンプルの組織学的診断も追加実施されるべきである．フルコナゾール耐性カンジダ属が文献上報告されており，フルコナゾール耐性カンジダ属が疑われる場合，感受性試験が必要である．抗真菌感受性試験は一般細菌の感受性試験と比べると十分に確立されておらず，利用法も十分に確立していない．

(参考文献 14)

投票結果
同意：96％，反対：2％，棄権：2％（強いコンセンサス）

Question 5

- 真菌性 PJI における最善の外科的治療法は？ 洗浄デブリドマン（I & D），一期的再置換術，二期的再置換術，あるいは切除関節形成術のどれか？

コンセンサス

文献上，真菌性 PJI においては二期的再置換術が推奨される．しかし，その成功率は細菌性 PJI より低い．（参考文献 1, 8, 10-26）

投票結果

同意：95%，反対：2%，棄権：3%（強いコンセンサス）

Question 6

- 真菌性 PJI 治療における最適（理想的）な抗真菌薬全身投与法は何か？（投与経路と種類と投与量）

コンセンサス

全身投与抗真菌薬として確立されているのは，アゾール系薬およびアムホテリシン製品の経口あるいは静脈投与，最低 6 週間である．ある種のカンジダ属はフルコナゾールに耐性を持つことが文献上報告されているので，微生物学者と協力のもと，感受性試験が行われるべきである．

（参考文献 1, 3, 8, 13, 15-17, 21, 22, 27-33）

投票結果

同意：93%，反対：5%，棄権：2%（強いコンセンサス）

Question 7

- 真菌性 PJI の段階的手術的治療において，セメントスペーサーにはどのような抗真菌薬あるいは抗細菌薬が投与されるべきか？ その推奨される投与量は？

コンセンサス

文献上，抗真菌薬は局所に高用量溶出する．しかし，臨床的有効性を立証する臨床研究はまだない．骨セメントに充填したリポソーム・アムホテシン B は，従来のアムホテシン B デオキシコール酸よりもはるかに溶出力がある．またアゾール系抗真菌薬の徐放性，特にボリコナゾールについては骨セメントからの徐放性についてのデータがある．抗真菌薬だけでなく，抗細菌薬も骨セメントに加えることを考慮する必要がある．

(参考文献 3, 18, 27, 29, 34-45)

投票結果
同意：94％, 反対：2％, 棄権：4％ (強いコンセンサス)

Question 8
- 真菌性 PJI をモニターし，再置換術のタイミングを決定するために推奨される検査は何か？

コンセンサス
真菌性 PJI モニターには，C 反応性タンパクおよび赤血球沈降速度が推奨される．検査結果を見て再置換術のタイミングを判断することはできない．(参考文献 28, 46)

投票結果
同意：89％, 反対：8％, 棄権：3％ (強いコンセンサス)

Question 9
- 真菌性 PJI 治療における全身性抗菌薬（抗真菌薬）の投与期間は？

コンセンサス
真菌性 PJI 治療の全身性抗菌薬（抗真菌薬）投与はインプラント抜去時（Stage 1）に開始されるべきで，少なくとも 6 週間継続するべきである．その後，臨床所見と検査所見に基づいて再置換術（Stage 2）の前にいったん中止する．再置換術後の抗真菌薬投与の継続期間について適切なデータはない．

(参考文献 47)

投票結果
同意：85％, 反対：10％, 棄権：5％ (強いコンセンサス)

【掲載されている論文】

Management of fungal or atypical periprosthetic joint infections.

Gebauer M, Frommelt L, Achan P, Board TN, Conway J, Griffin W, Heidari N, Kerr G, McLaren A, Nelson SB, Nijhof M, Zahar A.

J Arthroplasty. 2014 Feb；29（2 Suppl）：112-4. doi：10.1016/j.arth.2013.09.049. Epub 2013 Oct 1. No abstract available.

PMID：24360494

References:

1. Azzam K, Parvizi J, Jungkind D, et al. Microbiological, clinical, and surgical features of fungal prosthetic joint infections: a multi-institutional experience. J Bone Joint Surg Am. 2009;91 Suppl 6:142-149.
2. Kohli R, Hadley S. Fungal arthritis and osteomyelitis. Infect Dis Clin North Am. 2005;19(4):831-851.
3. Phelan DM, Osmon DR, Keating MR, Hanssen AD. Delayed reimplantation arthroplasty for candidal prosthetic joint infection: a report of 4 cases and review of the literature. Clin Infect Dis. 2002;34(7):930-938.
4. Darouiche RO, Hamill RJ, Musher DM, Young EJ, Harris RL. Periprosthetic candidal infections following arthroplasty. Rev Infect Dis. 1989;11(1):89-96.
5. Hennessy MJ. Infection of a total knee arthroplasty by Candida parapsilosis. A case report of successful treatment by joint reimplantation with a literature review. Am J Knee Surg. Summer 1996;9(3):133-136.
6. Koch AE. Candida albicans infection of a prosthetic knee replacement: a report and review of the literature. J Rheumatol. 1988;15(2):362-365.
7. Lambertus M, Thordarson D, Goetz MB. Fungal prosthetic arthritis: presentation of two cases and review of the literature. Rev Infect Dis. 1988;10(5):1038-1043.
8. Selmon GP, Slater RN, Shepperd JA, Wright EP. Successful 1-stage exchange total knee arthroplasty for fungal infection. J Arthroplasty. 1998;13(1):114-115.
9. Simonian PT, Brause BD, Wickiewicz TL. Candida infection after total knee arthroplasty. Management without resection or amphotericin B. J Arthroplasty. 1997;12(7):825-829.
10. Wada M, Baba H, Imura S. Prosthetic knee Candida parapsilosis infection. J Arthroplasty. 1998;13(4):479-482.
11. Austin KS, Testa NN, Luntz RK, Greene JB, Smiles S. Aspergillus infection of total knee arthroplasty presenting as a popliteal cyst. Case report and review of the literature. J Arthroplasty. 1992;7(3):311-314.
12. Badrul B, Ruslan G. Candida albicans infection of a prosthetic knee replacement: a case report. Med J Malaysia. 2000;55 Suppl C:93-96.
13. Brooks DH, Pupparo F. Successful salvage of a primary total knee arthroplasty infected with Candida parapsilosis. J Arthroplasty. 1998;13(6):707-712.
14. Cardinal E, Braunstein EM, Capello WN, Heck DA. Candida albicans infection of prosthetic joints. Orthopedics. 1996;19(3):247-251.
15. Ceffa R, Andreoni S, Borre S, et al. Mucoraceae infections of antibiotic-loaded cement spacers in the treatment of bacterial infections caused by knee arthroplasty. J Arthroplasty. 2002;17(2):235-238.
16. Dumaine V, Eyrolle L, Baixench MT, et al. Successful treatment of prosthetic knee Candida glabrata infection with caspofungin combined with flucytosine. Int J Antimicrob Agents. 2008;31(4):398-399.
17. Fukasawa N, Shirakura K. Candida arthritis after total knee arthroplasty--a case of successful treatment without prosthesis removal. Acta Orthop Scand. 1997;68(3):306-307.
18. Gaston G, Ogden J. Candida glabrata periprosthetic infection: a case report and literature review. J Arthroplasty. 2004;19(7):927-930.
19. Iskander MK, Khan MA. Candida infection of a prosthetic knee replacement. J Rheumatol. 1988;15(10):1594-1595.
20. Lackner M, De Man FH, Eygendaal D, et al. Severe prosthetic joint infection in an immunocompetent male patient due to a therapy refractory Pseudallescheria apiosperma. Mycoses 2011;54 Suppl 3:22-27.
21. Lazzarini L, Manfrin V, De Lalla F. Candidal prosthetic hip infection in a patient with previous candidal septic arthritis. J Arthroplasty. 2004;19(2):248-252.
22. Lerch K, Kalteis T, Schubert T, Lehn N, Grifka J. Prosthetic joint infections with osteomyelitis due to Candida albicans. Mycoses. 2003;46(11-12):462-466.
23. Levine M, Rehm SJ, Wilde AH. Infection with Candida albicans of a total knee arthroplasty. Case report and review of the literature. Clin Orthop Relat Res. 1988(226):235-239.
24. Lim EV, Stern PJ. Candida infection after implant arthroplasty. A case report. J Bone Joint Surg Am. 1986;68(1):143-145.
25. MacGregor RR, Schimmer BM, Steinberg ME. Results of combined amphotericin B-5-fluorcytosine therapy for prosthetic knee joint infected with Candida parapsilosis. J Rheumatol. 1979;6(4):451-455.
26. Nayeri F, Cameron R, Chryssanthou E, Johansson L, Soderstrom C. Candida glabrata prosthesis infection following pyelonephritis and septicaemia. Scand J Infect Dis. 1997;29(6):635-638.
27. Wu MH, Hsu KY. Candidal arthritis in revision knee arthroplasty successfully treated with sequential parenteral-oral fluconazole and amphotericin B-loaded cement spacer. Knee Surg Sports Traumatol Arthrosc. 2011;19(2):273-276.
28. Anagnostakos K, Kelm J, Schmitt E, Jung J. Fungal periprosthetic hip and knee joint

infections clinical experience with a 2-stage treatment protocol. J Arthroplasty. 2012;27(2):293-298.
29. Marra F, Robbins GM, Masri BA, et al. Amphotericin B-loaded bone cement to treat osteomyelitis caused by Candida albicans. Can J Surg. 2001;44(5):383-386.
30. Ruhnke M, Rickerts V, Cornely OA, et al. Diagnosis and therapy of Candida infections: joint recommendations of the German Speaking Mycological Society and the Paul-Ehrlich-Society for Chemotherapy. Mycoses. 2011;54(4):279-310.
31. Wyman J, McGough R, Limbird R. Fungal infection of a total knee prosthesis: successful treatment using articulating cement spacers and staged reimplantation. Orthopedics. 2002;25(12):1391-1394; discussion 1394.
32. Yang SH, Pao JL, Hang YS. Staged reimplantation of total knee arthroplasty after Candida infection. J Arthroplasty. 2001;16(4):529-532.
33. Yilmaz M, Mete B, Ozaras R, et al. Aspergillus fumigatus infection as a delayed manifestation of prosthetic knee arthroplasty and a review of the literature. Scand J Infect Dis. 2011;43(8):573-578.
34. Gottesman-Yekutieli T, Shwartz O, Edelman A, Hendel D, Dan M. Pseudallescheria boydii infection of a prosthetic hip joint--an uncommon infection in a rare location. Am J Med Sci. 2011;342(3):250-253.
35. Buranapanitkit B, Oungbho K, Ingviya N. The efficacy of hydroxyapatite composite impregnated with amphotericin B. Clin Orthop Relat Res. 2005(437):236-241.
36. Chandra J, Kuhn DM, Mukherjee PK, Hoyer LL, McCormick T, Ghannoum MA. Biofilm formation by the fungal pathogen Candida albicans: development, architecture, and drug resistance. J Bacteriol. 2001;183(18):5385-5394.
37. Deelstra JJ, Neut D, Jutte PC. Successful treatment of Candida albicans-infected total hip prosthesis with staged procedure using an antifungal-loaded cement spacer. J Arthroplasty. 2013;28(2):374 e375-378.
38. Goss B, Lutton C, Weinrauch P, Jabur M, Gillett G, Crawford R. Elution and mechanical properties of antifungal bone cement. J Arthroplasty. 2007;22(6):902-908.
39. Grimsrud C, Raven R, Fothergill AW, Kim HT. The in vitro elution characteristics of antifungal-loaded PMMA bone cement and calcium sulfate bone substitute. Orthopedics. 2011;34(8):e378-381.
40. Harmsen S, McLaren AC, Pauken C, McLemore R. Amphotericin B is cytotoxic at locally delivered concentrations. Clin Orthop Relat Res. 2011;469(11):3016-3021.
41. Rouse MS, Heijink A, Steckelberg JM, Patel R. Are anidulafungin or voriconazole released from polymethylmethacrylate in vitro? Clin Orthop Relat Res. 2011;469(5):1466-1469.
42. Sealy PI, Nguyen C, Tucci M, Benghuzzi H, Cleary JD. Delivery of antifungal agents using bioactive and nonbioactive bone cements. Ann Pharmacother. 2009;43(10):1606-1615.
43. Silverberg D, Kodali P, Dipersio J, Acus R, Askew M. In vitro analysis of antifungal impregnated polymethylmethacrylate bone cement. Clin Orthop Relat Res. 2002(403):228-231.
44. Cunningham B, McLaren AC, Pauken C, McLemore R. Liposomal formulation increases local delivery of amphotericin from bone cement: a pilot study. Clin Orthop Relat Res. 2012;470(10):2671-2676.
45. Miller RB, McLaren AC, Pauken C, Clarke HD, McLemore R. Voriconazole is delivered from antifungal-loaded bone cement. Clin Orthop Relat Res. 2013;471(1):195-200.
46. Ostrosky-Zeichner L, Alexander BD, Kett DH, et al. Multicenter clinical evaluation of the (1-->3) beta-D-glucan assay as an aid to diagnosis of fungal infections in humans. Clin Infect Dis. 2005;41(5):654-659.
47. Fabry K, Verheyden F, Nelen G. Infection of a total knee prosthesis by Candida glabrata: a case report. Acta Orthop Belg. 2005;71(1):119-121.

Question 1

- **What is the definition of fungal or atypical periprosthetic joint infection (PJI)?**

<u>Consensus:</u> A fungal or atypical PJI is an infection of a joint arthroplasty caused by fungi or atypical bacteria.

Delegate Vote

Agree: 89%, Disagree: 7%, Abstain: 4% (Strong Consensus)

Question 2

- **When should fungal organisms be considered as a cause of PJI?**

<u>Consensus:</u> A PJI caused by fungi can be considered if fungal pathogens are isolated from periprosthetic tissue cultures or joint aspirations in a patient who has other signs or symptoms of PJI, such as abnormal serology and joint aspiration parameters (neutrophil count and differential). If clinical symptoms raise suspicion for a fungal PJI, repeated joint aspiration may be needed to isolate the infecting organism.

Delegate Vote

Agree: 94%, Disagree: 4%, Abstain: 2% (Strong Consensus)

Question 3

- **Which host factors (concomitant disease and other factors) predispose to fungal PJI?**

<u>Consensus:</u> Predisposing host factors to fungal PJI are : immunosuppression (decreased cellular immunity, neutropenia, corticosteroids or other immunosuppressive drugs, history of organ transplantation, and acquired immunodeficiency syndrome), malignancy and/or the use of antineoplastic agents, drug abuse, prolonged use of antibiotics, presence of indwelling catheters (intravenous, urinary or parenteral hyperalimentation), diabetes mellitus, malnutrition, rheumatoid arthritis, history of multiple abdominal surgeries, severe burns, tuberculosis, and preceding bacterial infection of the prosthesis

Delegate Vote

Agree: 95%, Disagree: 2%, Abstain: 3% (Strong Consensus)

Question 4

- **When fungal organisms are considered, what specimens should be collected and additional diagnostic tools should be used and how should they be processed to optimize diagnosis?**

Consensus: Fungal selective media must be included and it should be observed that prolonged culture may be required. In specific cases one should expand diagnostic testing to include tissue samples for histological examination, especially in cases where there is a high index of clinical suspicion. Resistance of Candida species to fluconazole has been reported in the literature and so susceptibility testing may be requested when resistance to fluconazole is suspected based on isolated species. Antifungal susceptibility testing remains less well developed and utilized than antibacterial testing.

Delegate Vote

Agree: 96%, Disagree: 2%, Abstain: 2% (Strong Consensus)

Question 5

- **What is the best way to surgically manage fungal PJI∶ irrigation and debridement, one-stage exchange, two-stage exchange, or permanent resection arthroplasty?**

Consensus: On the basis of the current literature, two-stage exchange arthroplasty is the recommended treatment option to manage fungal PJI. However, the success rate is lower than that of bacterial cases.

Delegate Vote

Agree: 95%, Disagree: 2%, Abstain: 3% (Strong Consensus)

Question 6

- **What are the optimal systemic antifungals administered (type and dose) in the treatment of fungal PJI?**

Consensus: Well-established agents for a systemic treatment are the azoles and amphotericin products given either orally or intravenously for a minimum of 6 weeks. Resistance of certain Candida species to fluconazole has been reported in the literature and so susceptibility testing should be performed, in collaboration with the microbiologist

Delegate Vote
Agree: 93%, Disagree: 5%, Abstain: 2% (Strong Consensus)

Question 7

- **When treating fungal PJIs in a staged manner, which antifungal or antibacterial medications should be used for the cement spacer? What is the recommended dose?**

<u>Consensus:</u> Recent literature confirms that antifungal agents are released in high amounts for local delivery, but there are no clinical studies yet to document the clinical effectiveness. The use of liposomal amphotericin B, loaded in bone cement, has more than an order of magnitude greater release than conventional amphotericin B deoxycholate. There is also controlled release data for azole antifungals, with specific data on the elution of voriconazole from bone cement. There should be a consideration for adding an antibacterial to the bone cement for local delivery in addition to the antifungal.

Delegate Vote
Agree: 94%, Disagree: 2%, Abstain: 4% (Strong Consensus)

Question 8

- **Which investigations are recommended to monitor fungal PJI and determine timing of reimplantation?**

<u>Consensus:</u> C-reactive protein and erythrocyte sedimentation rate are recommended to monitor fungal PJI. There is no clear evidence for the timing of reimplantation based on laboratory tests.

Delegate Vote
Agree: 89%, Disagree: 8%, Abstain: 3% (Strong Consensus)

Question 9

- **What is the duration for systemic antimicrobial (antifungal) agent administration in the treatment of fungal PJI?**

<u>Consensus:</u> Systemic antimicrobial (antifungal) agent administration in the treatment of fungal PJI should be started at the time of removal of the implants (stage one) and continued for at least 6 weeks. It should then be stopped before reimplantation (stage two) the timing

of which is based on clinical judgment and laboratory tests. There are no good data to support antifungal agent administration after reimplantation.

Delegate Vote

Agree: 85%, Disagree: 10%, Abstain: 5% (Strong Consensus)

14 経口抗菌薬療法

Workgroup 14：Oral Antibiotic Therapy

Question 1

- 適切な外科治療を行いインプラントの温存を試みた急性（早期あるいは晩期）の人工関節周囲感染（PJI）に対して，投与すべき適切な経口抗菌薬，あるいは併用療法は？

コンセンサス

グラム陽性菌による PJI では，可能であればリファンピシンを含む処方が，グラム陰性菌によるものではフルオロキノロンが用いられるべきである．リファンピシンをいつ開始すべきかのコンセンサスは得られていない．（参考文献 1-47, 54）

投票結果

同意：87％，不同意：7％，棄権：6％（強いコンセンサス）

Question 2

- デブリドマンによるインプラント温存療法が行われた急性の PJI において，抗菌薬はどれくらいの期間投与するべきか？

コンセンサス

静脈内および経口投与の期間は未解決の問題であり，抗菌薬の投与期間を比較した臨床試験はない．

（参考文献 1, 3, 8, 13-22, 26, 45, 46, 48-55）

投票結果

同意：85％，不同意：11％，棄権：4％（強いコンセンサス）

Question 3

- 外科的治療が適切に行われなかったPJIの治療において，抗菌薬併用療法の役割は？

コンセンサス

慢性 PJI において，インプラントを抜去せずに抗菌薬を投与したり，デブリドマンを単独で施行することは推奨しない．

(参考文献 13, 56, 57)
投票結果
同意:84%,不同意:14%,棄権:2%(強いコンセンサス)

Question 4

- 抗菌薬による抑制療法はどのくらいの期間なされるべきか?

コンセンサス

抗菌薬による抑制療法の期間についてのコンセンサスは得られていない.治療は症例に応じて行われるべきであるとのコンセンサスがある.(参考文献 58-61)

投票結果
同意:94%,不同意:4%,棄権:2%(強いコンセンサス)

Question 5

- 細菌別に,どのような抗菌薬が抑制療法として利用できるか?

コンセンサス

抑制療法における適切な抗菌薬についてコンセンサスは得られていない.分離された細菌,特に関節穿刺あるいは外科的デブリドマンによって得られた深部組織検体の感受性パターンに基づいて抗菌薬は選択されるべきである.使用可能な抗菌薬リストとそれらの投与量を示す.

投票結果
同意:97%,不同意:3%,棄権:0%(強いコンセンサス)

人工関節周囲感染の治療に使われる主要な経口抗菌薬

抗菌薬名	生物学的利用性(%)	経口投与量	副作用
ペニシリンV†	60	0.5〜1 g/6〜8時間	皮疹，アナフィラキシー，クロストリジウム・ディフィシル関連下痢症
アモキシシリン	80	1 g/8時間‡	
アモキシシリン−クラブラン酸	75*	875〜125 mg/8時間	
クロキサシリン†	50〜70	0.5〜1 g/4〜6時間	
セファレキシン	>90	0.5〜1 g/6〜8時間‡	
セファドロキシル†	>90	0.5〜1 g/8〜12時間	
シプロフロキサシン	75	500〜750 mg/12時間‡	肝毒性，アキレス腱炎/腱断裂，非可逆的神経障害，クロストリジウム・ディフィシル関連下痢症
レボフロキサシン	>95	500〜750 mg/24時間‡	
クリンダマイシン	90	300 mg/8時間	消化器症状，クロストリジウム・ディフィシル関連下痢症
リファンピシン***	90**	10〜20 mg/kg/24〜12時間‡	肝毒性，皮疹，消化器症状
ドキシサイクリン	95	100 mg/12時間	皮膚色素沈着，肝毒性
ミノサイクリン	95	100 mg/12時間	
コントリモキサゾール（〜リメトプリム/スルファメトキサゾール）	90	160 mg/8〜12時間‡	血液学的異常（白血球減少，貧血），皮疹，クマリン系薬剤との併用を避ける
	90	800 mg/8〜12時間‡	
リネゾリド	100	600 mg/12時間	血液学的異常（血小板減少，貧血），三環系抗うつ薬との併用を避ける
フシジン酸****†	90	0.5〜1 g/8〜12時間	肝毒性
フルコナゾール	>90	400 mg/24時間	肝毒性，CYP3A4阻害

*クラブラン酸を基準として，**空腹時内服した場合，***通常併用使用される，****米国では使用できない．
†日本にはない剤形，‡国内で使用する際は保険適応量の確認が必要．

【掲載されている論文】

Oral antibiotic therapy.

O'Toole P, Osmon D, Soriano A, Berdal JE, Bostrum M, Franco-Cendejas R, Huang D, Nelson C, Nishisaka F, Salgado CD, Sawyer R, Segreti J, Senneville E, Zhang XL.

J Arthroplasty. 2014 Feb；29（2 Suppl）：115-8. doi: 10.1016/j.arth.2013.09.050. Epub 2013 Oct 1. No abstract available.

PMID：24360497

References:

1. Lora-Tamayo J, Murillo O, Iribarren JA, et al. A large multicenter study of methicillin-susceptible and methicillin-resistant Staphylococcus aureus prosthetic joint infections managed with implant retention. Clin Infect Dis. 2012;56(2):182-194.
2. Silva M, Tharani R, Schmalzried TP. Results of direct exchange or debridement of the infected total knee arthroplasty. Clin Orthop Relat Res. 2002;(404):125-131.
3. Achermann Y, Eigenmann K, Ledergerber B, et al. Factors associated with rifampin resistance in staphylococcal periprosthetic joint infections (PJI): a matched case-control study. Infection. 2013;41(2):431-437.
4. Sia IG, Berbari EF, Karchmer AW. Prosthetic joint infections. Infect Dis Clin North Am. 2005;19(4):885-914.
5. Berbari EF, Osmon DR, Duffy MC, et al. Outcome of prosthetic joint infection in patients with rheumatoid arthritis: the impact of medical and surgical therapy in 200 episodes. Clin Infect Dis. 2006;42(2):216-223.
6. Fehring TK, Odum SM, Berend KR, et al. Failure of irrigation and debridement for early postoperative periprosthetic infection. Clin Orthop Relat Res. 2012;471(1):250-257.
7. Baldoni D, Haschke M, Rajacic Z, Zimmerli W, Trampuz A. Linezolid alone or combined with rifampin against methicillin-resistant Staphylococcus aureus in experimental foreign-body infection. Antimicrob Agents Chemother. 2009;53(3):1142-1148.
8. Ceri H, Olson ME, Stremick C, Read RR, Morck D, Buret A. The Calgary Biofilm Device: new technology for rapid determination of antibiotic susceptibilities of bacterial biofilms. J Clin Microbiol. 1999;37(6):1771-1776.
9. Garrigos C, Murillo O, Euba G, et al. Efficacy of usual and high doses of daptomycin in combination with rifampin versus alternative therapies in experimental foreign-body infection by methicillin-resistant Staphylococcus aureus. Antimicrob Agents Chemother. 2010;54(12):5251-5256.
10. Monzon M, Oteiza C, Leiva J, Lamata M, Amorena B. Biofilm testing of Staphylococcus epidermidis clinical isolates: low performance of vancomycin in relation to other antibiotics. Diagn Microbiol Infect Dis. 2002;44(4):319-324.
11. Saleh-Mghir A, Muller-Serieys C, Dinh A, Massias L, Cremieux AC. Adjunctive rifampin is crucial to optimizing daptomycin efficacy against rabbit prosthetic joint infection due to methicillin-resistant Staphylococcus aureus. Antimicrob Agents Chemother. 2011;55(10):4589-4593.
12. Zimmerli W, Frei R, Widmer AF, Rajacic Z. Microbiological tests to predict treatment outcome in experimental device-related infections due to Staphylococcus aureus. J Antimicrob Chemother. 1994;33(5):959-967.
13. Barberan J, Aguilar L, Carroquino G, et al. Conservative treatment of staphylococcal prosthetic joint infections in elderly patients. Am J Med. 2006;119(11):993 e997-910.
14. Byren I, Bejon P, Atkins BL, et al. One hundred and twelve infected arthroplasties treated with 'DAIR' (debridement, antibiotics and implant retention): antibiotic duration and outcome. J Antimicrob Chemother. 2009;63(6):1264-1271.
15. Cobo J, Miguel LG, Euba G, et al. Early prosthetic joint infection: outcomes with debridement and implant retention followed by antibiotic therapy. Clin Microbiol Infect. 2011;17(11):1632-1637.
16. El Helou OC, Berbari EF, Lahr BD, et al. Efficacy and safety of rifampin containing regimen for staphylococcal prosthetic joint infections treated with debridement and retention. Eur J Clin Microbiol Infect Dis. 2010;29(8):961-967.
17. Giulieri SG, Graber P, Ochsner PE, Zimmerli W. Management of infection associated with total hip arthroplasty according to a treatment algorithm. Infection. 2004;32(4):222-228.

18. Laffer RR, Graber P, Ochsner PE, Zimmerli W. Outcome of prosthetic knee-associated infection: evaluation of 40 consecutive episodes at a single centre. Clin Microbiol Infect. 2006;12(5):433-439.
19. Senneville E, Joulie D, Legout L, et al. Outcome and predictors of treatment failure in total hip/knee prosthetic joint infections due to Staphylococcus aureus. Clin Infect Dis. 2011;53(4):334-340.
20. Soriano A, Garcia S, Bori G, et al. Treatment of acute post-surgical infection of joint arthroplasty. Clin Microbiol Infect. 2006;12(9):930-933.
21. Soriano A, Garcia S, Ortega M, et al. [Treatment of acute infection of total or partial hip arthroplasty with debridement and oral chemotherapy]. Med Clin (Barc). 2003;121(3):81-85.
22. Vilchez F, Martinez-Pastor JC, Garcia-Ramiro S, et al. Outcome and predictors of treatment failure in early post-surgical prosthetic joint infections due to Staphylococcus aureus treated with debridement. Clin Microbiol Infect. 2011;17(3):439-444.
23. Anderl JN, Zahller J, Roe F, Stewart PS. Role of nutrient limitation and stationary-phase existence in Klebsiella pneumoniae biofilm resistance to ampicillin and ciprofloxacin. Antimicrob Agents Chemother. 2003;47(4):1251-1256.
24. Nijland HM, Ruslami R, Suroto AJ, et al. Rifampicin reduces plasma concentrations of moxifloxacin in patients with tuberculosis. Clin Infect Dis. 2007;45(8):1001-1007.
25. Zeller V, Dzeing-Ella A, Kitzis MD, Ziza JM, Mamoudy P, Desplaces N. Continuous clindamycin infusion, an innovative approach to treating bone and joint infections. Antimicrob Agents Chemother. 2010;54(1):88-92.
26. Gandelman K, Zhu T, Fahmi OA, et al. Unexpected effect of rifampin on the pharmacokinetics of linezolid: in silico and in vitro approaches to explain its mechanism. J Clin Pharmacol. 2011;51(2):229-236.
27. Tornero E, Garcia-Oltra E, Garcia-Ramiro S, et al. Prosthetic joint infections due to Staphylococcus aureus and coagulase-negative staphylococci. Int J Artif Organs. 2012;35(10):884-892.
28. Bradbury T, Fehring TK, Taunton M, et al. The fate of acute methicillin-resistant Staphylococcus aureus periprosthetic knee infections treated by open debridement and retention of components. J Arthroplasty. 2009;24(6 Suppl):101-104.
29. Ferry T, Uckay I, Vaudaux P, et al. Risk factors for treatment failure in orthopedic device-related methicillin-resistant Staphylococcus aureus infection. Eur J Clin Microbiol Infect Dis. 2010;29(2):171-180.
30. Salgado CD, Dash S, Cantey JR, Marculescu CE. Higher risk of failure of methicillin-resistant Staphylococcus aureus prosthetic joint infections. Clin Orthop Relat Res. 2007;461:48-53.
31. Bassetti M, Vitale F, Melica G, et al. Linezolid in the treatment of Gram-positive prosthetic joint infections. J Antimicrob Chemother. 2005;55(3):387-390.
32. Gomez J, Canovas E, Banos V, et al. Linezolid plus rifampin as a salvage therapy in prosthetic joint infections treated without removing the implant. Antimicrob Agents Chemother. 2011;55(9):4308-4310.
33. Rao N, Hamilton CW. Efficacy and safety of linezolid for Gram-positive orthopedic infections: a prospective case series. Diagn Microbiol Infect Dis. 2007;59(2):173-179.
34. Rao N, Ziran BH, Hall RA, Santa ER. Successful treatment of chronic bone and joint infections with oral linezolid. Clin Orthop Relat Res. 2004;(427):67-71.
35. Razonable RR, Osmon DR, Steckelberg JM. Linezolid therapy for orthopedic infections. Mayo Clin Proc. 2004;79(9):1137-1144.
36. Soriano A, Gomez J, Gomez L, et al. Efficacy and tolerability of prolonged linezolid therapy in the treatment of orthopedic implant infections. Eur J Clin Microbiol Infect Dis. 2007;26(5):353-356.
37. Pea F, Furlanut M, Cojutti P, et al. Therapeutic drug monitoring of linezolid: a retrospective monocentric analysis. Antimicrob Agents Chemother. 2010;54(11):4605-4610.
38. Peel TN, Buising KL, Dowsey MM, et al. Outcome of debridement and retention in prosthetic joint infections by methicillin-resistant staphylococci, with special reference to rifampin and fusidic acid combination therapy. Antimicrob Agents Chemother. 2012;57(1):350-355.
39. Stein A, Bataille JF, Drancourt M, et al. Ambulatory treatment of multidrug-resistant Staphylococcus-infected orthopedic implants with high-dose oral co-trimoxazole (trimethoprim-sulfamethoxazole). Antimicrob Agents Chemother. 1998;42(12):3086-3091.
40. Wu WS, Chen CC, Chuang YC, et al. Efficacy of combination oral antimicrobial agents against biofilm-embedded methicillin-resistant Staphylococcus aureus. J Microbiol Immunol Infect. 2013;46(2):89-95.
41. Meehan AM, Osmon DR, Duffy MC, Hanssen AD, Keating MR. Outcome of penicillin-susceptible streptococcal prosthetic joint infection treated with debridement and retention of the prosthesis. Clin Infect Dis. 2003;36(7):845-849.
42. Odum SM, Fehring TK, Lombardi AV, et al. Irrigation and debridement for periprosthetic infections: does the organism matter? J Arthroplasty. 2011;26(6 Suppl):114-118.
43. El Helou OC, Berbari EF, Marculescu CE, et al. Outcome of enterococcal prosthetic joint infection: is combination systemic therapy superior to monotherapy? Clin Infect Dis.

2008;47(7):903-909.

44. Holmberg A, Morgelin M, Rasmussen M. Effectiveness of ciprofloxacin or linezolid in combination with rifampicin against Enterococcus faecalis in biofilms. J Antimicrob Chemother. 2012;67(2):433-439.

45. Aboltins CA, Dowsey MM, Buising KL, et al. Gram-negative prosthetic joint infection treated with debridement, prosthesis retention and antibiotic regimens including a fluoroquinolone. Clin Microbiol Infect. 2011;17(6):862-867.

46. Martinez-Pastor JC, Munoz-Mahamud E, Vilchez F, et al. Outcome of acute prosthetic joint infections due to gram-negative bacilli treated with open debridement and retention of the prosthesis. Antimicrob Agents Chemother. 2009;53(11):4772-4777.

47. San Juan R, Garcia-Reyne A, Caba P, et al. Safety and efficacy of moxifloxacin monotherapy for treatment of orthopedic implant-related staphylococcal infections. Antimicrob Agents Chemother. 2010;54(12):5161-5166.

48. Daver NG, Shelburne SA, Atmar RL, et al. Oral step-down therapy is comparable to intravenous therapy for Staphylococcus aureus osteomyelitis. J Infect. 2007;54(6):539-544.

49. Euba G, Murillo O, Fernandez-Sabe N, et al. Long-term follow-up trial of oral rifampin-cotrimoxazole combination versus intravenous cloxacillin in treatment of chronic staphylococcal osteomyelitis. Antimicrob Agents Chemother. 2009;53(6):2672-2676.

50. Karamanis EM, Matthaiou DK, Moraitis LI, Falagas ME. Fluoroquinolones versus beta-lactam based regimens for the treatment of osteomyelitis: a meta-analysis of randomized controlled trials. Spine (Phila Pa 1976). 2008;33(10):E297-304.

51. Osmon DR, Berbari EF, Berendt AR, et al. Diagnosis and management of prosthetic joint infection: clinical practice guidelines by the Infectious Diseases Society of America. Clin Infect Dis. 2013;56(1):e1-e25.

52. Zimmerli W, Trampuz A, Ochsner PE. Prosthetic-joint infections. N Engl J Med. 2004;351(16):1645-1654.

53. Edmiston CE, Jr., Goheen MP, Seabrook GR, et al. Impact of selective antimicrobial agents on staphylococcal adherence to biomedical devices. Am J Surg. 2006;192(3):344-354.

54. Bernard L, Legout L, Zurcher-Pfund L, et al. Six weeks of antibiotic treatment is sufficient following surgery for septic arthroplasty. J Infect. 2010;61(2):125-132.

55. Bejon P, Byren I, Atkins BL, et al. Serial measurement of the C-reactive protein is a poor predictor of treatment outcome in prosthetic joint infection. J Antimicrob Chemother. 2011;66(7):1590-1593.

56. Bengtson S, Knutson K. The infected knee arthroplasty. A 6-year follow-up of 357 cases. Acta Orthop Scand. 1991;62(4):301-311.

57. Koyonos L, Zmistowski B, Della Valle CJ, Parvizi J. Infection control rate of irrigation and debridement for periprosthetic joint infection. Clin Orthop Relat Res. 2011;469(11):3043-3048.

58. Lentino JR. Prosthetic joint infections: bane of orthopedists, challenge for infectious disease specialists. Clin Infect Dis. 2003;36(9):1157-1161.

59. Marculescu CE, Berbari EF, Hanssen AD, et al. Outcome of prosthetic joint infections treated with debridement and retention of components. Clin Infect Dis. 2006;42(4):471-478.

60. Rao N, Crossett LS, Sinha RK, Le Frock JL. Long-term suppression of infection in total joint arthroplasty. Clin Orthop Relat Res. 2003(414):55-60.

61. Segreti J, Nelson JA, Trenholme GM. Prolonged suppressive antibiotic therapy for infected orthopedic prostheses. Clin Infect Dis. 1998;27(4):711-713.

Question 1

- **What are the appropriate oral antibiotic or antibiotic combinations following adequate surgical treatment for acute (early or late) PJI in which the implant has been retained?**

<u>Consensus:</u> Regimens containing rifampicin, when feasible, should be used in gram-positive PJI and fluoroquinolones in gram-negative PJI. There is no consensus as to when rifampicin should be started.

Delegate Vote

Agree: 87%, Disagree: 7%, Abstain: 6% (Strong Consensus)

Question 2

- **How long should antibiotic treatment in acute PJI treated with debridement and retention of the implant be?**

<u>Consensus:</u> The duration of intravenous and oral treatment is a question that remains unsolved and there is no clinical trial comparing different durations of antibiotic treatment.

Delegate Vote

Agree: 85%, Disagree: 11%, Abstain: 4% (Strong Consensus)

Question 3

- **What is the role of antibiotic combinations for treatment of PJI managed without adequate surgical intervention?**

<u>Consensus:</u> We do not recommend administration of antibiotics and open debridement alone without removing the implant in chronic PJI.

Delegate Vote

Agree: 84%, Disagree: 14%, Abstain: 2% (Strong Consensus)

Question 4

- **How long should suppressive therapy be administered?**

<u>Consensus:</u> There is no consensus about the length of time that patients should receive suppressive antibiotic therapy, there is consensus that treatment should be individualized.

Delegate Vote

Agree: 94%, Disagree: 4%, Abstain: 2% (Strong Consensus)

Question 5

- **What antibiotics could be useful for suppressive treatment based on type of organism?**

Consensus: There is no consensus regarding appropriate antibiotics for suppression therapy. The antibiotic should be chosen according to the susceptibility pattern of the isolated microorganism, preferably obtained from deep samples by joint aspiration or surgical debridement. The list of potential antibiotics and their doses is provided.

Delegate Vote

Agree: 97%, Disagree: 3%, Abstain: 0% (Strong Consensus)

15 晩期人工関節周囲感染の予防

Workgroup 15：Prevention of Late PJI

Question 1
- 晩期人工関節周囲感染（PJI）の定義は？

コンセンサス
晩期 PJI は，人工関節置換術後，様々な期間経過した後に発生する PJI と定義される．晩期 PJI は，術後早期には臨床所見や画像所見を認めない初回の人工関節置換術に発生する PJI である．晩期 PJI のリスクファクターは PJI と同様である（Workgroup 1）．（参考文献 1-3）

投票結果
同意：56％，反対：39％，棄権：5％（弱いコンセンサス）

Question 2
- 晩期 PJI を診断するには何をすべきか？

コンセンサス
関節痛の訴えがあり晩期 PJI が疑われる患者の診断には，Workgroup 7 で提示されたアルゴリズムを使用するべきである．
（参考文献 5-45）

投票結果
同意：89％，反対：9％，棄権：2％（強いコンセンサス）

Question 3
- 予防的に投与する抗凝固剤の種類，投与量および投与期間は，人工関節全置換術（TJA）後の手術部位感染（SSI）の発生に影響するか？

コンセンサス
影響する．静脈血栓塞栓症予防のために投与する抗凝固剤の種類，投与量および投与期間は TJA 後の SSI 発生に影響する．
（参考文献 46-51）

投票結果
同意：76%，反対：9%，棄権：15%（強いコンセンサス）

Question 4

- TJA 後の患者にルーチンで歯科処置時の予防抗菌薬を投与するべきか？

コンセンサス

TJA 後の患者における歯科処置時の予防抗菌薬の使用は，患者のリスクファクターおよび施行される歯科治療の侵襲に基づいて個別化されるべきである．（参考文献 52-98）

投票結果
同意：81%，反対：16%，棄権：3%（強いコンセンサス）

コンセンサス

ハイリスク患者では，TJA 後は生涯にわたって歯科処置時の予防抗菌薬投与を推奨する．（参考文献 53，72，99-108）

コンセンサス

歯科処置の前に，下に示す用量で経口抗菌薬を単回投与することを推奨する．（参考文献 62，81，109-122）
—アモキシシリン 2 g，処置の 1 時間前．[81,109-114]
—アジスロマイシン 500 mg，処置の 30 分〜1 時間前．[115]
—セファクロル 1 g，処置の 1 時間前．[116]
—セファレキシン 2 g，処置の 30 分〜1 時間前．[115]
—クリンダマイシン 600 mg，処置の 1〜1.5 時間前．[109,115,117,118]
—エリスロマイシン 1.5 g，処置の 1〜1.5 時間前．[119,120]
—モキシフロキサシン 400 mg 処置の 1〜2 時間前．[109]
—ペニシリン 2 g，処置の 1 時間前．[62,113,121,122]

コンセンサス

歯科処置の前には，下に示す用量で経静脈的（IV），あるいは筋肉注射で抗菌薬を単回投与することを推奨する．
（参考文献 111，115，123，124）
—アンピシリン（IV）2 g，処置の 30 分〜1 時間前．
—セファゾリン（IV）1 g，処置の 30 分〜1 時間前．[115]
—セフロキシム（IV）1.5 g，処置の 10 分前．[123]
—セフトリアキソン（IV）1 g，処置の 30 分〜1 時間前．[115]
—テイコプラニン（IV）400 mg，処置の直前．[111,124]

Question 5

- 晩期 PJI のハイリスク患者は,ウイルス性疾患に罹患している間,予防抗菌薬を投与されるべきか?

コンセンサス

ウイルス性疾患に罹患した TJA 患者に対する経口抗菌薬の投与は不要である.(参考文献 125-134)

投票結果

同意:98%,反対:2%,棄権:0%(強いコンセンサス)

Question 6

- 大腸内視鏡検査などの内視鏡治療の際,晩期 PJI を予防するために,一過性の菌血症を最小化できるか?

コンセンサス

小手術に伴う一過性の菌血症の影響は,個々の患者,とりわけハイリスク患者に対する予防抗菌薬の投与によって最小化されうる.(参考文献 135-178)

投票結果

同意:85%,反対:13%,棄権:2%(強いコンセンサス)

Question 7

- 腸壁からの細菌の転移を減少させるために,薬草サプリメント,プロバイオティクス,および代替医療は役に立つか?

コンセンサス

晩期 PJI 予防を目的として腸壁からの細菌の転移を減少させるために,薬草サプリメント,プロバイオティクスや代替医療が有用であることを支持する十分なエビデンスはない.

(参考文献 179-198)

投票結果

同意:95%,反対:3%,棄権:2%(強いコンセンサス)

Question 8

- 無症候性の患者に対する術後のメチシリン耐性黄色ブドウ球菌(MRSA)保菌のモニタリングに意味はあるか?

コンセンサス

無症候性の患者における術後の MRSA 保菌のモニタリング

は不要である．(参考文献 199)
投票結果
同意：98％，反対：2％，棄権：0％（強いコンセンサス）

コンセンサス
次の人工関節置換術を行う前に，再度，黄色ブドウ球菌のスクリーニングと除菌を行うことを推奨する．(参考文献 200)

Question 9
- 晩期 PJI の関節外感染巣を特定する方法は？

コンセンサス
晩期 PJI に寄与する関節外感染巣は病歴聴取，詳細な身体所見，臨床検査，および感染の疑いがある部位の画像検査などで特定すべきである．(参考文献 150, 167, 169, 201-220)

投票結果
同意：92％，反対：3％，棄権：5％（強いコンセンサス）

Question 10
- TJA 後の発熱に対して，いつから精査を行うべきか？

コンセンサス
術直後における 38.5 度以上の熱発に対して，ルーチンでの熱源精査は不要である．しかし，術後 3 日たっても持続する発熱についての熱源精査は必要である．(参考文献 221-231)

投票結果
同意：81％，反対：15％，棄権：4％（強いコンセンサス）

【掲載されている論文】
Prevention of Late PJI.
Chen A, Haddad F, Lachiewicz P, Bolognesi M, Cortes LE, Franceschini M, Gallo J, Glynn A, Gonzalez Della Valle A, Gahramanov A, Khatod M, Lazarinis S, Lob G, Nana A, Ochsner P, Tuncay I, Winkler T, Zeng Y.
J Arthroplasty. 2014 Feb；29（2 Suppl）：119-28. doi：10.1016/j.arth.2013.09.051. Epub 2013 Oct 1. No abstract available.
PMID：24370487

References:

1. Coventry MB. Treatment of infections occurring in total hip surgery. Orthop Clin North Am. 1975;6(4):991-1003.
2. Garvin KL, Hanssen AD. Infection after total hip arthroplasty. Past, present, and future. J Bone Joint Surg Am. 1995;77(10):1576-1588.
3. McPherson EJ, Woodson C, Holtom P, Roidis N, Shufelt C, Patzakis M. Periprosthetic total hip infection: outcomes using a staging system. Clin Orthop Relat Res. 2002(403):8-15.
4. Senci P, Banderet F, Graber P, Zimmerli W. Clinical comparison between exogenous and haematogenous periprosthetic joint infections caused by Staphylococcus aureus. Clin Microbiol Infect. 2011;17(7):1098-1100.
5. Cipriano CA, Brown NM, Michael AM, Moric M, Sporer SM, Della Valle CJ. Serum and synovial fluid analysis for diagnosing chronic periprosthetic infection in patients with inflammatory arthritis. J Bone Joint Surg Am. 2012;94(7):594-600.
6. Chryssikos T, Parvizi J, Ghanem E, Newberg A, Zhuang H, Alavi A. FDG-PET imaging can diagnose periprosthetic infection of the hip. Clin Orthop Relat Res. 2008;466(6):1338-1342.
7. Delank KS, Schmidt M, Michael JW, Dietlein M, Schicha H, Eysel P. The implications of 18F-FDG PET for the diagnosis of endoprosthetic loosening and infection in hip and knee arthroplasty: results from a prospective, blinded study. BMC Musculoskelet Disord. 2006;7:20.
8. Gemmel F, Van den Wyngaert H, Love C, Welling MM, Gemmel P, Palestro CJ. Prosthetic joint infections: radionuclide state-of-the-art imaging. Eur J Nucl Med Mol Imaging. 2012;39(5) 892-909.
9. Glithero PR, Grigoris P, Harding LK, Hesslewood SR, McMinn DJ. White cell scans and infected joint replacements. Failure to detect chronic infection. J Bone Joint Surg Br. 1993;75(3):371-374.
10. Graute V, Feist M, Lehner S, et al. Detection of low-grade prosthetic joint infections using 99mTc-antigranulocyte SPECT/CT: initial clinical results. Eur J Nucl Med Mol Imaging. 2010;37(9):1751-1759.
11. Kobayashi N, Inaba Y, Choe H, et al. Use of F-18 fluoride PET to differentiate septic from aseptic loosening in total hip arthroplasty patients. Clin Nucl Med. 2011;36(11):e156-161.
12. Love C, Marwin SE, Tomas MB, et al. Diagnosing infection in the failed joint replacement: a comparison of coincidence detection 18F-FDG and 111In-labeled leukocyte/99mTc-sulfur colloid marrow imaging. J Nucl Med. 2004;45(11):1864-1871.
13. Magnuson JE, Brown ML, Hauser MF, Berquist TH, Fitzgerald RH, Jr., Klee GG. In-111-labeled leukocyte scintigraphy in suspected orthopedic prosthesis infection: comparison with other imaging modalities. Radiology. 1988;168(1):235-239.
14. Nagoya S, Kaya M, Sasaki M, Tateda K, Yamashita T. Diagnosis of peri-prosthetic infection at the hip using triple-phase bone scintigraphy. J Bone Joint Surg Br. 2008;90(2):140-144.
15. Savarino L, Baldini N, Tarabusi C, Pellacani A, Giunti A. Diagnosis of infection after total hip replacement. J Biomed Mater Res B Appl Biomater. 2004;70(1):139-145.
16. Scher DM, Pak K, Lonner JH, Finkel JE, Zuckerman JD, Di Cesare PE. The predictive value of indium-111 leukocyte scans in the diagnosis of infected total hip, knee, or resection arthroplasties. J Arthroplasty. 2000;15(3):295-300.
17. Segura AB, Munoz A, Brulles YR, et al. What is the role of bone scintigraphy in the diagnosis of infected joint prostheses? Nucl Med Commun. 2004;25(5):527-532.
18. Sousa R, Massada M, Pereira A, Fontes F, Amorim I, Oliveira A. Diagnostic accuracy of combined 99mTc-sulesomab and 99mTc-nanocolloid bone marrow imaging in detecting prosthetic joint infection. Nucl Med Commun. 2011;32(9):834-839.
19. Aggarwal VK, Higuera C, Deirmengian G, Parvizi J, Austin MS. Swab Cultures Are Not As Effective As Tissue Cultures for Diagnosis of Periprosthetic Joint Infection. Clin Orthop Relat Res. Apr 9 2013. Epub before print.
20. Tsaras G, Maduka-Ezeh A, Inwards CY, et al. Utility of intraoperative frozen section histopathology in the diagnosis of periprosthetic joint infection: a systematic review and meta-analysis. J Bone Joint Surg Am. 19;94(18):1700-1711.
21. Della Valle C, Parvizi J, Bauer TW, et al. American Academy of Orthopaedic Surgeons clinical practice guideline on: the diagnosis of periprosthetic joint infections of the hip and knee. J Bone Joint Surg Am. 20 20;93(14):1355-1357.
22. Parvizi J, Ghanem E, Menashe S, Barrack RL, Bauer TW. Periprosthetic infection: what are the diagnostic challenges? J Bone Joint Surg Am. 2006;88 Suppl 4:138-147.
23. Schinsky MF, Della Valle CJ, Sporer SM, Paprosky WG. Perioperative testing for joint infection in patients undergoing revision total hip arthroplasty. J Bone Joint Surg Am. 2008;90(9):1869-1875.
24. Spangehl MJ, Masri BA, O'Connell JX, Duncan CP. Prospective analysis of preoperative and intraoperative investigations for the diagnosis of infection at the sites of two hundred and two revision total hip arthroplasties. J Bone Joint Surg Am. 1999;81(5):672-683.
25. Spangehl MJ, Masterson E, Masri BA, O'Connell JX, Duncan CP. The role of intraoperative gram stain in the diagnosis of infection during revision total hip arthroplasty. J

Arthroplasty. 1999;14(8):952-956.
26. Deirmengian C, Hallab N, Tarabishy A, et al. Synovial fluid biomarkers for periprosthetic infection. Clin Orthop Relat Res. 2010;468(8):2017-2023.
27. Kersey R, Benjamin J, Marson B. White blood cell counts and differential in synovial fluid of aseptically failed total knee arthroplasty. J Arthroplasty. 2000;15(3):301-304.
28. Mason JB, Fehring TK, Odum SM, Griffin WL, Nussman DS. The value of white blood cell counts before revision total knee arthroplasty. J Arthroplasty. 2003;18(8):1038-1043.
29. Trampuz A, Hanssen AD, Osmon DR, Mandrekar J, Steckelberg JM, Patel R. Synovial fluid leukocyte count and differential for the diagnosis of prosthetic knee infection. Am J Med. 2004;117(8):556-562.
30. Della Valle CJ, Sporer SM, Jacobs JJ, Berger RA, Rosenberg AG, Paprosky WG. Preoperative testing for sepsis before revision total knee arthroplasty. J Arthroplasty. 2007;22(6 Suppl 2):90-93.
31. Ghanem E, Parvizi J, Burnett RS, et al. Cell count and differential of aspirated fluid in the diagnosis of infection at the site of total knee arthroplasty. J Bone Joint Surg Am. 2008;90(8):1637-1643.
32. Parvizi J, Ghanem E, Sharkey P, Aggarwal A, Burnett RS, Barrack RL. Diagnosis of infected total knee: findings of a multicenter database. Clin Orthop Relat Res. 2008;466(11):2628-2633.
33. Jacovides CL, Parvizi J, Adeli B, Jung KA. Molecular markers for diagnosis of periprosthetic joint infection. J Arthroplasty. 2011;26(6 Suppl):99-103 e101.
34. Parvizi J, Jacovides C, Antoci V, Ghanem E. Diagnosis of periprosthetic joint infection: the utility of a simple yet unappreciated enzyme. J Bone Joint Surg Am. 2011;93(24):2242-2248.
35. Schafer P, Fink B, Sandow D, Margull A, Berger I, Frommelt L. Prolonged bacterial culture to identify late periprosthetic joint infection: a promising strategy. Clin Infect Dis. 2008;47(11):1403-1409.
36. Fink B, Gebhard A, Fuerst M, Berger I, Schafer P. High diagnostic value of synovial biopsy in periprosthetic joint infection of the hip. Clin Orthop Relat Res. 2013;471(3):956-964.
37. Corvec S, Portillo ME, Pasticci BM, Borens O, Trampuz A. Epidemiology and new developments in the diagnosis of prosthetic joint infection. Int J Artif Organs. 2012;35(10):923-934.
38. Trampuz A, Piper KE, Jacobson MJ, et al. Sonication of removed hip and knee prostheses for diagnosis of infection. N Engl J Med. 2007;357(7):654-663.
39. De Man FH, Graber P, Luem M, Zimmerli W, Ochsner PE, Sendi P. Broad-range PCR in selected episodes of prosthetic joint infection. Infection. 2009;37(3):292-294.
40. Mariani BD, Levine MJ, Booth RE, Jr., Tuan RS. Development of a novel, rapid processing protocol for polymerase chain reaction-based detection of bacterial infections in synovial fluids. Mol Biotechnol. 1995;4(3):227-237.
41. Mariani BD, Martin DS, Levine MJ, Booth RE, Jr., Tuan RS. The Coventry Award. Polymerase chain reaction detection of bacterial infection in total knee arthroplasty. Clin Orthop Relat Res. 1996(331):11-22.
42. Levine MJ, Mariani BA, Tuan RS, Booth RE, Jr. Molecular genetic diagnosis of infected total joint arthroplasty. J Arthroplasty. 1995;10(1):93-94.
43. Bergin PF, Doppelt JD, Hamilton WG, et al. Detection of periprosthetic infections with use of ribosomal RNA-based polymerase chain reaction. J Bone Joint Surg Am. 2010;92(3):654-663.
44. Birmingham P, Helm JM, Manner PA, Tuan RS. Simulated joint infection assessment by rapid detection of live bacteria with real-time reverse transcription polymerase chain reaction. J Bone Joint Surg Am. 2008;90(3):602-608.
45. Cazanave C, Greenwood-Quaintance KE, Hanssen AD, et al. Rapid molecular microbiologic diagnosis of prosthetic joint infection. J Clin Microbiol. 2013;51(7):2280-2287.
46. Barber HM, Feil EJ, Galasko CS, et al. A comparative study of dextran-70, warfarin and low-dose heparin for the prophylaxis of thrombo-embolism following total hip replacement. Postgrad Med J. 1977;53(617):130-133.
47. Bozic KJ, Vail TP, Pekow PS, Maselli JH, Lindenauer PK, Auerbach AD. Does aspirin have a role in venous thromboembolism prophylaxis in total knee arthroplasty patients? J Arthroplasty. 2010;25(7):1053-1060.
48. Chin PL, Amin MS, Yang KY, Yeo SJ, Lo NN. Thromboembolic prophylaxis for total knee arthroplasty in Asian patients: a randomised controlled trial. J Orthop Surg (Hong Kong). 2009;17(1):1-5.
49. Asensio A, Antolin FJ, Sanchez-Garcia JM, et al. Timing of DVT prophylaxis and risk of postoperative knee prosthesis infection. Orthopedics. 2010;33(11):800.
50. Parvizi J, Ghanem E, Joshi A, Sharkey PF, Hozack WJ, Rothman RH. Does "excessive" anticoagulation predispose to periprosthetic infection? J Arthroplasty. 2007;22(6 Suppl 2):24-28.
51. Burnett RS, Clohisy JC, Wright RW, et al. Failure of the American College of Chest Physicians-1A protocol for lovenox in clinical outcomes for thromboembolic prophylaxis. J Arthroplasty. 2007;22(3):317-324.

52. Kurtz SM, Ong KL, Lau E, Bozic KJ, Berry D, Parvizi J. Prosthetic joint infection risk after TKA in the Medicare population. Clin Orthop Relat Res. 2010;468(1):52-56.
53. LaPorte DM, Waldman BJ, Mont MA, Hungerford DS. Infections associated with dental procedures in total hip arthroplasty. J Bone Joint Surg Br. 1999;81(1):56-59.
54. Ong KL, Kurtz SM, Lau E, Bozic KJ, Berry DJ, Parvizi J. Prosthetic joint infection risk after total hip arthroplasty in the Medicare population. J Arthroplasty. 2009;24(6 Suppl):105-109.
55. Berbari EF, Osmon DR, Carr A, et al. Dental procedures as risk factors for prosthetic hip or knee infection: a hospital-based prospective case-control study. Clin Infect Dis. 2010;50(1):8-16.
56. Skaar DD, O'Connor H, Hodges JS, Michalowicz BS. Dental procedures and subsequent prosthetic joint infections: findings from the Medicare Current Beneficiary Survey. J Am Dent Assoc. 2011;142(12):1343-1351.
57. Ali NT, Tremewen DR, Hay AJ, Wilkinson DJ. The occurrence of bacteraemia associated with the use of oral and nasopharyngeal airways. Anaesthesia. 1992;47(2):153-155.
58. Baumgartner JC, Heggers JP, Harrison JW. The incidence of bacteremias related to endodontic procedures. I. Nonsurgical endodontics. J Endod. 1976;2(5):135-140.
59. Bender IB, Seltzer S, Tashman S, Meloff G. Dental procedures in patients with rheumatic heart disease. Oral Surg Oral Med Oral Pathol. 1963;16:466-473.
60. Berger SA, Weitzman S, Edberg SC, Casey JI. Bacteremia after the use of an oral irrigation device. A controlled study in subjects with normal-appearing gingiva: comparison with use of toothbrush. Ann Intern Med. 1974;80(4):510-511.
61. Brown AR, Papasian CJ, Shultz P, Theisen FC, Shultz RE. Bacteremia and intraoral suture removal: can an antimicrobial rinse help? J Am Dent Assoc. 1998;129(10):1455-1461.
62. Casolari C, Neglia R, Forabosco A, Galetti R, Fabio U. Incidence of oral bacteremia and antimicrobial prophylaxis. J Chemother. 1989;1(4 Suppl):968-971.
63. Cherry M, Daly CG, Mitchell D, Highfield J. Effect of rinsing with povidone-iodine on bacteraemia due to scaling: a randomized-controlled trial. J Clin Periodontol. 2007;34(2):148-155.
64. Crasta K, Daly CG, Mitchell D, Curtis B, Stewart D, Heitz-Mayfield LJ. Bacteraemia due to dental flossing. J Clin Periodontol. 2009;36(4):323-332.
65. Daly C, Mitchell D, Grossberg D, Highfield J, Stewart D. Bacteraemia caused by periodontal probing. Aust Dent J. 1997;42(2):77-80.
66. Daly CG, Mitchell DH, Highfield JE, Grossberg DE, Stewart D. Bacteremia due to periodontal probing: a clinical and microbiological investigation. J Periodontol. 2001;72(2):210-214.
67. De Leo AA, Schoenknecht FD, Anderson MW, Peterson JC. The incidence of bacteremia following oral prophylaxis on pediatric patients. Oral Surg Oral Med Oral Pathol. 1974;37(1):36-45.
68. Dinner M, Tjeuw M, Artusio JF, Jr. Bacteremia as a complication of nasotracheal intubation Anesth Analg. 1987;66(5):460-462.
69. Enabuele OI, Aluyi HSA, Omokao O. Incidence of bacteraemia following teerh extraction at the dental clinic of the University of Benin Teaching Hospital. African Journal of Biotechnology. 2008;10:1390-1393.
70. Erverdi N, Kadir T, Ozkan H, Acar A. Investigation of bacteremia after orthodontic banding. Am J Orthod Dentofacial Orthop. 1999;116(6):687-690.
71. Felix JE, Rosen S, App GR. Detection of bacteremia after the use of an oral irrigation device in subjects with periodontitis. J Periodontol. 1971;42(12):785-787.
72. Forner L, Nielsen CH, Bendtzen K, Larsen T, Holmstrup P. Increased plasma levels of IL-6 in bacteremic periodontis patients after scaling. J Clin Periodontol. 2006;33(10):724-729.
73. Gurel HG, Basciftci FA, Arslan U. Transient bacteremia after removal of a bonded maxillary expansion appliance. Am J Orthod Dentofacial Orthop. 2009;135(2):190-193.
74. Hansen CP, Westh H, Brok KE, Jensen R, Bertelsen S. Bacteraemia following orotracheal intubation and oesophageal balloon dilatation. Thorax. 1989;44(8):684-685.
75. Heimdahl A, Hall G, Hedberg M, et al. Detection and quantitation by lysis-filtration of bacteremia after different oral surgical procedures. J Clin Microbiol. 1990;28(10):2205-2209.
76. Josefsson K, Heimdahl A, von Konow L, Nord CE. Effect of phenoxymethylpenicillin and erythromycin prophylaxis on anaerobic bacteraemia after oral surgery. J Antimicrob Chemother. 1985;16(2):243-251.
77. Khairat O. The non-aerobes of post-extraction bacteremia. J Dent Res. 1966;45(4):1191-1197.
78. King RC, Crawford JJ, Small EW. Bacteremia following intraoral suture removal. Oral Surg Oral Med Oral Pathol. 1988;65(1):23-28.
79. Lafaurie GI, Mayorga-Fayad I, Torres MF, et al. Periodontopathic microorganisms in peripheric blood after scaling and root planing. J Clin Periodontol. 2007;34(10):873-879.
80. Lineberger LT, De Marco TJ. Evaluation of transient bacteremia following routine periodontal procedures. J Periodontol. 1973;44(12):757-762.
81. Lockhart PB, Brennan MT, Sasser HC, Fox PC, Paster BJ, Bahrani-Mougeot FK. Bacteremia associated with toothbrushing and dental extraction. Circulation.

2008;117(24):3118-3125.
82. Lofthus JE, Waki MY, Jolkovsky DL, et al. Bacteremia following subgingival irrigation and scaling and root planing. J Periodontol. 1991;62(10):602-607.
83. Lucartorto FM, Franker CK, Maza J. Postscaling bacteremia in HIV-associated gingivitis and periodontitis. Oral Surg Oral Med Oral Pathol. 1992;73(5):550-554.
84. Morozumi T, Kubota T, Abe D, Shimizu T, Komatsu Y, Yoshie H. Effects of irrigation with an antiseptic and oral administration of azithromycin on bacteremia caused by scaling and root planing. J Periodontol. 2010;81(11):1555-1563.
85. Oncag O, Cokmez B, Aydemir S, Balcioglu T. Investigation of bacteremia following nasotracheal intubation. Paediatr Anaesth. 2005;15(3):194-198.
86. Pineiro A, Tomas I, Blanco J, Alvarez M, Seoane J, Diz P. Bacteraemia following dental implants' placement. Clin Oral Implants Res. 2010;21(9):913-918.
87. Ramadan AE, Zaki SA, Nour ZM. A study of transient bacteremia following the use of dental floss silk and interdental stimulators. Egypt Dent J. 1975;21(4):19-28.
88. Rogosa M, Hampp EG, Nevin TA, Wagner HN, Jr., Driscoll EJ, Baer PN. Blood sampling and cultural studies in the detection of postoperative bacteremias. J Am Dent Assoc. 1960;60:171-180.
89. Romans AR, App GR. Bacteremia, a result from oral irrigation in subjects with gingivitis. J Periodontol. 1971;42(12):757-760.
90. Savarrio L, Mackenzie D, Riggio M, Saunders WP, Bagg J. Detection of bacteraemias during non-surgicalroot canal treatment. J Dent. 2005;33(4):293-303.
91. Sconyers JR, Albers DD, Kelly R. Relationship of bacteremia to toothbrushing in clinically healthy patients. Gen Dent. 1979;27(3):51-52.
92. Sconyers JR, Crawford JJ, Moriarty JD. Relationship of bacteremia to toothbrushing in patients with periodontitis. J Am Dent Assoc. 1973;87(3):616-622.
93. Takai S, Kuriyama T, Yanagisawa M, Nakagawa K, Karasawa T. Incidence and bacteriology of bacteremia associated with various oral and maxillofacial surgical procedures. Oral Surg Oral Med Oral Pathol Oral Radiol Endod. 2005;99(3):292-298.
94. Valdes C, Tomas I, Alvarez M, Limeres J, Medina J, Diz P. The incidence of bacteraemia associated with tracheal intubation. Anaesthesia. 2008;63(6):588-592.
95. Wada K, Tomizawa M, Sasaki I. Study on bacteriemia in patients with pyorrhea alveolaris caused by surgical operations. J Nihon Univ Sch Dent. 1968;10(2):52-57.
96. Waki MY, Jolkovsky DL, Otomo-Corgel J, et al. Effects of subgingival irrigation on bacteremia following scaling and root planing. J Periodontol. 1990;61(7):405-411.
97. Wampole HS, Allen AL, Gross A. The incidence of transient bacteremia during periodontal dressing change. J Periodontol. 1978;49(9):462-464.
98. Wank HA, Levison ME, Rose LF, Cohen DW. A quantitative measurement of bacteremia and its relationship to plaque control. J Periodontol. 1976;47(12):683-686.
99. Friedlander AH. Antibiotic prophylaxis after total joint replacement. Hong Kong Med J. 2010;16(4):320; author reply 321.
100. Jacobson JJ, Patel B, Asher G, Woolliscroft JO, Schaberg D. Oral staphylococcus in older subjects with rheumatoid arthritis. J Am Geriatr Soc. 1997;45(5):590-593.
101. Poss R, Thornhill TS, Ewald FC, Thomas WH, Batte NJ, Sledge CB. Factors influencing the incidence and outcome of infection following total joint arthroplasty. Clin Orthop Relat Res. 1984(182):117-126.
102. Berbari EF, Hanssen AD, Duffy MC, et al. Risk factors for prosthetic joint infection: case-control study. Clin Infect Dis. 1998;27(5):1247-1254.
103. Jacobson JJ, Millard HD, Plezia R, Blankenship JR. Dental treatment and late prosthetic joint infections. Oral Surg Oral Med Oral Pathol. 1986;61(4):413-417.
104. Murray RP, Bourne MH, Fitzgerald RH, Jr. Metachronous infections in patients who have had more than one total joint arthroplasty. J Bone Joint Surg Am. 1991;73(10):1469-1474.
105. Nadlacan LM, Hirst P. Infected total knee replacement following a dental procedure in a severe haemophiliac. Knee. 2001;8(2):159-161.
106. Lockhart PB, Brennan MT, Thornhill M, et al. Poor oral hygiene as a risk factor for infective endocarditis-related bacteremia. J Am Dent Assoc. 2009;140(10):1238-1244.
107. Silver JG, Martin AW, McBride BC. Experimental transient bacteraemias in human subjects with varying degrees of plaque accumulation and gingival inflammation. J Clin Periodontol. 1977;4(2):92-99.
108. Bhanji S, Williams B, Sheller B, Elwood T, Mancl L. Transient bacteremia induced by toothbrushing a comparison of the Sonicare toothbrush with a conventional toothbrush. Pediatr Dent. 2002;24(4):295-299.
109. Diz Dios P, Tomas Carmona I, Limeres Posse J, Medina Henriquez J, Fernandez Feijoo J, Alvarez Fernandez M. Comparative efficacies of amoxicillin, clindamycin, and moxifloxacin in prevention of bacteremia following dental extractions. Antimicrob Agents Chemother. 2006;50(9):2996-3002.
110. Lockhart PB, Brennan MT, Kent ML, Norton HJ, Weinrib DA. Impact of amoxicillin prophylaxis on the incidence, nature, and duration of bacteremia in children after intubation and dental procedures. Circulation. 2004;109(23):2878-2884.

111. Maskell JP, Carter JL, Boyd RB, Williams RJ. Teicoplanin as a prophylactic antibiotic for dental bacteraemia. J Antimicrob Chemother. 1986;17(5):651-659.
112. Roberts GJ, Radford P, Holt R. Prophylaxis of dental bacteraemia with oral amoxycillin in children. Er Dent J. 1987;162(5):179-182.
113. Shanson DC, Cannon P, Wilks M. Amoxycillin compared with penicillin V for the prophylaxis of dental bacteraemia. J Antimicrob Chemother. 1978;4(5):431-436.
114. Vergis EN, Demas PN, Vaccarello SJ, Yu VL. Topical antibiotic prophylaxis for bacteraemia after dental extractions. Oral Surg Oral Med Oral Pathol Oral Radiol Endod. 2001;91(2):162-165.
115. Wilson W, Taubert KA, Gewitz M, et al. Prevention of infective endocarditis: guidelines from the American Heart Association: a guideline from the American Heart Association Rheumatic Fever, Endocarditis, and Kawasaki Disease Committee, Council on Cardiovascular Disease in the Young, and the Council on Clinical Cardiology, Council on Cardiovascular Surgery and Anesthesia, and the Quality of Care and Outcomes Research Interdisciplinary Working Group. Circulation. 2007;116(15):1736-1754.
116. Hall G, Heimdahl A, Nord CE. Effects of prophylactic administration of cefaclor on transient bacteremia after dental extraction. Eur J Clin Microbiol Infect Dis. 1996;15(8):646-649.
117. Aitken C, Cannell H, Sefton AM, et al. Comparative efficacy of oral doses of clindamycin and erythromycin in the prevention of bacteraemia. Br Dent J. 1995;178(11):418-422.
118. deVries J, Francis LE, Lang D. Control of post-extraction bacteraemias in the penicillin-hypersensitive patient. J Can Dent Assoc (Tor). 1972;38(2):63-66.
119. Cannell H, Kerawala C, Sefton AM, et al. Failure of two macrolide antibiotics to prevent post-extraction bacteraemia. Br Dent J. 1991;171(6):170-173.
120. Shanson DC, Akash S, Harris M, Tadayon M. Erythromycin stearate, 1.5 g, for the oral prophylaxis of streptococcal bacteraemia in patients undergoing dental extraction: efficacy and tolerance. J Antimicrob Chemother. 1985;15(1):83-90.
121. Head TW, Bentley KC, Millar EP, deVries JA. A comparative study of the effectiveness of metronidazole and penicillin V in eliminating anaerobes from postextraction bacteremias. Oral Surg Oral Med Oral Pathol. 1984;58(2):152-155.
122. Jokinen MA. Bacteremia following dental extraction and its prophylaxis. Suom Hammaslaak Toim. 1970;66(3):69-100.
123. Wahlmann U, Al-Nawas B, Jutte M, Wagner W. Clinical and microbiological efficacy of single dose cefuroxime prophylaxis for dental surgical procedures. Int J Antimicrob Agents. 1999;12(3):253-256.
124. Shanson DC, Shehata A, Tadayon M, Harris M. Comparison of intravenous teicoplanin with intramuscular amoxycillin for the prophylaxis of streptococcal bacteraemia in dental patients. J Antimicrob Chemother. 1987;20(1):85-93.
125. Lehman CR, Ries MD, Paiement GD, Davidson AB. Infection after total joint arthroplasty in patients with human immunodeficiency virus or intravenous drug use. J Arthroplasty. 2001;16(3):330-335.
126. Peersman G, Laskin R, Davis J, Peterson M. Infection in total knee replacement: a retrospective review of 6489 total knee replacements. Clin Orthop Relat Res. 2001;(392):15-23.
127. Pour AE, Matar WY, Jafari SM, Purtill JJ, Austin MS, Parvizi J. Total joint arthroplasty in patients with hepatitis C. J Bone Joint Surg Am. 2011;93(15):1448-1454.
128. Bozic KJ, Ong K, Lau E, et al. Estimating risk in Medicare patients with THA: an electronic risk calculator for periprosthetic joint infection and mortality. Clin Orthop Relat Res. 2013;471(2):574-583.
129. Bozic KJ, Lau E, Kurtz S, et al. Patient-related risk factors for periprosthetic joint infection and postoperative mortality following total hip arthroplasty in Medicare patients. J Bone Joint Surg Am. 2012;94(9):794-800.
130. Everhart JS, Altneu E, Calhoun JH. Medical Comorbidities Are Independent Preoperative Risk Factors for Surgical Infection After Total Joint Arthroplasty. Clin Orthop Relat Res. Mar 22 2013. Epub before print.
131. Fulido L, Ghanem E, Joshi A, Purtill JJ, Parvizi J. Periprosthetic joint infection: the incidence, timing, and predisposing factors. Clin Orthop Relat Res. 2008;466(7):1710-1715.
132. Young J, De Sutter A, Merenstein D, et al. Antibiotics for adults with clinically diagnosed acute rhinosinusitis: a meta-analysis of individual patient data. Lancet. 2008;371(9616):908-914.
133. Reyes H, Guiscafre H, Munoz O, Perez-Cuevas R, Martinez H, Gutierrez G. Antibiotic noncompliance and waste in upper respiratory infections and acute diarrhea. J Clin Epidemiol. 1997;50(11):1297-1304.
134. Okeke IN, Lamikanra A, Edelman R. Socioeconomic and behavioral factors leading to acquired bacterial resistance to antibiotics in developing countries. Emerg Infect Dis. 1999;5(1):18-27.
135. LeFrock JL, Ellis CA, Turchik JB, Weinstein L. Transient bacteremia associated with sigmoidoscopy. N Engl J Med. 1973;289(9):467-469.
136. Coughlin GP, Butler RN, Alp MH, Grant AK. Colonoscopy and bacteraemia. Gut. 1977;18(8):678-679.
137. Dickman MD, Farrell R, Higgs RH, et al. Colonoscopy associated bacteremia. Surg

Gynecol Obstet. 1976;142(2):173-176.
138. Norfleet RG, Mulholland DD, Mitchell PD, Philo J, Walters EW. Does bacteremia follow colonoscopy? Gastroenterology. 1976;70(1):20-21.
139. Geraci K, Simfendorfer C, Rosenthal M. Does bacteraemia follow colonoscopy. Gastroenterology. 1976;70:1189.
140. Leiberman TR. Bacteraemia and fibreoptic endoscopy. Gastrointest Endosc. 1976;23:36-37.
141. Kumar S, Abcarian H, Prasad ML, Lakshmanan S. Bacteremia associated with lower gastrointestinal endoscopy, fact or fiction? I. Colonoscopy. Dis Colon Rectum. 1982;25(2):131-134.
142. Kumar S, Abcarian H, Prasad ML, Lakshmanan S. Bacteremia associated with lower gastrointestinal endoscopy: fact or fiction? II. Proctosigmoidoscopy. Dis Colon Rectum. 1983;26(1):22-24.
143. Hirota WK, Petersen K, Baron TH, et al. Guidelines for antibiotic prophylaxis for GI endoscopy. Gastrointest Endosc. 2003;58(4):475-482.
144. Practice parameters for antibiotic prophylaxis to prevent infective endocarditis or infected prosthesis during colon and rectal endoscopy. The Standards Task Force. The American Society of Colon and Rectal Surgeons. Dis Colon Rectum. 2000;43(9):1193.
145. Meyer GW, Artis AL. Antibiotic prophylaxis for orthopedic prostheses and GI procedures: report of a survey. Am J Gastroenterol. 1997;92(6):989-991.
146. Barragan Casas JM, Hernandez Hernandez JM, Garcinuno Jimenez MA, et al. Bacteremia caused by digestive system endoscopy. Rev Esp Enferm Dig. 1999;91(2):105-116.
147. Nelson DB. Infectious disease complications of GI endoscopy: Part I, endogenous infections. Gastrointest Endosc. 2003;57(4):546-556.
148. Spach DH, Silverstein FE, Stamm WE. Transmission of infection by gastrointestinal endoscopy and bronchoscopy. Ann Intern Med. 1993;118(2):117-128.
149. Nelson DB. Infection control during gastrointestinal endoscopy. J Lab Clin Med. 2003;141(3):159-167.
150. Cornelius LK, Reddix RN, Jr., Carpenter JL. Periprosthetic knee joint infection following colonoscopy. A case report. J Bone Joint Surg Am. 2003;85-A(12):2434-2436.
151. Zuckerman GR, O'Brien J, Halsted R. Antibiotic prophylaxis in patients with infectious risk factors undergoing gastrointestinal endoscopic procedures. Gastrointest Endosc. 1994;40(5):538-543.
152. Schlaeffer F, Riesenberg K, Mikolich D, Sikuler E, Niv Y. Serious bacterial infections after endoscopic procedures. Arch Intern Med. 1996;156(5):572-574.
153. Coelho-Prabhu N, Oxentenko AS, Osmon DR, et al. Increased risk of prosthetic joint infection associated with esophago-gastro-duodenoscopy with biopsy. Acta Orthop. 2013;84(1):82-86.
154. Bac DJ, van Blankenstein M, de Marie S, Fieren MW. Peritonitis following endoscopic polypectomy in a peritoneal dialysis patient: the need for antibiotic prophylaxis. Infection. 1994;22(3):220-221.
155. Lin YC, Lin WP, Huang JY, Lee SY. Polymicrobial peritonitis following colonoscopic polypectomy in a peritoneal dialysis patient. Intern Med. 2012;51(14):1841-1843.
156. Dajani AS, Taubert KA, Wilson W, et al. Prevention of bacterial endocarditis: recommendations by the American Heart Association. Clin Infect Dis. 1997;25(6):1448-1458.
157. Ainscow DA, Denham RA. The risk of haematogenous infection in total joint replacements. J Bone Joint Surg Br. 1984;66(4):580-582.
158. Chihara S, Popovich KJ, Weinstein RA, Hota B. Staphylococcus aureus bacteriuria as a prognosticator for outcome of Staphylococcus aureus bacteremia: a case-control study. BMC Infect Dis. 2010;10:225.
159. Muder RR, Brennen C, Rihs JD, et al. Isolation of Staphylococcus aureus from the urinary tract: association of isolation with symptomatic urinary tract infection and subsequent staphylococcal bacteremia. Clin Infect Dis. 2006;42(1):46-50.
160. Bhanot N, Sahud AG, Sepkowitz D. Best practice policy statement on urologic surgery antimicrobial prophylaxis. Urology. 2009;74(1):236-237.
161. Sullivan NM, Sutter VL, Carter WT, Attebery HR, Finegold SM. Bacteremia after genitourinary tract manipulation: bacteriological aspects and evaluation of various blood culture systems. Appl Microbiol. 1972;23(6):1101-1106.
162. Breslin JA, Turner BI, Faber RB, Rhamy RK. Anaerobic infection as a consequence of transrectal prostatic biopsy. J Urol. 1978;120(4):502-503.
163. Edson RS, Van Scoy RE, Leary FJ. Gram-negative bacteremia after transrectal needle biopsy of the prostate. Mayo Clin Proc. 1980;55(8):489-491.
164. Gross M, Winkler H, Pitlik S, Weinberger M. Unexpected candidemia complicating ureteroscopy and urinary stenting. Eur J Clin Microbiol Infect Dis. 1998;17(8):583-586.
165. Hedelin H, Claesson BE, Wilpart A. Febrile reactions after transrectal ultrasound-guided prostatic biopsy: a retrospective study. Scand J Urol Nephrol. 2011;45(6):393-396.
166. Thompson PM, Talbot RW, Packham DA, Dulake C. Transrectal biopsy of the prostate and bacteraemia. Br J Surg. 1980;67(2):127-128.

167. Thompson PM, Pryor JP, Williams JP, et al. The problem of infection after prostatic biopsy: the case for the transperineal approach. Br J Urol. 1982;54(6):736-740.
168. Zani EL, Clark OA, Rodrigues Netto N, Jr. Antibiotic prophylaxis for transrectal prostate biopsy. Cochrane Database Syst Rev. 2011(5):CD006576.
169. Pepke W, Lehner B, Bekeredjian-Ding I, Egermann M. Haematogenous infection of a total knee arthroplasty with Klebsiella pneumoniae. BMJ Case Rep. 2013;2013.
170. Madsen PO, Larsen EH, Dorflinger T. Infectious complications after instrumentation of urinary tract. Urology. 1985;26(1 Suppl):15-17.
171. Vivien A, Lazard T, Rauss A, Laisne MJ, Bonnet F. Infection after transurethral resection of the prostate: variation among centers and correlation with a long-lasting surgical procedure. Association pour la Recherche en Anesthesie-Reanimation. Eur Urol. 1998;33(4):365-369.
172. Roth RA, Beckmann CF. Complications of extracorporeal shock-wave lithotripsy and percutaneous nephrolithotomy. Urol Clin North Am. 1988;15(2):155-166.
173. Zimhony O, Goland S, Malnick SD, Singer D, Geltner D. Enterococcal endocarditis after extracorporeal shock wave lithotripsy for nephrolithiasis. Postgrad Med J. 1996;72(843):51-52.
174. Tiossi CL, Rodrigues FO, Santos AR, Franken RA, Mimica L, Tedesco JJ. [Bacteremia induced by labor. Is prophylaxis for infective endocarditis necessary?]. Arq Bras Cardiol. 1994;62(2):91-94.
175. Murray S, Hickey JB, Houang E. Significant bacteremia associated with replacement of intrauterine contraceptive device. Am J Obstet Gynecol. 1987;156(3):698-700.
176. Silverman NS, Sullivan MW, Jungkind DL, Weinblatt V, Beavis K, Wapner RJ. Incidence of bacteremia associated with chorionic villus sampling. Obstet Gynecol. 1994;84(6):1021-1024.
177. Wolf JS, Jr., Bennett CJ, Dmochowski RR, Hollenbeck BK, Pearle MS, Schaeffer AJ. Best practice policy statement on urologic surgery antimicrobial prophylaxis. J Urol. 2008;179(4):1379-1390.
178. American College of Onstetricians and Gynecologists Committee on Obstetric Practice. ACOG Committee Opinion No. 421, November 2008: antibiotic prophylaxis for infective endocarditis. Obstet Gynecol. 2008;112(5):1193-1194.
179. Schimpl G, Pesendorfer P, Steinwender G, Feierl G, Ratschek M, Hollwarth ME. The effect of vitamin C and vitamin E supplementation on bacterial translocation in chronic portal hypertensive and common-bile-duct-ligated rats. Eur Surg Res. 1997;29(3):187-194.
180. Gianotti L, Alexander JW, Gennari R, Pyles T, Babcock GF. Oral glutamine decreases bacterial translocation and improves survival in experimental gut-origin sepsis. JPEN J Parenter Enteral Nutr. 1995;19(1):69-74.
181. Zhang W, Frankel WL, Bain A, Choi D, Klurfeld DM, Rombeau JL. Glutamine reduces bacterial translocation after small bowel transplantation in cyclosporine-treated rats. J Surg Res. 1995;58(2):159-164.
182. White JS, Hoper M, Parks RW, Clements WD, Diamond T. Glutamine improves intestinal barrier function in experimental biliary obstruction. Eur Surg Res. 2005;37(6):342-347.
183. Noth R, Hasler R, Stuber E, et al. Oral glutamine supplementation improves intestinal permeability dysfunction in a murine acute graft-vs.-host disease model. Am J Physiol Gastrointest Liver Physiol. 2013;304(7):G646-654.
184. Gurbuz AT, Kunzelman J, Ratzer EE. Supplemental dietary arginine accelerates intestinal mucosal regeneration and enhances bacterial clearance following radiation enteritis in rats. J Surg Res. 1998;74(2):149-154.
185. Karatepe O, Acet E, Battal M, et al. Effects of glutamine and curcumin on bacterial translocation in jaundiced rats. World J Gastroenterol. 2010;16(34):4313-4320.
186. Huang CW, Lee TT, Shih YC, Yu B. Effects of dietary supplementation of Chinese medicinal herbs on polymorphonuclear neutrophil immune activity and small intestinal morphology in weanling pigs. J Anim Physiol Anim Nutr (Berl). 2012;96(2):285-294.
187. Bose S, Song MY, Nam JK, Lee MJ, Kim H. In vitro and in vivo protective effects of fermented preparations of dietary herbs against lipopolysaccharide insult. Food Chem. 2012;134(2):758-765.
188. Fabia R, Ar'Rajab A, Willen R, et al. Effects of phosphatidylcholine and phosphatidylinositol on acetic-acid-induced colitis in the rat. Digestion. 1992;53(1-2):35-44.
189. Wang XD, Andersson R, Soltesz V, Wang WQ, Ar'Rajab A, Bengmark S. Phospholipids prevent enteric bacterial translocation in the early stage of experimental acute liver failure in the rat. Scand J Gastroenterol. 1994;29(12):1117-1121.
190. Mangiante G, Canepari P, Colucci G, et al. [A probiotic as an antagonist of bacterial translocation in experimental pancreatitis]. Chir Ital. 1999;51(3):221-226.
191. Mao Y, Nobaek S, Kasravi B, et al. The effects of Lactobacillus strains and oat fiber on methotrexate-induced enterocolitis in rats. Gastroenterology. 1996;111(2):334-344.
192. Berg R, Bernasconi P, Fowler D, Gautreaux M. Inhibition of Candida albicans translocation from the gastrointestinal tract of mice by oral administration of Saccharomyces boulardii. J Infect Dis. 1993;168(5):1314-1318.
193. Caetano JA, Parames MT, Babo MJ, et al. Immunopharmological effects of Saccharomyces boulardii in healthy human volunteers. Int J Immunopharmacol. 1986;8(3):245-259.

194. Catanzarro JA, Green L. Mirobial ecology and probitoics in human medicine (Part II). Alt Med Rev. 1997;2:245-259.
195. Tang ZF, Ling YB, Lin N, Hao Z, Xu RY. Glutamine and recombinant human growth hormone protect intestinal barrier function following portal hypertension surgery. World J Gastroenterol. 2007;13(15):2223-2228.
196. Berg RD. Bacterial translocation from the gastrointestinal tract. J Med. 1992;23(3-4):217-244.
197. Spaeth G, Berg RD, Specian RD, Deitch EA. Food without fiber promotes bacterial translocation from the gut. Surgery. 1990;108(2):240-246; discussion 246-247.
198. Spaeth G, Specian RD, Berg RD, Deitch EA. Bulk prevents bacterial translocation induced by the oral administration of total parenteral nutrition solution. JPEN J Parenter Enteral Nutr. 1990;14(5):442-447.
199. Economedes DM, Deirmengian GK, Deirmengian CA. Staphylococcus aureus Colonization among Arthroplasty Patients Previously Treated by a Decolonization Protocol: A Pilot Study. Clin Orthop Relat Res. Mar 5 2013. Epub before print.
200. Immerman I, Ramos NL, Katz GM, Hutzler LH, Phillips MS, Bosco JA, 3rd. The persistence of Staphylococcus aureus decolonization after mupirocin and topical chlorhexidine: implications for patients requiring multiple or delayed procedures. J Arthroplasty. 2012;27(6):870-876.
201. Rodriguez D, Pigrau C, Euba G, et al. Acute haematogenous prosthetic joint infection: prospective evaluation of medical and surgical management. Clin Microbiol Infect. 2010;16(12):1789-1795.
202. Schmalzried TP, Amstutz HC, Au MK, Dorey FJ. Etiology of deep sepsis in total hip arthroplasty. The significance of hematogenous and recurrent infections. Clin Orthop Relat Res. 1992(280):200-207.
203. Strazzeri JC, Anzel S. Infected total hip arthroplasty due to Actinomyces israelii after dental extraction. A case report. Clin Orthop Relat Res. 1986(210):128-131.
204. Wust J, Steiger U, Vuong H, Zbinden R. Infection of a hip prosthesis by Actinomyces naeslundii. J Clin Microbiol. 2000;38(2):929-930.
205. Meehan AM, Osmon DR, Duffy MC, Hanssen AD, Keating MR. Outcome of penicillin-susceptible streptococcal prosthetic joint infection treated with debridement and retention of the prosthesis. Clin Infect Dis. 2003;36(7):845-849.
206. Sapico FL, Liquete JA, Sarma RJ. Bone and joint infections in patients with infective endocarditis: review of a 4-year experience. Clin Infect Dis. 1996;22(5):783-787.
207. Han Z, Burnham CA, Clohisy J, Babcock H. Mycoplasma pneumoniae periprosthetic joint infection identified by 16S ribosomal RNA gene amplification and sequencing: a case report. J Bone Joint Surg Am. 2011;93(18):e103.
208. Cordero-Ampuero J, de Dios M. What are the risk factors for infection in hemiarthroplasties and total hip arthroplasties? Clin Orthop Relat Res. 2010;468(12):3268-3277.
209. Fabry K, Verheyden F, Nelen G. Infection of a total knee prosthesis by Candida glabrata: a case report. Acta Orthop Belg. 2005;71(1):119-121.
210. Szabados F, Anders A, Kaase M, et al. Late Periprosthetic Joint Infection due to Staphylococcus lugdunensis Identified by Matrix-Assisted Laser Desorption/Ionisation Time of Flight Mass Spectrometry: A Case Report and Review of the Literature. Case Rep Med. 2011;2011:608919.
211. O'Brien JP, Goldenberg DL, Rice PA. Disseminated gonococcal infection: a prospective analysis of 49 patients and a review of pathophysiology and immune mechanisms. Medicine (Baltimore). 1983;62(6):395-406.
212. Ollivere BJ, Ellahee N, Logan K, Miller-Jones JC, Allen PW. Asymptomatic urinary tract colonisation predisposes to superficial wound infection in elective orthopaedic surgery. Int Orthop. 2009;33(3):847-850.
213. Brumfitt W. Urinary Cell Counts and Their Value. J Clin Pathol. 1965;18:550-555.
214. Trautner BW. Asymptomatic bacteriuria: when the treatment is worse than the disease. Nat Rev Urol. 1997;9(2):85-93.
215. Drancourt M, Argenson JN, Tissot Dupont H, Aubaniac JM, Raoult D. Psoriasis is a risk factor for hip-prosthesis infection. Eur J Epidemiol. 1997;13(2):205-207.
216. Beyer CA, Hanssen AD, Lewallen DG, Pittelkow MR. Primary total knee arthroplasty in patients with psoriasis. J Bone Joint Surg Br. 1991;73(2):258-259.
217. Iofin I, Levine B, Badlani N, Klein GR, Jaffe WL. Psoriatic arthritis and arthroplasty: a review of the literature. Bull NYU Hosp Jt Dis. 2008;66(1):41-48.
218. Zaman R, Abbas M, Burd E. Late prosthetic hip joint infection with Actinomyces israelii in an intravenous drug user: case report and literature review. J Clin Microbiol. 2002;40(11):4391-4392.
219. Pascual A, Fleer A, Westerdaal NA, Verhoef J. Modulation of adherence of coagulase-negative staphylococci to Teflon catheters in vitro. Eur J Clin Microbiol. 1986;5(5):518-522.
220. Raad I, Darouiche R. Catheter-related septicemia: risk reduction. Infect Med. 1996;13:807-823.

221. Athanassious C, Samad A, Avery A, Cohen J, Chalnick D. Evaluation of fever in the immediate postoperative period in patients who underwent total joint arthroplasty. J Arthroplasty. 2011;26(8):1404-1408.
222. Czaplicki AP, Borger JE, Politi JR, Chambers BT, Taylor BC. Evaluation of postoperative fever and leukocytosis in patients after total hip and knee arthroplasty. J Arthroplasty. 2011;26(8):1387-1389.
223. Summersell PC, Turnbull A, Long G, et al. Temperature trends in total hip arthroplasty: a retrospective study. J Arthroplasty. 2003;18(4):426-429.
224. Andres BM, Taub DD, Gurkan I, Wenz JF. Postoperative fever after total knee arthroplasty: the role of cytokines. Clin Orthop Relat Res. 2003(415):221-231.
225. Kennedy JG, Rodgers WB, Zurakowski D, et al. Pyrexia after total knee replacement. A cause for concern? Am J Orthop (Belle Mead NJ). 1997;26(8):549-552, 554.
226. Guinn S, Castro FP, Jr., Garcia R, Barrack RL. Fever following total knee arthroplasty. Am J Knee Surg. Summer 1999;12(3):161-164.
227. Shaw JA, Chung R. Febrile response after knee and hip arthroplasty. Clin Orthop Relat Res. 1999(367):181-189.
228. Ghosh S, Charity RM, Haidar SG, Singh BK. Pyrexia following total knee replacement. Knee. 2006;13(4):324-327.
229. Anderson JT, Osland JD. Blood cultures for evaluation of fever after total joint arthroplasty. Am J Orthop (Belle Mead NJ). 2009;38(8):E134-136.
230. Tai TW, Chang CW, Lin CJ, Lai KA, Yang CY. Elevated temperature trends after total knee arthroplasty. Orthopedics. 2009;32(12):886.
231. Ward DT, Hansen EN, Takemoto SK, Bozic KJ. Cost and effectiveness of postoperative fever diagnostic evaluation in total joint arthroplasty patients. J Arthroplasty. 2010;25(6 Suppl):43-48.

Question 1

- **What is the definition of a late periprosthetic joint infection (PJI)?**

Consensus: Late PJI can be defined as a PJI that develops at a variable length of time after an index arthroplasty procedure. The late PJI occurs after an initially successful index procedure with no clinical or radiographic signs of PJI. Risk factors for late PJI are similar to those described for PJI (Workgroup 1).

Delegate Vote

Agree: 56%, Disagree: 39%, Abstain: 5% (Weak Consensus)

Question 2

- **Which diagnostic procedures have to be done to verify late PJI?**

Consensus: The workup of patients with painful joint and suspected (late) PJI should follow the algorithm provided in Workgroup 7.

Delegate Vote

Agree: 89%, Disagree: 9%, Abstain: 2% (Strong Consensus)

Question 3

- **Does the type, dose, and length of anticoagulation for prophylaxis influence the incidence of surgical site infection (SSI) following total joint arthroplasty (TJA)?**

Consensus: Yes. The type, dose, and length of administration of anticoagulation drugs for prophylaxis against venous thromboembolism influence the incidence of SSI following TJA.

Delegate Vote

Agree: 76%, Disagree: 9%, Abstain: 15% (Strong Consensus)

Question 4

- **Should a patient with TJA be given routine dental antibiotic prophylaxis?**

Consensus: The use of dental antibiotic prophylaxis in patients with TJA should be individualized based on patient risk factors and the complexity of the dental procedure to be performed.

Delegate Vote

Agree: 81%, Disagree: 16%, Abstain: 3% (Strong Consensus)

Consensus: We recommend that high-risk patients receive lifetime dental antibiotic prophylaxis after TJA.

Consensus: We recommend that an oral antibiotic be given at the following dosages for only one dose prior to dental procedures.

Consensus: We recommend that one of the following intravenous (IV) or intramuscular antibiotics be given at the following dosages for only one dose prior to dental procedures.

Question 5

- **Should patients at high risk of late PJI be given prophylactic antibiotics during viral illnesses?**

Consensus: There is no role for the administration of oral antibiotics to patients with TJA who develop viral illnesses.

Delegate Vote

Agree: 98%, Disagree: 2%, Abstain: 0% (Strong Consensus)

Question 6

- **Can transient bactermia be minimized during endoscopic procedures such as colonoscopy to prevent late PJI?**

Consensus: The influence of transient bacteremia can be minimized during minor surgical procedures by administering prophylactic antibiotics to individualized patients and especially to high-risk patients.

Delegate Vote

Agree: 85%, Disagree: 13%, Abstain: 2% (Strong Consensus)

Question 7

- **What is the role of herbal supplements, probiotics, and alternative medicine in decreasing translocation of bacteria across the intestinal wall?**

Consensus: There is insufficient evidence that supports the use of herbal supplements, probiotics, and alternative medicine to decrease translocation of bacteria across the intestinal wall to prevent late PJIs.

Delegate Vote
Agree: 95%, Disagree: 3%, Abstain: 2% (Strong Consensus)

Question 8

- **Is there a role for post-surgical monitoring of methicillin-resistant Staphylococcus (MRSA) colonization in the asymptomatic patient?**

Consensus: We recommend against post-surgical monitoring of MRSA colonization in the asymptomatic patient.

Delegate Vote
Agree: 98%, Disagree: 2%, Abstain: 0% (Strong Consensus)

Consensus: We recommend that patients undergo repeat screening for *Staphylococcus aureus* and decolonization prior to additional arthroplasty.

Question 9

- **What are the methods to identify extra-articular sources of late PJI?**

Consensus: Extra-articular sources that contribute to late PJI should be identified by obtaining history, performing a thorough physical exam, laboratory testing, and imaging of suspected areas of infection.

Delegate Vote
Agree: 92%, Disagree: 3%, Abstain: 5% (Strong Consensus)

Question 10

- **When should further workup for postoperative fevers be performed after TJA?**

Consensus: We recommend against the routine workup of fevers greater than 38.5℃ in the immediate postoperative period. However, the workup of persistent fevers after postoperative day 3 may be warranted.

Delegate Vote
Agree: 81%, Disagree: 15%, Abstain: 4% (Strong Consensus)

"International Consensus Meeting on Periprosthetic Joint Infection" に参加して

2013年8月に米国フィラデルフィアで開催された"International Consensus Meeting on Periprosthetic Joint Infection"に参加するという貴重な機会をいただきました．私が担当したWorkgroupは本冊子でも翻訳に携わったWorkgroup 7の人工関節周囲感染（PJI）における診断に関するグループであり，会議の数ヵ月前からweb上での議論をもとにQuestionとそれに対する回答，根拠となる文献的考察などの文書作成が行われました．全体会議前日の各グループ会議では私の留学時代の恩師であるThomas Bauer先生が司会を務められたため個人的には助かりましたが，白熱した議論に圧倒されたことが思い出されます．全体会議当日も実に多くの国より参加者が集結し，一つ一つの質問に対するコンセンサスを確認するという作業が行われまし

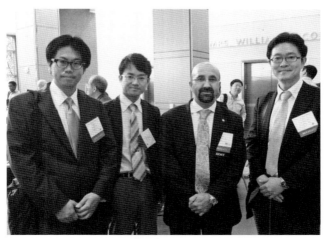

（左より，横浜市大から齋藤教授の代理として出席した小林秀郎，筆者，Parvizi先生，山田浩司先生）

た.その後,この会議のリーダーである Javad Parvizi 先生のご自宅で懇親パーティーが開かれ,本冊子の編集者であられる山田浩司先生らとともに大変楽しいひとときを過ごさせていただきました.

　PJI に関しては予防,診断,治療のいずれにおいてもさらなる研究が必要であり,今後も微力ながらこの分野の発展に貢献できればと思います.今回はこのような貴重な機会をいただき誠にありがとうございました.

横浜市立大学医学部整形外科
小林直実

あとがき

　Musculoskeletal Infection Society（MSIS）元会長の Javad Parvizi 教授と European Bone and Joint Infection Society（EBJIS）元会長の Thorsten Gehrke 教授の惜しみのない努力と熱意により，全世界の英知を結集し，2013 年夏に整形外科領域としてその規模・質ともに前代未聞のコンセンサスステートメントが完成した．人工関節置換術の術後合併症として最も重要である人工関節周囲感染（Periprosthetic Joint Infection：PJI）のマネージメントをテーマとした壮大なプロジェクトであり，すでに世界十数か国で翻訳が行われており，世界中の整形外科医の道標となっている．国内においても，手術部位感染に関わる多数の文献や学会報告などで引用されており，2015 年に刊行された骨・関節術後感染予防ガイドライン改訂版の作成においても重要な情報源となり，その影響力は計り知れない．

　PJI マネージメントは，医師だけでなく多くの医療従事者の協力なくして良い結果は得られない．邦訳版は，少しでも多くの関係者に本コンセンサスの内容をより正確に理解いただくために重要なツールになると考え，多くの方々にご協力いただき丁寧な翻訳を心がけた．一人でも多くの患者様へ，少しでも高いレベルの医療を提供するために，是非多くの関係者にご活用いただければと思っている．

　本コンセンサスの目標は，PJI マネージメントに関して臨床上問題となる様々な状況に対して何かしら指針を作成することである．PJI 診療を大きく 15 のテーマに分け，特に判断に困る状況を厳選し，200 以上の設問に対して其々のワーキンググループを中心にその指針をまとめ上げた．本コンセンサスは，整形外科医だけでなく感染症内科，病理学，細菌学，薬理学，核医学，リウマチ科，筋骨格系を専門とした放射線科，皮膚科，麻酔科など様々な専門家が集まり，3500 を超える文献の引用と，約 25000 通ものメール交換を経て，途方もない時間と労力をかけ作成された．本領域では群を抜いた情報量となっている．

　残念ながら，PJI 診療においてエビデンスレベルの高い研究

はまだまだ限られている．多くの局面において，医学的根拠は十分と言えない．しかしながら，一度感染が起これば，それは待ったなしであり，我々は限られた時間と情報の中で最善と思われる医療行為を適切に判断し，適宜実践していく必要がある．本合併症の発生割合は決して高くなく，経験豊富な術者も少ない．限られたエビデンスと経験の中での判断は必然的に非常に難しいものとなる．どこまでエビデンスがあるのか？　また，エビデンスがないのであれば世界的に標準と考えられる対策はあるのか？　これらの疑問を一冊でカバーできる本があれば，それほど有用なものはない．本コンセンサスは，まさにこのような要望にお応えする待望の一冊と言える．

　本書は現場での使いやすさを優先し，国際コンセンサスのjustificationの部分は割愛した．コンセンサスの原文は，MSISのホームページからいつでも無料でダウンロードできる[1]．より詳細な情報については，原文を適宜ご参照いただきたい．

　最後に，本書作成をサポートいただいたParvizi教授，Gehrke教授，編集や翻訳作業でご尽力いただいた訳者の皆様，三輪様，荻原様，宮内様，CBR関係者の皆様にこの場をお借りして，厚く御礼申し上げたい．

---

1) Proceedings of the International Consensus Meeting on Periprosthetic Joint Infection, 2013.
   http://www.msis-na.org/wp-content/themes/msis-temp/pdf/ism-periprosthetic-joint-information.pdf

2016年4月吉日

関東労災病院整形外科・脊椎外科
山田浩司

和文索引

あ

アゾール系 187
アゾール系薬 187
アミノグリコシド 25
アムホテリシン 187
アルギン酸塩 125
アルコール 15
アルゴリズム 108, 203
アンチバイオグラム 139

い

イソキサゾリルペニシリン 23
一期的（人工関節）再置換術 167, 175
一期的再置換術 167, 175, 176, 187
インプラントの温存 195

え

栄養失調症 1
栄養不良 185
エリスロポエチン 84
炎症性関節症 110
炎症マーカー 166

お

黄色ブドウ球菌 206
汚染細菌量 49
温風式加温ブランケット 53

か

塊状他家骨移植 30
核医学画像診断 114
カッティングガイド 56
カルバペネム耐性腸球菌 31
カンジダ属 186, 187
患者体温管理 53
感受性 186, 187, 196
関節液細胞数 111
関節鏡検査 155

関節固定術 177
関節穿刺 4, 154, 168, 185, 196
関節内（局所）抗菌薬投与 157, 167
関節リウマチ 186
乾癬 16
感染性関節炎既往 4

き

器械台 55
吸引ドレーン 85
吸引の先 56
急性期PJI 109, 110, 155, 195
休薬期間 166
銀含浸ドレッシング材 125

く

クリンダマイシン 24
グルコン酸クロルヘキシジン（CHG） 15

け

経験的抗菌薬投与 27
経口抗菌薬 165, 195, 205
血腫 154
血清C反応性タンパク（CRP） 107, 109
血清学的検査 4
ゲンタマイシン 140

こ

抗凝固剤 203
抗菌薬 5
抗菌薬感受性 113
抗菌薬含有（骨）セメント 26, 27, 95
抗菌薬含有セメントスペーサー 142
抗菌薬含有ポリメタクリル酸メチル（ABX-PMMA）セメント 95
抗菌薬投与期間 165, 166, 167

抗菌薬の長期投与　156
抗菌薬の併用療法　25
抗菌薬の予防投与　112
抗菌薬パウダー　97
口腔衛生　2
抗酸菌（AFB）　111
抗真菌感受性試験　186
抗真菌薬　187, 188
骨欠損　97
骨セメント　5
コンピューター断層撮影（CT）　113

さ

再置換術　30, 112, 135, 136, 166, 167, 168, 176, 188

し

紫外線照射　51
歯科処置時の予防抗菌薬　204
磁気共鳴画像法（MRI）　113
自己血回収（装置）　82, 84
自己血製剤　59
自己血貯血　85
自己血輸血　81, 82
自己免疫性疾患　30
疾患修飾薬　3
膝関節固定術　176, 177
湿疹　16
市販されているスペーサー　138, 139
周術期抗菌薬　127
手指衛生　54
手術時間　52
手術用安全チェックリスト　59
術衣　52
出血量　28
術後ドレーン　26
術後予防抗菌薬投与　27
術者が手作りした可動性のあるスペーサー　138, 139
術中培養　5
術野消毒　15

摺動面　96
消毒薬　15, 17
初回人工関節置換術　30, 128
除菌　2, 15, 206
除毛　16
真菌　111, 112, 168, 185, 186
真菌性PJI　187, 188
人工関節型スペーサー　135, 136, 137, 138
人工関節再置換術　95, 97, 177
人工関節の温存　153
人工関節抜去後　165
人工股関節全置換術（THA）　81, 96, 136, 154
人工膝関節周囲感染　135
人工膝関節全置換術（TKA）　81, 154
人工挿入物　95, 96, 98
人工物　23
浸出が持続する創　126, 127

す

スクリーニング　2, 3, 25, 29
ステープル　59, 128

せ

生物学的マーカー　166
脊髄麻酔　81, 82
赤血球数　111
赤血球沈降速度　107, 109, 188
切除関節形成術　175, 177, 187
切断術　177
セファゾリン　23
セファロスポリン　23, 24, 25
セフロキシム　23
セメントレス人工関節　97
洗浄　58, 154
洗浄デブリドマン　126, 153, 187
全身除菌　15
全身排気スーツ　50
全身麻酔　81, 82

そ

早期 PJI 155, 195
早期感染 153
創閉鎖法 128
層流換気 49, 50

た

大規模な再建 30
第二期の手術 27
タイムアウト 59
多形核好中球の割合 107, 109
多血小板血漿（PRP） 84
多剤耐性アシネトバクター 31
脱毛 16
タブレット 52
単純 X 線 113

ち

遅発性 PJI 110
超音波処理 113
長時間手術 28, 81

て

手洗い 17
低栄養 127
テイコプラニン 24, 29
剃毛 16
手袋 54, 55
デブリドマン 195, 196
電気メス 56
電子機器 52

と

同種血輸血 81, 83
糖尿病 1, 30, 127, 185
トブラマイシン 140
トラネキサム酸（TA） 83
ドレープ 57, 58
ドレーン 26, 83

に

二期的再置換術 84, 85, 135, 136, 137, 175, 176, 187
尿検査 3, 26, 107
尿路カテーテル 26
尿路感染症（UTI） 3, 26

ね

粘着ドレープ 57

の

膿盆 56
ノート型パソコン 52

は

バイオクリーンルーム 49, 50
ハイドロキシアパタイト 95
ハイドロファイバー 125
培養陰性の PJI 168
培養期間 111
ハイリスク 25, 95, 205
白血球（WBC） 107, 109
白血球エステラーゼ 107
白血球濃度 111
白血球分析 111
晩期 PJI 195, 203, 205, 206
晩期血行性感染 153
晩期人工関節周囲感染 203
半減期 28
バンコマイシン 23, 24, 25, 29, 97, 140

ひ

比色定量試験 107
非人工関節型スペーサー 135, 136, 137, 138
非定型細菌 185
非定型的人工関節周囲感染 185
皮内テスト 24
皮膚潰瘍 16
皮膚除菌 15

皮膚病変 16
標準予防策（standard precautions） 54
病理組織所見 107
貧血 84, 127

ふ

フィブリン糊 84
フルオロキノロン 23, 195
フルコナゾール 186, 187
分子生物学的手法 113

へ

米国整形外科学会 108
閉鎖法 59
併用療法 25, 195
ペニシリン 24

ほ

縫合 128
縫合糸 59
補液量 28
ボリコナゾール 187
ポリメラーゼ連鎖反応（PCR） 113

ま

麻酔法 81
マスク 51, 52
慢性 PJI 195

む

無菌性ゆるみ 112

め

メガプロステーシス 29, 96

メス刃 55
メタル・オン・メタル 96
メチシリン感受性黄色ブドウ球菌 2
メチシリン耐性黄色ブドウ球菌 2, 25
滅菌ドレープ 57
免疫不全 1, 30
免疫抑制 3, 185

や

薬物動態 28
薬用石鹸 15

ゆ

輸血 81

よ

ヨード含有粘着ドレープ 57
抑制療法 196
予防抗菌薬 23, 24, 26, 27, 28, 29, 30, 31, 59, 205

ら

ライトハンドル 50
落下細菌 49

り

リスク 4, 52, 53, 81, 82, 96
リスクファクター 1, 155, 203, 204
リファンピシン 166, 167, 195
リファンピン 166, 167, 195

ろ

瘻孔 107, 153, 175

欧文索引

A

AAOS 108
acid-fast bacillus (AFB) 111, 112
acute PJI 109, 110, 155, 195
adhesive drape 57
AFB 111, 112
algorithm 108, 203
allogeneic transfusion 81, 83
American Academy of Orthopaedic Surgeons (AAOS) 108
aminoglycosides 25
amphotericin 187
amputation 177
antibiotic cement spacer 142
antibiotic powder 97
antibiotic sensitivity 113
Antibiotic-impregnated cement 26, 95
Antibiotic-laden bone cement 27
Antibiotics 5
anticoagulation 203
antifungal medication (agents) 187, 188
antiseptic 15, 17
antiseptic soap 15
arthrodesis 177
articulating spacers 135, 136, 137, 138
atypical FJI 185
autoimmune disease 30
autologous blood donation 85
autologous transfusion 81, 82
azoles 187

B

bearing surface 96
blood transfusion 81
body exhaust suits 50
bone defect 97

bone deficiency 97

C

C-reative protein (CRP) 110, 188
Candida species 186, 187
carbapenem resistant *enterobacteriaceae* 31
cephalosporin 23, 24, 25
chlorhexidine gluconate (CHG) 15
chronic PJI 110, 195
clindamycin 24
computed tomography (CT) 113
CRP 110, 188
cutting guide 56
C反応性タンパク 188

D

debridement 195, 196
decolonization 2, 15, 206
dental antibiotic prophylaxis 204
diabetes (mellitus) 1, 30, 127, 185
disease-modifying agent 3
drain 26, 83
dual antibiotics 25

E

eczema 16
electrocautery 56
empiric antibiotic 27
erythrocyte sedimentation rate (ESR) 107, 109, 188
erythropoietin 84
ESR 110
extended antibiotic 156

F

FAW ブランケット 53
fibrin glue 84
fluconazole 186, 187
fluoroquinolones 23, 195

forced air warming (FAW) blanket 53
fungal PJI 187, 188
fungus 111, 112, 168, 185, 186

G

general anesthesia 81, 82
gentamicin 140

H

hair removal 16
hand hyiene 54
histological analysis 107
holiday period 166

I

I & D 126, 127, 153, 154, 155, 156, 157, 187
immunosuppressant medication 3, 185
immunosuppression disease 1, 30
intraoperative culture 5
iodine-impregnated skin incise drape 57
irrigation 58, 154
irrigation and debridement (I & D) 126, 127, 153, 154, 155, 156, 157, 187

J

joint aspiration 4, 154, 168, 185, 196

K

knee arthrodesis 176, 177
knife blade 55

L

Laminar air flow 49, 50
Laminar flow room 49, 50
late hematogenous infection 153
late PJI 195, 203, 205, 206
leukocyte esterase 107
light handle 50

M

magnetic resonance imaging (MRI) 113
major (orthopaedic) reconstruction 30
mega-prosthesis 29, 96
metal-on-metal 96, 111
methicillin-resistant *Staphylococcus aureus* (MRSA) 2, 3, 25, 29, 166, 168
methicillin-sensitive *Staphylococcus aureus* (MSSA) 2, 3
MRSA 2, 3, 25, 29, 166, 168
MRSA carriers 29
MRSA colonization 205
MRSA 保菌 205
MRSA 保菌者 29
MSSA 2, 3
multi-drug resistant Acinetobacter spp 31

N

neuraxial anesthesia (blockade) 81, 82
normothermia 53
nuclear imaging 114

O

one-stage exchange arthroplasty 167, 175, 176, 187
oral hygiene 2

P

PCR 法 113
penicillin allergy 24
Perioperative antibiotics prophylaxis 23, 24, 26, 27, 28, 29, 30, 31, 59, 205
persistent (wound) drainage 125, 126, 127
pharmacokinetics 28
plain radiograph 113
platelet-rich plasma (PRP) 84

PMMA セメント　96
PMN%　107, 109, 110
polymerase chain reaction (PCR)　113
polymorphonuclear neutrophil percentage (PMN%)　107, 109, 110
postoperative antibiotic　27
preoperateive skin cleansing　15
Propionibacterium acnes　107
Prosthesis　95, 96, 98
PRP　84
psoriasis　16

R

reimplantation　30, 112, 135, 136, 166, 167, 168, 176, 188
resection arthroplasty　175, 177, 187
revision procedure　30, 112, 135, 166, 167, 168, 176, 188
revision (joint) arthroplasty　95, 97, 177
rheumatoid arthritis　186
rifampicin　166, 167, 195
rifampin　166, 167, 195
risk　4, 52, 53, 81, 82, 96
risk factors　1, 155, 203, 204

S

scarpel blade　55
second stage procedure　27, 84, 85, 135, 136, 137, 175, 176, 187
single-stage exchange (arthroplasty)　167, 175, 176, 187
sinus tract　107, 153, 175
skin lesion　16
sonication　113
space suits　50
splash basin　56
standard precaution　54
staple　59, 128
suction drain　85
suppressive therapy (treatment)　196

surgical safety checklist　59
surgical skin preparation　15
susceptibility testing　186, 187, 196
suture　128

T

TA　83
teicoplanin　24, 29
THA　81, 96, 136, 154
time-out　59
TJA 後の発熱　206
TKA　81, 135, 154
tobramycin　140
total hip arthroplasty (THA)　81, 96, 136, 154
total knee arthroplasty (TKA)　81, 135, 154
tranexamic acid (TA)　83
two-stage exchange (arthroplasty)　27, 84, 85, 135, 136, 137, 175, 176, 187

U

ultraviolet (UV) light　51
universal screening　2, 3, 25, 29
urinary catheter　26
urinary tract infection (UTI)　3, 26
urine screening　3, 26, 107
UV　51
UV ライト　51

V

vancomycin　23, 24, 25, 29, 97, 140
vancomycin powder　97
voriconazole　187

W

WBC 数　107, 109, 110, 111, 112
white blood cell (WBC)　107, 109, 110, 111, 112

人工関節周囲感染対策における国際コンセンサス
── 204 の設問とコンセンサス

2016 年 4 月 30 日　第 1 版第 1 刷Ⓒ

編　　　集	山田浩司(やまだこうじ)
発 行 人	三輪　敏
発 行 所	株式会社シービーアール
	東京都文京区本郷 3-32-6　〒 113-0033
	☎(03)5840-7561　(代)　Fax(03)3816-5630
	E-mail／info@cbr-pub.com
	ISBN 978-4-908083-10-5　C3047
	定価は裏表紙に表示
印 刷 製 本	三報社印刷株式会社
	Ⓒ Koji Yamada 2016

本書の内容の無断複写・複製・転載は，著作権・出版権の侵害となることがありますのでご注意ください．

JCOPY　＜(社)出版者著作権管理機構　委託出版物＞

本書の無断複製は著作権法上での例外を除き禁じられています．
複製される場合は，そのつど事前に，(社)出版者著作権管理機構
(電話 03-3513-6969, FAX 03-3513-6979, e-mail: info@jcopy.or jp)の許諾を得てください．